STUDIES IN HOMOSEXUALITY

Edited with
Introductions by

Wayne R. Dynes
Hunter College, City University
of New York

and Stephen Donaldson

Contents of Series

VOLUME IX

Homosexuality and Medicine, Health, and Science

Edited with Introductions by
Wayne R. Dynes
Hunter College, City University of New York
and Stephen Donaldson

Routledge
Taylor & Francis Group
LONDON AND NEW YORK

First published 1992 by Garland Publishing, Inc.

Published 2019 by Routledge
2 Park Square, Milton Park, Abingdon, Oxon OX14 4RN
52 Vanderbilt Avenue, New York, NY 10017

Routledge is an imprint of the Taylor & Francis Group, an informa business

Library of Congress Cataloging-in-Publication Data

Homosexuality and medicine, health, and science / edited by Wayne R. Dynes and Stephen Donaldson.
p. cm. — (Studies in homosexuality ; v. 9)
A collection of articles from 20th century scholarly journals.
Includes bibliographical references.
ISBN 0-8153-0554-0
1. Homosexuality—Research. 2. Homosexuality—Psychological aspects.
3. Gays—Identity. 4. Gays—Health and hygiene. 5. AIDS (Disease)—Research.
I. Dynes, Wayne R. II. Donaldson, Stephen. III. Title: Homosexuality and medicine, health and science. IV. Series.
HQ76.25.C6738 1992
305.9'0664—dc20

92-13993
CIP

ISBN 13: 978-0-8153-0554-5 (hbk)

General Introduction

Over the past quarter century powerful currents of research and writing on homosexuality, lesbianism, and bisexuality have rippled through widening channels, finding outlets in scores of journals affiliated with more than a dozen disciplines. While this increase in the volume of publications signals a welcome lessening of the taboo on the subject and a growing sense of its importance, this profusion makes it difficult for even specialists to monitor the progress of scholarship in its many domains. Much of the key material in this area has appeared in hard-to-locate and often unlikely appearing academic periodicals, which have escaped even diligent indexers and bibliographers. Moreover, not a few of these journals appeared in very limited issues and cannot be found today even in the larger research libraries.

To make more accessible to the reader the classic, the pioneering, and the most recent outstanding articles of scholarly work in a wide variety of disciplines, this series gathers a selection of such articles, reprinting them in thirteen volumes organized by discipline. Sifting through thousands of journal articles, the editors have chosen for republication works of scholarly distinction without attempting to impose any uniform ideological perspective on a field still characterized by lively controversies. Dates of original publication of the selections included in these volumes span the twentieth century, from Erich Bethe's landmark 1907 article on Dorian pederasty in *Rheinisches Museum* to current articles embodying the latest techniques of archival research and conceptual analysis. In some cases, it has been impossible to obtain permission to reprint material we felt worth inclusion; Haworth Press, for example, declined to permit republication of any articles from the *Journal of Homosexuality*. Fortunately, that periodical is widely available so that its absence does not detract from our goal of furnishing important but hard-to-find research.

The earlier situation in which work on homosexuality typically found its home in the social sciences and in medicine has significantly broadened, with important work in history, the humanities, and the arts. Attention has also shifted from the isolated individual to the interaction of the gay/lesbian/bi person with his/her peers. Increased attention has also been devoted to cultural representations in novels and poetry, films and popular music.

Each individual volume brings together the best article-length scholarship on homosexuality from that discipline and will save the specialist a great deal of time and effort. Each volume is self-contained; at the same time, the entire series is designed so that the reader seeking a broad understanding of the phenomena of homosexualities and their cultural, literary, and historical manifestations can make profitable use of the volumes representing other disciplines.

The introduction to each volume examines the history of the discipline(s) represented and its approaches to the study of homosexuality, critiques the development of research in the field, notes milestones in the evolution of thought and research, raises methodological issues, discusses conceptual questions, and suggests directions for future investigation and developments in the field. These introductions allow the reader from outside the discipline to survey and appreciate the issues raised. At the same time specialists will find a constructive critique of the state of their discipline as well as an appreciation of its contributions to the overall development of gay, lesbian, and bisexual scholarship. Appended to each introduction is a survey bibliography of important book-length works in that field.

Introduction

At the end of the nineteenth century, the pioneers of the German homosexual rights movement looked to science as a liberating force. With its rigor and "objective" methodology, science (which, many believed, was certain to demonstrate the biological basis of homosexuality) would, in an ironic reversal of the traditional demonology, exorcise the ghosts of Christian bigotry and medieval superstition, showing everyone the pointlessness of treating homosexuals as inferior sinners and criminals.

The twentieth century, however, has produced numerous examples of science as a tool of oppression. In the early and middle parts of the century, some scientists did undermine earlier misconceptions, but many more reinforced popular attitudes and all too many proved themselves willing to support schemes for the eradication of homosexuality—and in Nazi Germany, of the homosexuals as well—through social and psychological engineering.

Medicine in particular embraced concepts of homosexuality as a disease, providing the rationale for further discrimination; its offspring, psychiatry, proved every bit as hostile as the Christian establishment.

Towards the middle of the present century, however, and just as psychiatric theories of homosexual pathology were reaching their apogee of influence, another, less subjective, branch of science, biology, in the person of entomologist Alfred C. Kinsey, came riding to the rescue.

Quantification Efforts

Kinsey's massive investigation, which reached the world through his 1948 volume *Sexual Behavior in the Human Male* (followed in 1953 by the female volume), not only shocked the general public with its high incidence rates for homosexuality, but established a new standard of objective language to describe homosexuality. Discarding even such vague terms as "homosexual," "heterosexual," and "bisexual" in favor of a continuum of sexual orientation and practice, Kinsey created a seven-step numerical scale to measure the proportions of heterosexual and homosexual "outlets" in the behavior of white Americans. (The continuum concept, while joining the vocabulary of scholars as more accurate than simple binary or even triadic classificatory schemes, never became popular among activists, possibly because it did not lend itself to a politics of "gay and lesbian identity.") Kinsey's training as an entomologist was no doubt instrumental in his ability to discard conventional viewpoints in order to examine sexual events with the same dispassion he employed in studying gall wasps.

The tradition of objectivity in the study of homosexuality which Kinsey established in the United States suffered first as a result of massive opposition to his work in the conservative fifties, and more recently from the other side as a result of an overriding commitment to political objectives among activist-oriented scholars who came to dominate the subject in many disciplines. Nevertheless it has become more and more the norm for scientific research. Today Kinsey's quest for objective measurements of sexual phenomena continues with new techniques such as plethysmography, which records the engorgement of blood vessels in the pelvic area due to sexual arousal, and electroencephalographic recording of brain waves ("evoked potentials") in response to erotic stimuli.

The Czech researcher Kurt Freund first used plethysmography in determining that aversion therapy to change sexual orientation was not productive. Plethysmography is useful in quantifying such areas as sexual orientation, changes in sexuality with age, and the discrepancies between biological reactions and conscious reporting by the subject.

Brain researchers have also used electrode recording of evoked potentials to measure sexual orientation independent of conscious reports. After discovering that the anticipation of pleasure produces a characteristic electrical pattern in the brain, neuroscientists measured the strength of this reaction in response to visual images.

Both techniques could potentially be of use to repressive governments or private organizations in invading the privacy of people's sexual feelings or thoughts, and thus they raise issues of ethical application, so far more for hypothetical future misuse than for present research, which relies on volunteers.

A new entry in the field is neuroanatomy, where Simon LeVay's pioneering work at the Salk Institute measuring variations in very small brain structures has aroused both intense interest and considerable scepticism.

Another area in which scientific objectivity has begun to make itself felt is genetic and hormonal studies, though here the methodologies are more complicated and the results more controversial. Twin studies, however, appear to have made considerable progress in establishing solid data pointing to genetic factors.

Work in these areas, combined with theoretical studies in sociobiology, has occasioned a revival of interest in biological explanations of homosexuality. The ground for this revival was broken by the Kinsey Institute, which, using path analysis techniques, discredited the major psychiatric theories of homosexual etiology.

Perhaps science is, a century late, finally beginning to fulfill the role the founders of the gay rights movement predicted for it.

Medical Theory

Medical theorists have concerned themselves with homosexuality since classical antiquity, when writers associated with the Hippocratic and Aristotelian schools formulated different physiological explanations for the rare cases of adults who crossed the boundaries of traditional gender behavior; neither school thought that pederastic behavior required such explanations. The Greeks, whose model of homosexuality was age-differentiated, thought the gender-differentiated and androphilic types to be abnormal, thus displaying the tendency towards cultural bias which has characterized medical theory in this area for millennia.

Beginning with the Renaissance, medicine acquired a forensic tradition which sought physical evidence for the crime of sodomy. Under the cloak of psychiatry, this forensic tradition produced the modern Western concept of sexual orientation in the latter nineteenth century.

Meanwhile theorists had ascribed homosexuality to degenerative diseases of the nervous system, moral insanity, erotic monomania, and sexual inversion.

The modern medical theories of homosexuality (which seldom went beyond the androphilic type familiar to modern middle-class northern Europeans) originated in an unsuccessful attempt on behalf of defendants to attack criminal sanctions, but then turned against their sponsors, becoming vehicles to deny the legitimacy of homosexual expression. Eventually the United States went so far as to bar homosexual immigration on medical grounds as a psychiatric pathology. Thus the strategy of defense against the medieval sodomy laws opened the door to a new and in many ways more pernicious enemy, cloaked in the mantle of "science."

Beginning in the mid-1960s, however, gay rights advocates vigorously attacked these theories, beginning with logical arguments and proceeding through pickets and demonstrations (1968 on) to the use of disruptive tactics at psychiatric conventions. They succeeded in persuading the American Psychiatric Association to remove homosexuality from its list of mental diseases in 1973, a decision confirmed in a subsequent mail ballot of APA members. This reform finally (and quietly) reached the United Nations-sponsored World Health Organization in 1992.

Biology and Etiology

The medical theorists did not stop to consider the question of homosexuality in animals, assuming as they did that human homosexuality was "unnatural." Ethologists beginning with Konrad Lorenz, however, following a path blazed long ago by Aristotle, have observed homosexual behaviors in fish, birds, lizards, goats, dogs, monkeys, dolphins, and many other species; often this appears to be related to dominance contests among males; for females no such correlation has suggested itself.

The presence of homosexuality—especially exclusive long-term homosexuality in humans—poses an outstanding theoretical problem to evolutionary biology, which is rooted in Darwinian concepts of reproductive fitness. This challenge, supported by findings that sexual orientation does tend somewhat to run in families, and strongly among genetically identical twins, has elicited various responses from sociobiologists. G. Evelyn Hutchinson developed a theory of heterozygote advantage, which may apply best to bisexuality, in 1959. James D. Weinrich developed kin selection theory to account for gender-differentiated types of homosexuality in 1976; a later essay by Weinrich is included herein. Other types of homosexuality, such as the Greek pederastic model, situational homosexuality, adolescent experimentation, and dominance-enforcement, do not have significant effects on marriage and reproductive rates and thus do not pose such puzzles for evolutionary theorists. Modern androphilia (usually reciprocal relations between two adults, both identified with the same gender and of formally equal status) remains the most difficult case, but it may be too recent a development as a common type for Darwinian selection to have had significant effects.

Twin studies of homosexuality go back to Franz J. Kallmann's pioneering, but flawed, 1951 research with monozygotic (genetically identical) twins, which found startlingly complete concordance for sexual orientation of the twin pairs. Taken as a whole, twin studies show that identical male twins, sharing the same genes, whether raised together or apart, ordinarily share the same sexual orientation. Fraternal twins, on the other hand, with only half their genes in common, whether raised together or apart are far less likely than identical twins to develop similar sexual orientations. Even fraternal twins raised apart, however, are more likely to show similar sexual orientations than mere chance would indicate. Further confirmation of these findings appeared in a major study published in late 1991 by J. Michael Bailey and Richard C. Pillard. In addition to showing that environment alone cannot account for the development of male homosexuality, the studies cast doubt on theories of prenatal hormonal factors in the mother's womb, since such theories cannot account for the greater concordance of sexual orientation of identical twins as against fraternal ones, each pair being subject to the same hormonal influences.

A 1985 study of identical twins reared apart by Elke D. Eckert and others (included herein) concluded that "it is hard to deny genetic factors an etiological role" in the formation of male homosexuality. Eckert suggested on the basis of a comparison of male and female twin pairs that lesbianism may have entirely different, non-genetic, roots. He did find a significant difference in the age of first menstruation between the heterosexual and lesbian members of a pair of twins, with the lesbians maturing later; Eckert noted no differences in the age of puberty in the male twins.

The debate over the etiology of homosexuality—or more accurately, the etiologies of various types of homosexuality, any common denominator other than some type of same-sex behavior having yet to appear—has had serious consequences for the ways society treats the people who exhibit such phenomena. These can range from burning sodomites at the stake for their willful sins through compulsory electroshock therapy for psychopathic inverts and a resigned acceptance of homosexuality as the unalterable condition of homosexuals to seeing homosexuality as one in a repertoire of many normal human sexual behaviors, one not associated with any particular character or personality traits, much less a fixed identity.

While the etiological issues remain a subject of intense interest, progress in this area will require not only dispassionate scientific objectivity (as rare among gay activists as among their opponents) but a recognition of assorted types of homosexuality, an integration of disciplines, a cross-cultural perspective, a recognition that sexual patterns may change over an individual lifetime as well as over centuries within societies, and a willingness to accept empirical evidence instead of reliance on abstract theorizing alone.

Health Care

Turning to health care, which with the spread of the AIDS epidemic has become of primary importance to the gay community, one should first note that the particular medical concerns of gay men and lesbians did not become a subject for discussion until the 1970s, and the organizers of health care systems did not acknowledge or accommodate the gay or lesbian patient. For a discussion of lesbian medicine, see the article by Susan R. Johnson and J. L. Palermo; on the male homosexual see the article by Michael W. Ross; both are included herein.

Only in recent years have health care providers who are themselves homosexual become visible, but today gay and lesbian medicine has become a recognizable specialty among physicians, and there are professional associations of gay and lesbian physicians, nurses, and other health workers. One of the consequences of the general lack of a gay-oriented medical practice has been a turn to medical self-help, most notably in the case of such organizations as New York's Gay Men's Health Crisis.

Students of alcoholism have long maintained that the rate of alcohol abuse is higher among male and female homosexuals than among the general population; for most Americans the gay bar is the central homosexual social institution. Various and often conflicting theories have sought to account for this. Recent therapy has tended to focus on adaptational responses to a homophobic environment, encouraging gay alcoholics to enter treatment programs where they are encouraged to be themselves. Articles on alcoholism and homosexuals are included from Stephen Israelstam and Sylvia Lambert and from Edward Small and Barry Leach.

Other drug use among homosexuals has drawn less attention. It appears that the illegal status of various substances has had less of a deterrent effect among those whose sexual life was illegal to start with, leading to widespread scepticism about government pronouncements concerning the use of one's own body to perform victimless crimes. Living in a subculture which already included an aura of illicit pleasure, gays and lesbians proved hospitable to "recreational" drug use in the 1960s and 1970s. Use of nitrate inhalants, marijuana, snortable cocaine, and hallucinogens was widespread, though the gay subculture has apparently generally avoided the more destructive drugs such as opiates, crack, methamphetamines, barbiturates, and PCP. Nicotine addiction has followed patterns in the general culture. See articles by Ellen Herman and John A. Newmeyer, included herein.

Until the 1980s, the main health concerns of gay and bisexual men (and to a diminishing extent, of bisexual women and lesbians) were the conventional sexually transmitted diseases, gonorrhea and syphilis, which were reputedly more common among male homosexuals than in the general population. Antibiotics are effective against both, but awareness and diagnosis do not always come easy when the gonococcus bacteria lodges in the rectum (it does not survive in the mouth) or remains asymptomatic, or when the initial manifestations of syphilis go unrecognized. Genital herpes occasioned considerable alarm in the late 1970s, but turned out to be chiefly a problem for heterosexuals.

Due to its spread through anal-oral contact, infectious hepatitis affected ten times as many gay as straight men until a vaccine proved effective in the early 1980s.

Concerns developed around physical traumas associated with the practice of inserting a fist inside the rectum ("fisting"), a practice which appears to have drastically declined since the 1970s.

Also controversial was the use of legal amyl or butyl nitrate inhalants ("poppers") during the sex act, a habit which was once widespread among homosexuals but never caught on among heterosexuals. Apart from occasional transient headaches and cautions over their use by elderly heart patients (for whom they were originally devised as vasodilators), these inhalants were considered harmless. Then in 1986 a sensational book by John Lauritsen and Hank Wilson suggested that they caused or contributed to AIDS, leading to legal restrictions in some states and a drastic decline in use. Conclusive evidence for this claim has not developed, however, and AIDS has gone on to strike down vast numbers of non-users; thus a low residual level of use by sceptical gay men in major urban centers continues.

AIDS

The Acquired Immunodeficiency Syndrome (AIDS) first came to public awareness in the early 1980s as a mysterious and fatal disease which seemed to afflict only homosexuals, hence it acquired a reputation as a "gay disease," a misconception which lingered in the public mind long after it had disappeared from the health professions.

The ravages of AIDS among the gay male community are too well known to require elaboration here; the fact that the bulk of the articles in this volume are concerned with the epidemic speaks for itself. At the beginning of the closing decade of the century this scourge showed no sign of abating, though the rate of increase in cases among homosexuals showed a significant decline (presumably due to changes in sexual practices which also reduced the incidence of venereal disease), the opportunistic infections which usually caused death were under better control, new experimental drug programs were on the way, and hope existed for an eventual post-infection "vaccine" which, if it would not eliminate the HIV virus that was linked to the disease, at least might keep it harmless. Researchers suggested that newly infected people should no longer expect a necessarily fatal outcome, but rather a disability comparable to, say, diabetes, which could be kept under control through continuous surveillance and treatment. Twelve years after the first cases became known, it remained unclear what percentage of those infected with the virus would develop "full-blown" AIDS or what the eventual mortality rate was; such progression seems to have occurred in most but not all cases of early infection.

While the scientific establishment has accepted the evidence for the Human Immunodeficiency Virus (HIV) as the primary causal agent, and information about the workings of that virus had multiplied many times over after a decade of intensive research, others remained unconvinced. Conspiracy theorists continue to believe that the agent, whatever it is, was unleashed from government laboratories. A growing body of opinion among professionals now suggests that the HIV virus is a necessary but not sufficient causal agent, requiring as yet unknown (though sometimes strongly suspected for epidemeological reasons, such as the presence of other sexually transmitted diseases) co-factors for its activation, virulence, and for disease progression.

Understanding of the progress of HIV infection has much improved, though major gaps in knowledge remain despite intense research efforts. New diagnostic tests have established general correlations between various levels of T4-cell counts and the progression from asymptomatic infection (which may last years or even a lifetime) through ARC (AIDS-Related Complex) to full-blown AIDS, and the controversial drug AZT has been prescribed even for asymptomatic HIV-positives in an effort to retard this progressive deterioration.

The usually fatal prognosis and lack of conventional treatments have encouraged persons with HIV infection or AIDS symptoms to experiment with a wide range of unconventional methods, new and unproven drugs, and holistic programs, some of which have claimed to be able to cure the disease. The desperation of the stricken patient facilitates exploitation and quackery, but exploration of many of the "alternative" non-allopathic medical techniques (such as acupuncture, megavitamins, and herbal remedies) has been quietly encouraged by medical professionals who have little else to offer and who believe that these methods would at least not harm the patient; the net result is a growing familiarity among the gay male community with holistic systems of health care and a scepticism regarding the commitment of the medical establishment to explore any remedies which do not promise major profits for the pharmaceuticals industry.

The political questions surrounding the AIDS epidemic and the response to it have generated considerable debate, with gay activists charging that the American government was slow to react to the crisis because it appeared at first to kill only homosexuals and then drug addicts. This perception was aided by pronouncements from conservative leaders close to the Reagan White House that AIDS was "God's punishment" for homosexuals. Certainly the crisis has had profound effects on the homosexual movement and on public awareness of and opinion with respect to homosexuality. Impatience with government agencies dealing with the epidemic has spawned a new wave of militancy and even civil disobedience on the part of such groups as ACT UP, while public and internal debate has focused on serious questions about funding for research, treatment, and disabled victims and on the very lengthy approval process for new drugs. Changes in this process, stimulated by the AIDS crisis, have taken place as reluctant government agencies responded to the public and political pressure to make experimental drugs available to patients who had little left to lose. A patient self-medication movement is another by-product of the approval process.

AIDS has also had major effects on homosexual behavior, though documentation for this conclusion is spotty and based primarily on a decline in venereal diseases and anecdotal evidence. The major consequences appear to be a decline in anal intercourse, especially without condoms, a greater reluctance on the part of heterosexuals to engage in homosexual acts, a decline in promiscuity in favor of monogamous pairs, and an increase in mutual masturbation (often via telephone).

For the most part, lesbians have remained medically unaffected, though the lesbian community has been very active in efforts to help victims of the disease. The epidemic, which could have driven a wedge between male and female homosexuals, has instead served to bring them together in a common cause.

Bisexuality, which was almost becoming chic in the mid-1970s, appeared as a dangerous source of contagion to the heterosexual majority and hence became heavily stigmatized even as its extent became more obvious. The bisexual movement, which had shown a preponderance of men in the seventies, reemerged from the eighties with female leadership and mostly female rank-and-file.

The rate of "coming out" and adoption of a homosexual identity seems to have slowed among healthy males, while death and disease "outed" many celebrities, but little or no documentation on these effects has been forthcoming.

Another area in which AIDS has had major consequences has been in the public awareness of homosexuality. The last mass media taboos in the West against mentioning homosexuality have all fallen, so that it has become virtually impossible for a Westerner to come to adulthood thinking he is the only one with same-sex desires, as often happened in previous eras. On the contrary, homosexual AIDS victims seem to be everywhere, often confounding stereotypical assumptions in the process. The most "macho" occupations and ethnic groups, the most rural settlements, the most conservative priests and politicians, have all offered up their victims for public examination. Terms like *anal intercourse* have appeared in television news programs and family newspapers, while "lovers" and "companions" have become a standard feature of obituaries.

Nonetheless, mass media squeamishness about particular sexual techniques combined with a conservative American government's inclination to suppress all homosexual activity and innate cautiousness on the part of health professionals have prevented media coverage of the stark difference in transmission danger between unprotected anal and oral activities. The latter are at least far less risky than the former, and may well be virtually risk-free, but studies tending to exculpate oral transmission gathered publicity only in parts of the gay press, not in media directed at the general public or in government-sponsored publications in the United States. The Canadian government, on the other hand, has included such information in its AIDS education program. Another important area of information which has been similarly neglected is the fact that anal transmission of the virus normally goes from penis to anus rather than vice versa.

Homophobia appears to have increased in the wake of the epidemic, with the incidence of violent assaults against homosexuals reportedly rising in the United States, prompting the formation of gay vigilante groups and agitation for "hate crimes" legislation in several areas. The movement for gay rights and for decriminalization appeared to have lost momentum for a decade, in part because the attentions of the gay community have been focused on AIDS and in part because of growing public resistance. On the other hand, Congress adopted federal legislation protecting the civil rights of those infected with the HIV virus, in marked contrast to its treatment of gay rights bills, which have never even reached the committee hearing stage.

The Christian religious establishment has reacted to the epidemic in predictable ways, with liberals emphasizing compassion for the victims and conservative fundamentalists preaching God's plague on the sodomites.

The decimation of the gay male community has had major effects in the cultural sphere, not only through the loss of key creative talents but through the refocusing of cultural attention on the disease and its consequences through innumerable books, films, plays, songs, and benefits. Notable also has been the revival of a long-dormant folk art in the Names Project Quilt, begun in 1987.

AIDS has also taken its toll on gay institutions, resulting in the closing of gay baths around the U.S. and in a major reduction in the number of gay bars.

Tourism has been affected, especially "sex tourism" in the Third World, and some countries have required HIV testing of visitors; the United States sought to exclude HIV-positive persons from entry altogether.

Legal questions relating to discrimination against persons with AIDS and HIV-positives have multiplied, with the U.S. government adopting antidiscrimination legislation based on classification of AIDS as a "handicap" in 1990. Many gay males have lost employment and/or housing as a result of public hysteria over AIDS contagion. Proposals for quarantines and camps continue to surface, though as yet they have not come near adoption as public policy.

The counseling professions have also been affected in major ways, having to deal with numerous consequences of AIDS, including depression, grief, and paranoia; social workers have become involved on a major scale in the living problems of homosexuals suffering simultaneously from the ravages of the disease and from the rejection of a fearful and homophobic public.

Public health and epidemiological needs for reliable information on risky sexual behavior has highlighted the absence of such data and focused attention on the need for further empirical research, which has made little progress since the 1947 Kinsey report. In 1990 and 1991 conservatives in Congress blocked a project for a new survey of American sexual behavior sponsored by public health agencies.

New ethical and sometimes legal issues have arisen in connection with hypothetical vaccine trials, the confidentiality of HIV testing, and the moral obligations of infected persons with respect to sexual partners.

While the United States has shown the greatest number of cases of homosexual transmission of AIDS, the number of men afflicted in other countries as a result of homosexual acts is steadily growing (while the proportion of new cases due to heterosexual transmission, usually from man to woman, rises both in the United States and abroad). In general, these nations have looked to the U.S. for leadership on this issue. France has taken a prominent role in the international research effort, and Britain in the area of public education. In central Africa, AIDS appears to be spread mostly heterosexually and has become a demographic catastrophe comparable to the medieval plagues of Europe.

Major funding problems loom for the treatment of the ever-increasing number of AIDS patients, who are already overloading health care systems in major American cities. Often deserted by insurance companies and employers, persons with AIDS may have little to contribute financially to their intensive and expensive care. At the same time, financially hard-pressed state and city governments are under intense pressure to cut back on Medicaid funding and disability benefits. In the future, this sad fact may prompt triage application and the lowering of standards of treatment, developments which may show the consequences of homophobia on the part of the taxpaying public.

The slow but progressive spread of AIDS to the heterosexual citizenry of the United States may transform the landscape of public concern dramatically, as would the development of either a preventive vaccine or a successful (at least in terms of preventing illness) treatment. Eventually, though perhaps decades off, the epidemic will take its course and recede in medical importance, but in many ways it has already drastically altered the history of homosexuality, and these changes will reverberate into the future for a long time to come.

Bibliography

Bayer, Ronald. *Private Acts, Social Consequences: AIDS and the Politics of Public Health.* New York: Free Press, 1989.

Carter, Erica, and Simon Watney, eds. *Taking Liberties: AIDS and Cultural Politics.* London: Serpent's Tail, 1989.

Celli, Giogio. *L'omosessualità negli animali.* Milan: Longanesi, 1973.

Crimp, Douglas, ed. *AIDS: Cultural Analysis/Cultural Activism.* Cambridge, Mass.: MIT Press, 1988.

Dalton, Harlon L., and Scott Burris. *AIDS and the Law: A Guide to the Public.* New Haven: Yale University Press, 1987.

Dilley, James W., Cheri Pies, and Michael Helquist, eds. *Face to Face: A Guide to AIDS Counseling.* Berkeley: Celestial Arts, 1989.

Fee, Elizabeth, and Daniel M. Fox, eds. *AIDS: The Burden of History.* Berkeley: University of California Press, 1988.

Gong, Victor, ed. *AIDS: Facts and Issues.* New Brunswick, N.J.: Rutgers University Press, 1986.

Lauritsen, John, and Hank Wilson. *Death Rush: Poppers and AIDS.* New York: Pagan Press, 1986.

Levine, Paula L. et al., eds. *The Psychosocial Aspects of AIDS: An Annotated Bibliography,* New York: Garland Publishing, 1990.

McCormack, Thomas P. *The AIDS Benefit Handbook.* New Haven: Yale University Press, 1990.

Malinowski, H. Robert, and Gerald J. Perry. *AIDS Information Sourcebook.* 2nd ed. Phoenix, Ariz.: Oryx Press, 1989.

Meldrum, Julian. *AIDS through the British Media*. London: AIDS Action Group, 1984.

Miller, Alan V. *Gays and Acquired Immune Deficiency Syndrome*. 2nd ed. Toronto: Canadian Gay Archives, 1983.

Nelkin, Dorothy, David P. Willis, and Scott V. Parris, eds. *A Disease of Society: Cultural & Institutional Responses to AIDS*. New York: Cambridge University Press, 1991.

Nichols, Eve K. *Mobilizing Against AIDS: The Unfinished Story of a Virus*. Cambridge, Mass.: Harvard University Press, 1986.

Nussbaum, Bruce. *Good Intentions: How Big Business and the Medical Establishment Are Corrupting the Fight Against AIDS*. New York: Atlantic Monthly Press, 1990.

O'Donnell, Mary, et al. *Lesbian Health Matters!* Santa Cruz, Calif.: Santa Cruz Women's Health Collective, 1979.

Ostrow, David G., ed. *Sexually Transmitted Diseases in Homosexual Men*. New York: Plenum, 1983.

Panem, Sandra. *The AIDS Bureaucracy*. Cambridge, Mass.: Harvard University Press, 1988.

Patton, Cindy. *Sex and Germs: The Politics of AIDS*. Boston: South End Press, 1985; Idem. *Inventing AIDS*. New York: Routledge, 1990.

Pomeroy, Wardell B. *Dr. Kinsey and the Institute for Sex Research*. New York: Harper & Row, 1972.

Puterbaugh, Geoff, ed. *Twins and Homosexuality: A Casebook*. New York: Garland Publishing, 1990.

Schwaber, Fern A., and Michael Shernoff, eds. *Sourcebook on Lesbian/Gay Health Care*. New York: National Gay Health Education Foundation, 1984.

Shilts, Randy. *And the Band Played On: Politics, People and the AIDS Epidemic*. New York: St. Martin's, 1987.

Weinrich, James D. *Sexual Landscapes: Why We Love Whom We Love*. New York: Charles Scribner's Sons, 1987.

Ziebold, Thomas, and John Mongeon, eds. *Gay and Sober*. New York: Harrington Press, 1985.

Contents

Archives of Sexual Behavior, Vol. 5, No. 6, 1976

Homosexual Behavior in a Laboratory Group of Stumptail Monkeys (*Macaca arctoides*)[1]: Forms, Contexts, and Possible Social Functions[2]

Suzanne Chevalier-Skolnikoff, Ph.D.[3]

Observations of stumptail monkeys revealed frequent prolonged, intensive genital stimulation between individuals of the same sex, both males and females, adults and infants. These homosexual interactions occurred in positive emotional contexts, were accompanied by positive emotional facial expressions, and often were evidently elicited by the observation of heterosexual behavior. Infants' first copulations were performed with adults of the same or opposite sex who actively aided them. This suggests that homosexual and heterosexual encounters function as training for adult sexual roles, and that homosexual behavior is a basic primate pattern not exclusive to man.

Key Words: homosexual behavior; *Macaca arctoides;* macaque; socialization; monkey.

INTRODUCTION

It is commonly thought that human sexual behavior is unique in its variability, diversity of sexual objects, and freedom from current physiological

This research was supported in part by the Interdisciplinary Training Program, Langley Porter Neuropsychiatric Institute, University of California, San Francisco, and by United States Public Health Service Training Grant MH-7082, from the National Institutes of Public Health.

[1] The stumptail macaque, *Macaca arctoides*, was formerly designated *Macaca speciosa* I. Geoffroy, 1926. For nomenclature, see Fooden (1967a,b) and International Commission on Zoological Nomenclature (1970).

[2] This article was part of the symposium "Biological and Cultural Bases of Sex Role Differentiation," presented at the Meetings of the American Association for the Advancement of Science, December 1971, in Philadelphia.

[3] Department of Anthropology, Stanford University, Stanford, California 94305, and the George Williams Hooper Foundation, University of California, San Francisco, California.

state. Actually, sexual behavior in nonhuman primates shares some of these qualities often ascribed exclusively to man. Studies on the nature of human sexual behavior from Ellis in 1896 to Kinsey in the 1940s and 1950s and Masters and Johnson in the 1960s and 1970s have described the prominence of both "normal" and "perverted" sexual behavior in preadolescents and in adults. The data on stumptail monkeys presented here help to place the determinants of human sexual behavior and sexual role into a broader primate perspective. They indicate that these kinds of sexual behaviors occur in infants and adults of primate species other than man, and are probably basic primate behavioral patterns.

In the course of a year-long study, 36 homosexual encounters were recorded in one laboratory group of ten stumptail monkeys (*Macaca arctoides*) living in a social group. Whether the frequency of homosexual behavior seen in this group is typical of the species is not known. However, my brief observations of a captive colony of *M. arctoides* at the University of California, Berkeley, and observations by Kling (1972) of two other colony groups at Rutgers Medical School, also revealed frequent homosexual encounters, suggesting that stumptail macaques may have a propensity for such behavior. On the other hand, Bertrand's (1969) descriptions of genital rubbing during "bullying," genital manipulation, and mounting behavior between various sex-age combinations in her groups of stumptail macaques may or may not have involved the prolonged, intensive genital stimulation between like-sexed individuals defined here as homosexual behavior. Female mounting occurred in only one of her groups, suggesting that this behavior might be a cultural tradition, as paternal care of infants evidently is in Japanese macaques (*Macaca fuscata*) (Itani, 1959).

In a comparative study on captive and free-ranging hamadryas baboons (*Papio hamadryas*), Kummer and Kurt (1965) found that the behavioral repertoires of the two groups were quite similar, although the frequencies of behavior, including some sexual behavior, were different in the two groups. Rowell (1967) also found such similarities in repertoires and differences in frequencies in wild and caged anubis baboons (*P. anubis*). Accordingly, it appears that behavior observed in the laboratory does reflect the behavioral range of the species, although the frequencies with which a particular behavior occurs in the wild may be altered by captivity.

The present study offers an opportunity to examine the homosexual potentials of nonhuman primates in terms of the forms of their behavior, to examine the conditions under which this kind of behavior occurs, and to investigate the possible social functions of the behavior.

Homosexual behavior in primates has been reported before, both in the laboratory and in the wild (Beach, 1949, and Ford and Beach, 1952, have reviewed homosexual behavior in mammals), but such reports are rare. Previous investigations have usually focused on brief mounts, or they have considered brief mounts and prolonged homosexual interactions together. Brief mounts generally have been found to correlate contextually with dominance interactions (Bernstein, 1970; Maslow, 1936; Talmage-Riggs and Anschel, 1973; Wickler, 1973; Zuckerman, 1932). There has been little study of the contexts of these formally different prolonged homosexual interactions.

The most detailed accounts of primate homosexual behavior, evidently incorporating prolonged genital stimulation, were reported by Hamilton (1914) and Kempf (1917). The same animals, 28 monkeys of three species – rhesus (*Macaca mulatta*), irus macaques (*M. fascicularis*), and baboons (unspecified) – were studied. The groups were composed of animals of both sexes, housed in cages about 18 ft high by 4 ft wide by 5 ft deep, although the animals were often released to roam at large. In these groups, male homosexual copulations were frequent and often included anal intromission and ejaculation. Extensive manual genital stimulation was also reported. Hamilton noted that homosexual behavior was particularly prevalent in immatures, and Kempf postulated that a specific homosexual stage ontogenetically precedes the heterosexual phase of life. Kempf also noted that the homosexual behavior he observed appeared to be strongly affected by dominance relationships, and that the subordinate animal gained social protection, while the dominant received sexual rewards.

Carpenter (1942) reported that among free-ranging rhesus monkeys (*Macaca mulatta*) at Cayo Santiago, an island off the coast of Puerto Rico, mountings with pelvic thrusts – which may have involved prolonged genital stimulation – occurred between eight of 150 females. Carpenter (and also Beach, 1949) suggested that homosexual behavior might be a substitute for heterosexual coitus. This has been postulated particularly for females who might be sexually attracted to other females in estrus (the period of sexual receptivity when ovulation generally occurs) or might themselves turn to other females during their early estrus period when they might not yet be of interest to males. Gordon and Bernstein's (1973) experimental study of captive male rhesus monkeys also suggests that male homosexual behavior is a substitute for heterosexual coitus in rhesus monkeys.

Hanby and Brown (1974), in a study on the development of sociosexual behavior in a captive group of approximately 100 Japanese macaques (*Macaca fuscata*) living in a 2-acre corral, present data on male-male and female-female mountings, some of which evidently involved prolonged genital stimulation. They found that in infants up to 1½ years of age male-male mounting, usually accompanied by pelvic thrusts, occurred with approximately the same frequency as male-female mounting. Most of these infantile homosexual mounts (70%) occurred in the context of play; the rest (about 27%) occurred in the context of "proximity" or "contact," while only 3% occurred in aggressive contexts. Among animals over 1½ years of age, male-male mountings occurred most frequently in the nonbreeding season. About half the time, these nonbreeding season mounts occurred without pelvic tnrusts and did not occur in series or lead to ejaculation as breeding season mounts often did. These relatively brief adult male mountings usually occurred after one male simply approached, or was approached by, another male. Female-female mounting was much less frequent than male-male mounting, and, unlike male-male mounting, occurred mostly during the breeding season, with adult females (over 3½ years) responsible for most of the female-female mounting. Female-female mountings were generally accompanied by pelvic thrusts and occurred in series and must have been of relatively long duration. Female-female mountings characteristically occurred in a context of close proximity, the pair usually walking around together or sitting in contact for long periods of time before and after the mounting.

Bingham (1928) reported an incident in which, after a period of masturbation on the part of one captive female chimpanzee (*Pan troglodytes*), she and another female chimp engaged in a series of embraces and then turned their faces in opposite directions and, standing on all fours, pushed their buttocks together and pushed and slid about in this manner for a short interval (p. 124). Sade (1968) reported one incident of male homosexual behavior in free-ranging rhesus monkeys (*Macaca mulatta*) between brothers at Cayo Santiago. This relationship included anal intromission and ejaculation (Sade, 1971). Morris (1970) reported on a long-term homosexual relationship between two young captive male orangutans (*Pongo pygmaeus*), which included frequent anal intercourse. This incident is of particular interest, for the experience resulted in an evidently irreversible reproductively abnormal behavioral pattern in one of the animals. When this orang was later paired with a female, he would only perform anal intercourse with her.

Similarly, Erwin and Maple (1976) report that a pair of male rhesus monkeys *(Macaca mulatta)* reared in a laboratory with exclusive social access to each other during their second year of life performed prolonged reciprocal mounting with anal penetration. Erwin and Maple suggest that the relationship between them was primarily based on mutual affection. However, while these males preferred each other to females as mounting partners, both males did perform adequately with both familiar and unfamiliar female partners.

METHODS

This study is based on 500 hr of observation of stumptail macaques made from September 1967 to September 1968 at the Primates Laboratory of the Department of Psychiatry, Stanford University School of Medicine. The monkeys were living in a social group housed in an indoor colony cage 18 ft long by 12 ft wide by 7 ft high. The group consisted of ten animals: one adult male, one subadult male, four adult females, one subadult female, and three infants (one male and two female) who were born into the group and were observed during their first 6 months of life (see Table 1). The adults were born in the wild. The group was formed 1 year before the initiation of the observations reported here, and,

Table I. Composition of the Stanford Group of Stumptail Macaques

Identification No.	Age, sex	Parity	Reproductive condition	Dominance status
1	Fully mature male		Breeding	1
2	Adult female	Probably primiparous	Pregnant, lactating	2
3	Adult female	Primiparous	Cycling, pregnant, cycling	6
4	Adult female	Primiparous	Cycling, pregnant, lactating	4
54	Adult female	Multiparous	Lactating	9
5	Subadult male		Breeding	8
6	Subadult female	Nulliparous	Cycling	7
2-1	Infant female			3
3-1	Infant male			5
54-2	Infant female			10

consequently, these observations reflect the behavior of animals in a well-integrated group.

Two observational methods were employed during the study. About 425 hr of qualitative observations were made on the whole group of animals, with running notes being taken on the animals' various activities. Not all sexual interactions that occurred during these observations were recorded, since it was not possible to simultaneously record all the activities. The sexual encounters were recorded in longhand, and care was taken to consider the total behavior of the particular animal(s) being observed, as well as to note sequential behaviors and interactions between animals.

A total of 75 hr of time-sampled quantitative observations were made, focusing on one animal at a time. All the sexual encounters in which focus animals were involved were recorded. Most of these data were recorded on checklists. Behavior was recorded according to the different body parts involved, including facial behavior, and according to the different sensory modes in which communications occurred. Prolonged interaction between like-sexed animals, involving intensive stimulation of at least one of the participating animals, was considered a homosexual encounter. Mounts and their various components were timed with a stopwatch. (See Chevalier-Skolnikoff, 1975, for a more detailed description of methods.)

FINDINGS

Homosexual Behavior Among Males

Thirteen incidents of male homosexual behavior were recorded during this study. All three males participated in male homosexual encounters. Such encounters occurred between two of the three potential pairs of males: the adult and subadult males, and the subadult and infant males.

Unlike heterosexual copulations, which were relatively stereotyped in form, male homosexual behavior was extremely varied. In the heterosexual encounters observed during this study, either the male or the female approached the potential mate, looking at the other with a direct gaze often accompanied by positive facial expressions, such as the lip-smacking, puckered-lips, or square-mouthed expressions (see Chevalier-Skolnikoff, 1974a, Fig. 1a-c). The female then presented her rear to the male, who, after a brief oral or manual examination of the female's genitals, mounted her from behind. In the mounted position, he grasped her loins with his hands and her legs with his feet (see Chevalier-Skolnikoff, 1974a, Fig. 2b). The copulation lasted an average of 2.8 min and consisted of three phases — a preejaculatory phase, an ejaculatory phase, and a post-ejaculatory phase. During the preejaculatory phase, which lasted about 1 min, the male executed about 60 pelvic thrusts. The ejaculatory phase was distinguished by a pause followed by stiffening of the body and muscular spasms and was accompanied by a characteristic intense frowning round-mouthed facial expression and rhythmic expiration vocalizations (see Chevalier-Skolnikoff, 1974a, Fig. 1d). The postejaculatory phase lasted about 2 min, during which the pair remained united. (For further descriptions of the heterosexual copulation pattern in this species, see Bertrand, 1969; Blurton-Jones and Trollope, 1968; Chevalier-Skolnikoff, 1975; Lemmon and Oakes, 1967. See also Kanagawa *et al.*, 1972, on the copulatory behavior of vasectomized males, whose behavior differs from that described in the other studies.)

Male homosexual encounters included prolonged manual genital stimulation, sometimes mutual; oral genital stimulation (fellatio), also sometimes mutual; dorsal mountings with pelvic thrusts and, occasionally, anal intromission. Some encounters consisted of sequences involving several methods of stimulation. No ejaculations, or evidence of orgasm were observed in this study during male homosexual encounters.

Homosexual manual genital stimulation was effected in one of three ways (see Table II): In association with mountings, the animal who was being mounted would reach back and manipulate the genitals of the mounting animal (see Chevalier-Skolnikoff, 1974a, Fig. 3a), holding his partner's penis in one hand and moving his hand back and forth along the shaft, or one monkey presented to a second monkey, who manually stimulated the presenting animal. In the case of mutual stimulation, the partners would present simultaneously, thereby bringing their genitals together and, standing rump to rump, would reach back and simultaneously manipulate each other's genitals (see Chevalier-Skolnikoff, 1974a, Fig. 3b).

Oral genital stimulation also occurred in several fashions (see Table II). One male might present and the second animal would orally stimulate the first, licking the presenting monkey's penis or taking his penis in his mouth and evidently sucking on it as he stood behind him. Or the second monkey might mount the first in a peculiar fashion that permitted him to simultaneously orally stimu-

Table II. Methods of Stimulation Recorded in Male Homosexual Encounters

Method of stimulation	Number of incidents recorded[a]
Mounting with pelvic thrusts, the mounter stimulating himself by rubbing his penis against the animal mounted	5
Mounting with intromission and pelvic thrusts	1
Mounting with oral stimulation of animal mounted	2
Mounting with mutual oral stimulation	2
Mounting with manual stimulation of mounter by animal mounted	4
Presentation, with the second male orally stimulating the presenting male	2
Presentation, with the second male manually stimulating the presenting male	1
Mutual presentations with mutual manual stimulation	2

[a] Some encounters involved several methods of stimulation occurring in sequence; consequently, the numbers of incidents add up to more than 13 (the number of encounters recorded).

late his partner (see Chevalier-Skolnikoff, 1974a, Fig. 3c). On some occasions, while being stimulated in the manner just described, the mounted animal simultaneously bent his head under his own body, thereby reaching the genitals of the mounting animal, orally stimulating them (see Chevalier-Skolnikoff, 1974a, Fig. 3d).

The single recorded case[4] of anal intromission occurred as follows:

> Stanford, 8/19/68, 11:45 a.m. (Description from notes.) The subadult male, No. 5, presents to the five-month-old infant male, No. 3-1, reaching back toward the infant with one hand. The infant mounts the subadult. The subadult manipulates the infant's penis with the extended hand while the infant remains awkwardly mounted too low on the subadult. The subadult ceases the genital manipulation and pushes the infant's posterior up toward his anal region and, with his hand, guides the infant's penis into his anus. The infant makes about three pelvic thrusts, and the subadult pulls the infant down from his mounted position. The infant starts to leave. He returns, and the subadult draws him to his ventrum and embraces him. The subadult grooms the infant.

As in the above incident, hugs and embraces, often accompanied by the excited teeth-chattering expression, frequently followed male homosexual encounters.

[4] Several cases of anal intromission were observed; only one was recorded.

The positive facial expressions generally associated with heterosexual copulations also accompanied various phases of the male homosexual encounters.

In all male homosexual encounters, one member of the pair assumed the sexual role carried out by the opposite sex in heterosexual coitus. In two incidents, both monkeys took on female sexual roles (they simultaneously presented and manipulated each other's genitals). On the 11 other occasions, only one animal took on a female role. The subordinate animal, who was the subadult male, No. 5, in both male pairings, took the female role ten times and a male role three times. The infant, No. 3-1 (who was dominant[5] over the subadult, probably because of the high dominance status of his adoptive[6] mother), enacted a female role five times and a male role seven times. The adult male, No. 1, the most dominant male in the group, never assumed a female role. There seemed to be a definite relationship between dominance status and sexual role in these male homosexual interactions. The more dominant the animal, the more frequently he adopted a male sexual role.

The settings and contexts of homosexual behavior were examined to gain some understanding of the social determinants and functions of homosexual behavior. The one recorded incident of prolonged oral genital stimulation between the adult male (No. 1) and subadult male (No. 5) took place at the beginning of the study. At that time, the subadult male was still sexually immature, as evidenced by the absence of observed ejaculations during heterosexual copulations.

The two monkeys had a strong affectional tie. The subadult was very submissive toward the adult and frequently addressed subordinate gestures toward him, such as subordinate presentation. The adult was always friendly and protective of the subadult, generally taking his part in aggressive encounters. The two often spent rest and sleep periods huddled together, the subadult with his back up against the ventrum of the adult, who sat with his arms around the younger animal, often holding the subadult's penis in one hand. Such behavior has also been observed between males in colony groups of stumptail monkeys at Davis (Lindburg, 1969).

During active periods, the adult male often approached the subadult from the rear and briefly examined his genitals. Such behavior is common in stumptail macaques. Males often examine the genitals of other males as part of their dominance behavior, and they also examine females both in dominance and in

[5] The infant's dominance was manifested by his ability to displace the subadult male or to take food from in front of him.

[6] Female No. 4, the infant male No. 3-1's adoptive mother, was the second most dominant adult female in the group. His biological mother, No. 3, was relatively subordinate. Six days before No. 3-1 was born, female No. 4 gave birth to an infant who was stillborn or died within 12 hr after birth. When No. 3-1 was first seen, within 5 hr after birth, he was being carried by female No. 4, rather than by his biological mother, female No. 3. Evidently female No. 4 had taken him from the more subordinate mother, female No. 3. Female No. 4 cared for No. 3-1 and nursed him throughout the study.

sexual interactions. Adults of both sexes routinely direct such behavior toward infants (Bertrand, 1969; personal observations). However, these incidents between the adult and subadult male were accompanied by the positive facial expressions that generally accompany precopulatory sexual examinations, rather than the threat expressions that often accompany dominance mounts, and they were also accompanied by the intensely excited teeth-chattering expression. Furthermore, these examinations were frequently followed by embraces and affectionate mutual mouth nibbles.

It was in this social setting, on a day in which the patterns of huddling while holding the penis and anogenital examination were particularly evident between the two animals, that after one of the usually brief anogenital examinations, the adult male proceeded to orally stimulate the genitals of the subadult for a prolonged interval. The two animals subsequently embraced and then huddled in their characteristic manner, the adult holding the subadult's penis in one hand. Approximately 1½ months after the above encounter, the subadult male began showing evidence of sexual maturity: heterosexual copulations were accompanied by ejaculation, his face began to assume the adult red sexual coloration, his browridges became heavier, and his canine teeth perceptibly increased in length. At this point, the relationship between the two males became less intense, and, although they remained amicable until the end of the study, they soon ceased their frequent embraces and mutual mouth nibbles and their characteristic huddling pattern.

Male homosexual encounters occurred most frequently between the subadult male (No. 5) (who by this time was probably sexually mature) and the infant male (No. 3-1). They, too, occurred in the context of an intensely positive emotional relationship. From the time the infant was approximately 5 weeks of age, the subadult male spent much time with him. By the infant's ninth week, the subadult male gave the infant routine parental care (which males characteristically do in this species, despite its seeming incongruence with the male sexual role). This parental care consisted of carrying, grooming, and holding the infant. He also played with the infant, which mothers tend not to do. During active periods of the day, the infant often was held and carried by the subadult male as much as by his mother. The first sexual interactions between these two animals were observed during the infant's fifth week, when the infant performed rudimentary mounts on the subadult male. During the infant's fourth month, his homosexual behavior with the subadult male became more elaborate. At this point, the two animals began to engage in oral and manual genital stimulation as well as mounting. During his fifth month, the infant was observed to achieve anal intromission (with pelvic thrusts, but without ejaculation or evidence of orgasm) with the aid of his partner (see, for example, the preceding quote from notes). This sexual aspect of the relationship between these two animals continued to be important until the end of the study when the infant was 6 months old.

An examination of the immediate contexts in which male homosexual encounters occurred reveals that only one of the 13 recorded incidents took place during or after an aggressive interaction. Five occurred in friendly contexts, such as after grooming or after embraces between the two monkeys. Eight of the 13 encounters took place on days in which a female in the group was evidently in estrus[7] and much heterosexual sexual activity was occurring (see Table III).

The males, including the infant, often appeared to become sexually aroused by this heterosexual activity prior to the homosexual encounters. On some occasions, the male involved in the heterosexual encounter became one of the principals in the homosexual encounter. This suggests that it was not the absence of an estrous female that led to the male homosexual encounters. Michael (1969) reported evidence that pheromones, or smell stimuli, from the estrous female rhesus monkey (*Macaca mulatta*) are involved in eliciting male sexual behavior. Although it is possible that pheromones are involved in eliciting the homosexual behavior reported here, homosexual relationships between the male stumptails were always an aspect of more generalized close affectional ties that were evidently rewarding to both the parties involved. In the relationship between the adult and subadult males, the adult gained reassertion of dominance while the subadult gained social protection. In the subadult-infant pair, the more dominant infant received parental care, and both parties gained play partners. All animals benefited at least on occasion in terms of sexual stimulation and general affective rewards.

Homosexual Behavior Among Females

Only adult and subadult females manifested homosexual behavior. Unlike male homosexual behavior, female homosexual behavior was rather stereotyped in form. One female mounted another by actually climbing on top of her, grasp-

[7]The term "estrus" refers to the period near the time of ovulation during which a female mammal is sexually receptive. In this study, estrus was inferred behaviorally from observations of females repeatedly initiating or submitting to copulations, since external signs of estrus, such as genital swelling or reddening, rarely occur in this species (Trollope and Blurton-Jones, 1970; personal observations). This interpretation of copulatory behavior indicating female estrus was often substantiated by the observation of its occurrence at approximately monthly intervals over several months in particular females. However, it could not be established that all the copulatory behavior of all the females occurred in monthly cycles, and some copulatory sequences may have occurred when females were not in estrus, or at least not ovulating. Bertrand's (1969) observations of females copulating during menstruation support this latter possibility, as do the experimental studies by Slob *et al.* (1974), who found that intact females copulated throughout their cycles, and that ovariectomized females continued to copulate, although at somewhat lower frequencies than prior to surgery. These data on copulations occurring out of ovulation phase suggest that copulatory behavior is more independent of hormonal cycles in stumptail monkeys than in most or all other primate species, with the exception of human beings.

ing the mounted female's shoulders with her hands and her hips with her feet. Subsequently, by thrusting, she rubbed her genitals on the rump of her mount (see Chevalier-Skolnikoff, 1974a, Fig. 2a). The mounting female was thereby genitally stimulated but the mounted female was not. Despite this lack of stimulation for the mounted female, she generally appeared to be very excited, and both animals usually made intense, friendly facial expressions before, during, and after the mounting.

Female mountings were of approximately the same duration as heterosexual copulations (around 2 or 3 min), and the phases were parallel. During the first phase, the mounting animal made a great number of pelvic thrusts, about the same number as the male makes in heterosexual copulations. On three recorded occasions, the mounting female (the most dominant female in each case) evidently reached orgasm, for she displayed all the behaviors characteristic of males during orgasm – pausing after the series of thrusts, stiffening, and then displaying muscular body spasms accompanied by the frowning round-mouthed expression and rhythmic expiration vocalizations. Extended postejaculatory phases, as seen in males during heterosexual copulations, were not observed, although the female having the orgasm did remain mounted during the period in which she made the characteristic orgasmic facial expression and vocalization. As in the case of male homosexual encounters, females often embraced after these homosexual mountings.

Evidence of orgasm in nonhuman female mammals has been reported (e.g., Zumpe and Michael, 1968; Burton, 1971; Fox and Fox, 1971), but no studies have described complete and obvious naturally occurring orgasmic patterns such as those observed in this study. Interestingly, all the obvious female orgasms observed here occurred during homosexual interactions. However, there is evidence that orgasms may also occur during heterosexual coitus (Chevalier-Skolnikoff, 1971, 1974a).

Four of the five adult and subadult females participated in female homosexual encounters; the most subordinate female (No. 54) was not involved. However, only two of the females (Nos. 2 and 4) ever took the male roles, and these were the two most dominant females; in every instance, the mounting female was dominant over the one being mounted. Every female in the group had one or two other females with whom she interacted most frequently (e.g., groomed, huddled). Some pairings changed over time, and others remained quite stable. As in the case of male homosexual interactions, females tended to mount other females with whom they had these close affectional ties. The most subordinate female in the group was also the most solitary animal with the weakest affectional bonds with other group members. She did not take part in any prolonged homosexual interactions, although she was frequently briefly mounted by adult females – often after being chased and bitten – in dominance interactions.

Despite the consistently higher dominance position of the mounting females, only two of the 23 female homosexual mountings occurred in aggressive

Table III. Contexts in Which Homosexual Encounters Occurred

Context	Number of encounters occurring in the various contexts[a]	
	Males (13 encounters)	Females (23 encounters)
Aggressive [e.g., immediately (within seconds) after a fight]	1	2
"Friendly" (e.g., immediately after grooming or after approaches that culminate in embraces)	5	1
Sexual (e.g., during or immediately after or between heterosexual copulations)	8	14
Context unknown	–	6

[a]Numbers of encounters occurring in particular contexts do not necessarily add up to the number of encounters, for some encounters occurred in two simultaneous contexts.

contexts (see Table III). These two cases occurred immediately after fights within the group. Female stumptails customarily embrace each other, briefly mount each other, or make half-mounts after group fights (personal observations), and Bertrand (1969) reported genital rubbing during "bullying" episodes. One might therefore expect to see homosexual behavior in such a context. However, most homosexual behavior observed during this study did not occur in or immediately following aggressive situations. One of the 23 mountings occurred in a generally friendly context, and 14 occurred in sexual contexts. In all the 14 cases occurring in sexual contexts, a female other than the mounting female was evidently in estrus, for she was repeatedly soliciting copulation and being mounted by one of the males prior to the homosexual encounter. In four cases, the female who was mounted homosexually was the female in estrus. In the other ten cases, females not in estrus were mounted. In no case was the mounting female in estrus, nor was she ever observed to come into estrus within 2 days of a homosexual encounter. Furthermore, in every case, the mounting female was lactating. These data indicate that, in most cases, prior heterosexual copulations were the immediate precursor to female homosexual activity. For example, observations were made during a series of eight complete copulations, each culminating in ejaculation, between the adult male and subadult female which were followed by a female-female homosexual encounter. The following are excerpts from the sequence:

Stanford, 4/25/68, 4:40 p.m. The subadult female (No. 6) presents to the adult male (No. 1), turning her head back to look at him over her shoulder with a direct gaze. The male mounts and obtains intromission and begins making pelvic thrusts, with a [friendly] square-mouthed expression on his face. Adult female No. 3 approaches with a square-mouthed expression and dances excitedly about, looking at the copulating couple. After 51 pelvic thrusts and 1 minute 46 seconds, the adult male ejaculates, pauses and then shows muscular spasms accompanied by the frowning round-mouthed look and rhythmic expiration vocalizations. The pair remains united during the 1 minute 47 seconds of the postejaculatory phase. The male dismounts, and the subadult female leaves.

4:57 The subadult female presents to the adult male, turning her head and looking back at him over her shoulder. The adult female (No. 2) approaches and presents to the adult male, looking back at him between her spread legs. The male ignores both females.

5:02 The subadult female and the adult male copulate again. While the couple is thus occupied, an adult female (No. 54) approaches the copulating pair and presents to the adult male; he ignores her.

5:11 The subadult female and the male copulate again. Adult females No. 2, No. 3, and No. 54 and the six-month-old infant female, No. 2-1, all approach excitedly. The infant has a square-mouthed expression. Female No. 2 alternately directs open-mouthed stare expressions [threats] at the copulating subadult female, and lip-smacking [friendly] expressions and teeth-chattering [excited friendly but nervous] expressions and squeaks at the adult male.

Shortly after: The female No. 2 approaches female No. 3, mounts her, and rubs her genitals on No. 3's rump. Female No. 2 dismounts from No. 3 and approaches and mounts female No. 4 and rubs her genitals on No. 4's rump. (No orgasm occured during either of these homosexual encounters.)

The observations of female homosexual behavior support some of the conclusions based on male homosexual behavior. First, homosexual behavior is not exclusive to infants and, in fact, the female infants did not participate at all. Second, it often appears to be directly elicited by observing sexual interactions. Third, it occurs between animals with close affectional ties (although this factor is less salient in females than in males). Fourth, dominance relationships are reflected in the homosexual interactions, although dominance need not be a primary elicitor of the behavior. They also indicate that neither the male nor the female form of sexual behavior is necessarily directly dependent on an estrous hormonal state in a female.[8]

DISCUSSION: SOME POSSIBLE FUNCTIONS OF HOMOSEXUAL BEHAVIOR

Homosexual behavior has often been considered "abnormal," or deviant and unadaptive, since it does not obviously serve the reproductive function. However, these observations of male, female, and infantile homosexual behavior in stumptail macaques, as well as reports in the literature of homosexual behavior in free-ranging macaques, suggest that homosexual behavior in nonhuman primates may not be abnormal and may foster general social cohesion.

[8] See Beach (1968) for a summary article on the available evidence on the factors involved in the control of mounting behavior in female mammals. See also Eaton (1973), Dixson *et al.* (1973), and Saayman (1973) on hormonal determinants of mating behavior in female primates.

In this study, prolonged homosexual encounters occurred between animals with strong affectional bonds, as manifested by their frequent grooming and huddling together, and supporting each other in dominance interactions with other monkeys. The sexual interactions in the homosexual dyads, especially between males, appeared to underscore these animals' close affectional ties. These data suggest that prolonged homosexual encounters usually differ functionally (represent the assertion of affectional ties) from brief homosexual mountings, which represent an assertion of dominance.

Male and female homosexual behavior in this study often followed prior heterosexual activity in the group. This suggests that copulating animals emit some sort of stimulus to other animals watching them. In females, the correlation was especially high. Since monkeys of this species do copulate when females are out of ovulatory phase, the viewing of heterosexual coitus is a likely elicitor. Furthermore, since the females who initiated homosexual activities apparently were not in the ovulatory phases of their cycles, their homosexual behavior evidently was not elicited directly by estrous hormonal states.

The work of Harlow and his coworkers (e.g., Harlow, 1960, 1961; Harlow and Harlow, 1962; Harlow and Zimmerman, 1959) on rhesus monkeys, *Macaca mulatta,* has stressed the significance of peer contact and, particularly, play in the development of adult sexual behavior. In this study, also, contact with peers was one setting in which rudimentary sexual activity was observed. However, in this mixed-aged social group, early male infantile sexual behavior occurred not only during interactions with other infants of both sexes but with adults as well (see Chevalier-Skolnikoff, 1974b). The assistance provided by adults of both sexes to infants during sexual activity suggests that homosexual and heterosexual encounters with adults as well as with infants function as training for adult sexual roles. However, long-term, exclusively homosexual experience, as cited by Morris (1970) in the case of the male orangutan, may result in a reproductively abnormal adult sexual role.

Several conclusions can be drawn from this study that have general bearing on the whole view of the evolution of sexual behavior:

1. Homosexual behavior is not exclusive to man. Consequently, homosexual behavior is not dependent on exclusively human biology, or on human capacity for culture or learning.
2. Nonhuman primate sexual interactions, like those of man, can be variable in form.
3. Homosexual behavior in nonhuman primates is not limited to any specific age period, and primates probably have the capacity for both male and female sexual roles throughout their lives.

Other conclusions and inferences from this study may or may not be generalizable:

1. Homosexual behavior occurs between individuals who have strong positive emotional ties.

2. Homosexual interactions most often follow and appear to be elicited by viewing heterosexual activities.
3. Homosexual behavior, like heterosexual copulation, does not appear to be dependent on an estrous hormonal state in stumptail females, although it was observed in adult but not in infant females.
4. Homosexual behavior between animals with strong positive emotional ties, in sexual contexts, with prolonged genital stimulation effected by various means and sometimes culminating in orgasm, subjectively appears to be pleasurable and sexually stimulating to the animals involved, as the term "erotic" implies for formally similar behavior in man.
5. For infants, both heterosexual and homosexual interactions, with peers and with adults, may be training for adult sexual roles.

ACKNOWLEDGMENTS

I wish to express thanks to David Hamburg and R. C. Boelkins, Directors of the Primates Laboratory of the Department of Psychiatry, Stanford University School of Medicine, who kindly provided the animals and laboratory facilities for this study. I thank Frank Beach for his helpful comments on an earlier version of this article. I thank Julie Pesonen, Janice Andersen, and Harriett Lukes for their assistance in the preparation of the manuscript.

REFERENCES

Beach, F. A. (1949). A cross-species survey of mammalian sexual behavior. *Proc. Am. Psychopathol. Assoc.* 38: 52-78.

Beach, F. A. (1968). Factors involved in the control of mounting behavior by female mammals. In Diamond, M. (ed.), *Perspectives in Reproduction and Sexual Behavior*, Indiana University Press, Bloomington, Ind.

Bernstein, I. S. (1970). Primate status hierarchies. In Rosenblum, L. A. (ed.), *Primate Behavior: Developments in Field and Laboratory Research*, Vol. 1, Academic Press, New York.

Bertrand, M. (1969). *The Behavioral Repertoire of the Stumptail Macaque: A Descriptive and Comparative Study*, Vol. 11 of *Bibliotheca Primatologica*, Karger, Basel.

Bingham, H. C. (1928). Sex development in apes. *Comp. Psychol. Monogr.* 5: 1-165.

Blurton-Jones, N. G., and Trollope, J. (1968). Social behavior of stumptailed macaques in captivity. *Primates* 9: 365-394.

Burton, F. D. (1971). Sexual climax in female *Macaca mulatta*. In *Proceedings of the Third International Congress of Primatology, 1970*, Vol. 2, Karger, Basel, pp. 180-191.

Carpenter, C. R. (1942). Sexual behavior of free ranging rhesus monkeys (*Macaca mulatta*): Specimens, procedures and behavioral characteristics of estrus. *J. Comp. Psychol.* 33: 113-162. (Reprinted in Carpenter, C. R. (ed.), *Naturalistic Behavior of Nonhuman Primates*, Pennsylvania State University Press, University Park, Pa., 1964.)

Chevalier-Skolnikoff, S. (1971). The female sexual response in stumptail monkeys (*Macaca speciosa*) and its broad implications for female mammalian sexuality. Paper presented at the American Anthropological Association Annual Meetings, New York, November 1971.

Chevalier-Skolnikoff, S. (1974a). Male-female, female-female, and male-male sexual behavior in the stumptail monkey, with special attention to the female orgasm. *Arch. Sex. Behav.* 3: 95-116.

Chevalier-Skolnikoff, S. (1974b). *The Ontogeny of Communication in the Stumptail Macaqe* (Macaca arctoides), Vol. 2 of *Contributions to Primatology*, Karger, Basel.

Chevalier-Skolnikoff, S. (1975). Heterosexual copulatory patterns in stumptail macaques *(Macaca arctoides)* and in other macaque species. *Arch. Sex. Behav.* 4: 199-220.

Dixson, A. F., Everitt, B. J., Herbert, J., Rugman, S. M., and Scruton, D. M. (1973). Hormonal and other determinants of sexual attractiveness and receptivity in rhesus and talapoin monkeys. In Phoenix, C. H. (ed.), *Primate Reproductive Behavior, Symposia of the Fourth International Congress of Primatology, Portland, Ore., August 15-18, 1972*, Vol. 2, Karger, Basel.

Eaton, G. G. (1973). Social and endocrine determinants of sexual behavior in simian and prosimian females. In Phoenix, C. H. (ed.), *Primate Reproductive Behavior, Symposia of the Fourth International Congress of Primatology, Portland, Ore., August 15-18, 1972*, Vol. 2, Karger, Basel.

Ellis, H. (1896). *Studies in the Psychology of Sex*, reprinted in 1936, Vols. I and II, Random House, Modern Library, New York.

Erwin, J., and Maple, T. (1976). Ambisexual behavior with male-male anal penetration in male rhesus monkeys. *Arch. Sex. Behav.* 5: 9-14.

Fooden, J. (1967a). Identification of the stump-tailed monkey, *Macaca speciosa* I, Geoffroy, 1826. *Folia Primatol.* 5: 153-164.

Fooden, J. (1967b). *Macaca fuscata* (Blyth, 1875): Proposed conservation as the name for the Japanese macaque (mammalia) Z. N. (S) 1802. *Bull. Zool. Nomenclature* 24: 250-251.

Ford, C. S., and Beach F. A. (1952). *Patterns of Sexual Behavior*, Eyre and Spotteswoode, London.

Fox, C. A., and Fox, B. (1971). A comparative study of coital physiology with special reference to the sexual climax. *J. Reprod. Fertil.* 24: 319-336.

Gordon, T. P., and Bernstein, I. S. (1973). Seasonal variation in sexual behavior of all-male rhesus troops. *Am. J. Phys. Anthropol.* 38: 221-225.

Hamilton, G. V. (1914). A study of sexual tendencies in monkeys and baboons. *J. Anim. Behav.* 4: 295-318.

Hanby, J. P., and Brown, C. E. (1974). Development of sociosexual behaviours in Japanese macaques, *Macaca fuscata*. *Behaviour* 49: 152-196.

Harlow H. F. (1960). Primary affectional patterns in primates. *J. Orthopsychiat.* 30: 676-684.

Harlow, H. F. (1961). The development of affectional patterns in infant monkeys. In Foss, B. M. (ed.), *Determinants of Infant Behaviour I*, Wiley, New York.

Harlow, H. F., and Harlow, M. K. (1962). Social deprivation in monkeys. *Sci. Am.* 207: 136-146.

Harlow, H. F., and Zimmerman, R. R. (1959). Affectional responses in the infant monkey. *Science* 130: 421-432.

International Commission on Zoological Nomenclature (1970). Opinion 920. *Bull. Zool. Nomenclature* 27: 77-78.

Itani, J. (1959). Paternal care in the wild Japanese monkey, *Macaca fuscata fuscata*. *Primates* 2: 61-93.

Kanagawa, H., Hafez, E. S. E., Nawar, M. N., and Jaszczak, St. (1972). Patterns of sexual behavior and anatomy of copulatory organs in macaques. *Z. Tierpsychol.* 31: 449-460.

Kempf, E. J. (1917). The social and sexual behavior of infrahuman primates with some comparable facts in human behavior. *Psychoanal. Rev.* 4: 127-154.

Kinsey, A. C., Pomeroy, W. B., and Martin, C. E. (1948). *Sexual Behavior in the Human Male*, Saunders, Philadelphia.

Kinsey, A. C., Pomeroy, W. B., Martin, C. E., and Gebhard, P. H. (1953). *Sexual Behavior in the Human Female*, Saunders, Philadelphia.

Kling, A. (1972). Personal communication.
Kummer, H., and Kurt, F. (1965). A comparison of social behavior in captive and wild hamadryas baboons. In Vagtborg, H. (ed.), *The Baboon in Medical Research,* University of Texas Press, Austin, Tex.
Lemmon, W. B., and Oakes, E. (1967). "Tieing" between stumptailed macaques during mating. *Lab. Primate Newsletter* 6: 14-15.
Lindburg, D. (1969). Personal communication.
Maslow, A. H. (1936). The role of dominance in the social and sexual behavior of infrahuman primates. I. Observations at Vilas Park Zoo. *J. Genet. Psychol.* 47: 261-338.
Masters, W. H., and Johnson, V. E. (1966). *Human Sexual Response,* Little, Brown, Boston.
Masters, W. H., and Johnson, V. E. (1970). *Human Sexual Inadequacy,* Little, Brown, Boston.
Michael, R. P. (1969). The role of pheromones in the communication of primate behavior. In *Proceedings of the Second International Congress of Primatology, Atlanta, Georgia, 1968,* Vol. 1, Karger, Basel, pp. 101-107.
Morris, D. (1970). The response of animals to a restricted environment. In Morris, D. (ed.), *Patterns of Reproductive Behavior,* McGraw-Hill, New York, pp. 490-511.
Ploog, D. W. (1967). The behavior of squirrel monkeys (*Saimiri sciureus*) as revealed by sociometry, bioacoustics, and brain stimulation. In Altmann, S. A. (ed.), *Social Communication Among Primates,* University of Chicago Press, Chicago, pp. 149-184.
Rowell, T. E. (1967). A quantitative comparison of the behavior of a wild and caged baboon group. *Anim. Behav.* 15: 499-509.
Saayman, G. S. (1973). Effects of ovarian hormones on the sexual skin and behavior of ovariectomized baboons (*Papio ursinus*) under free-ranging conditions. In Phoenix, C. H. (ed.), *Primate Reproductive Behavior, Symposia of the Fourth International Congress of Primatology, Portland, Ore., August 15-18, 1972,* Vol. 2, Karger, Basel.
Sade, D. S. (1968). Inhibition of son-mother mating among free-ranging rhesus monkeys. In Masserman, J. H. (ed.), *Animal and Human: Science and Psychoanalysis 12,* Grune and Stratton, New York, pp. 18-38.
Slob, A. K., Goy, R. W., Weigand, S. J., and Scheffler, G. (1974). Gonadal hormones and behaviour in the stumptail macaque (*Macaca arctoides*) under laboratory conditions: A preliminary report. *J. Endocrinol.* 64: 38.
Talmage-Riggs, G., and Anschel, S. (1973). Homosexual behavior and dominance hierarchy in a group of captive female squirrel monkeys (*Saimiri sciureus*). *Folia Primatol.* 19: 61-72.
Trollope, J., and Blurton-Jones, N. G. (1970). Breeding the stumptailed macaque, *Macaca arctoides. Lab. Anim.* 4: 161-169.
Wickler, W. (1973). *The Sexual Code: The Social Behavior of Animals and Men* (trans. by F. Garne), Anchor Press/Doubleday, Garden City, N.Y.
Zuckerman, S. (1932). *The Social Life of Monkeys and Apes,* K. Paul, Trench, Trubner, London.
Zumpe, D., and Michael, R. P. (1968). The clutching reaction and orgasm in the female rhesus monkey (*Macaca mulatta*). *J. Endocrinol.* 40: 117-123.

WHAT DOES GOD HAVE TO DO WITH IT?

The meaning of AIDS

DENNIS M. DOYLE

The title of the U.S. Catholic bishops' document, "The Many Faces of AIDS," highlights what a multi-faceted disease we are up against. AIDS is an illness, an epidemic, a killer, a threat, a news event, a mystery. In its commingling of sex, death, and drugs, AIDS strikes fear and fascination into our hearts. Our reactions to AIDS are complex and often anything but level-headed. The social phenomenon of AIDS breaks down our minds' defense systems and gives free rein to the deep-seated fears of even the most well-adjusted among us. AIDS is the great American Rorschach test, a dark blot whose interpretations may say more about the interpreter than about the picture being interpreted.

A recent Times Mirror Gallup Poll revealed that 42.5 percent of those surveyed think that AIDS might be a punishment from God for immoral sexual behavior (*Newsweek*, February 1, 1988). Presumably, about 57.5 percent find that pretty hard to believe. How could anyone see the hand of God in the pain of human beings? What about the people who acquired AIDS from blood transfusions or while in the womb? Is the fact that lesbians are currently the lowest risk group for AIDS a sign of God's favor?

And yet for the 42.5 percent who said yes, the connection may seem obvious. Since the question asked whether AIDS *might* be a punishment from God, isn't it outrageously presumptuous to suggest that God has nothing to do with AIDS? Didn't God send the angel of death to kill the firstborn of the Egyptians when the pharaoh refused to let God's people go? Didn't C.S. Lewis explain how pain can come as a gift from God to move us from sin to grace? Is it simply a coincidence that the two highest risk groups, nonmonogamous homosexuals and intravenous drug abusers, are engaged in activities that traditionally carry the admonishment of religious authorities?

It is clear that the social phenomenon of AIDS raises not just ethical questions but fundamental theological questions. Even the poll results are as interesting for what they suggest about people's attitudes toward God as for what they suggest about people's attitudes toward AIDS.

A reading of some of the popular literature on the ultimate meaning of AIDS reveals a complex picture. There are as many positions about how God acts in the world and, consequently, what AIDS means, as there are commentators. Each commentator is operating with basic theological presuppositions, whether explicit or implicit. An examination of several approaches to the question of how God acts in the world will serve as a vehicle for introducing some current literature about the meaning of AIDS.

The following models are intended to provide a general backdrop against which to understand the presuppositions

DENNIS M. DOYLE *teaches religious studies at the University of Dayton where he specializes in ecclesiology and pastoral ministry.*

of various interpretations of AIDS in its relationship to God. They are not intended to be either inclusive of all possible positions or free of overlap. The terms "interventionist" and "intentional" are taken from John Shea's *Stories of God* (Thomas More Press, 1978), though what Shea means by them differs somewhat from my usage here.

Beliefs about AIDS and Divine Activity:

• *Interventionist.* Stresses divine omnipotence, with an emphasis on God's occasional breaking into the natural order of things to accomplish special purposes.

This approach underlies the position of Charles Stanley, former president of the Southern Baptist Convention. Stanley is quoted in the *Los Angeles Times* (January 24, 1986) saying, "AIDS is God indicating his displeasure toward a sinful lifestyle."

Why would Stanley say this?

Imagine that you believe the Bible is inspired by God in a way that it is factually inerrant. You read the stories of God wiping out the world of Noah, putting plagues upon the Egyptians, sending the Israelites into captivity, striking dead Ananias and Sapphira, and on and on. You know well that God's wrath can be made manifest in this life and that justice is thereby done. You know also that in your fundamentalist reading of the Bible homosexual behavior is consistently and clearly condemned.

From this perspective it would be silly not to suspect strongly that God is directly behind AIDS. The argument that some victims are clearly "innocent" is unconvincing, for the Scriptures put no constraints upon God to have everything work out justly in this life. That the punishment of one group spills over onto others does not mean that God cannot be the cause.

• *Natural Consequences.* Believes that God is the primary cause of all, but there exist secondary chains of causality. Divine justice is structured into the universe such that ultimately one pays the price of one's transgressions.

This approach can be found in the position of Gene Antonio in *The AIDS Cover-Up? The Real and Alarming Facts about AIDS* (Ignatius Press, 1986). Antonio draws a connection between the onset of AIDS and the widespread violations of biblical injunctions against homosexuality and bestiality. He chastises the "self-appointed prophets of nihilism and pansexual libertinism who have succeeded in fostering the conditions leading to the biological and social downfall of society. . . . With AIDS, the horrendous physiological consequences of their deathstyle can no longer be concealed." Antonio laments that "the Pied Pipers of the homosexual liberation movement have led hundreds of thousands, perhaps millions, of young bathhouse habitués to an impending AIDS death."

Similar presuppositions are reflected in the position taken by the Vatican representative to the United Nations, Archbishop Justo Mullor, in a speech given to the World Health Organization in May, 1987 when he said that AIDS, although not directly caused by God, is the result of disturbances in human ecology due to a "suicidal permissiveness geared to anarchistic pleasures." This manifests one way of understanding: what you sow you reap. The universe is structured in such a way that sooner or later you will pay; official Catholic teaching is clear about the immorality of homosexual activity and drug abuse.

As with the interventionist position, it is not logically necessary that there be a one-to-one correspondence between those who are "guilty" and those who are punished. It is only necessary that there be a fairly high correlation. God is not directly zapping people. Secondary causes are at work in such a way as to achieve the ultimate ends of divine providence.

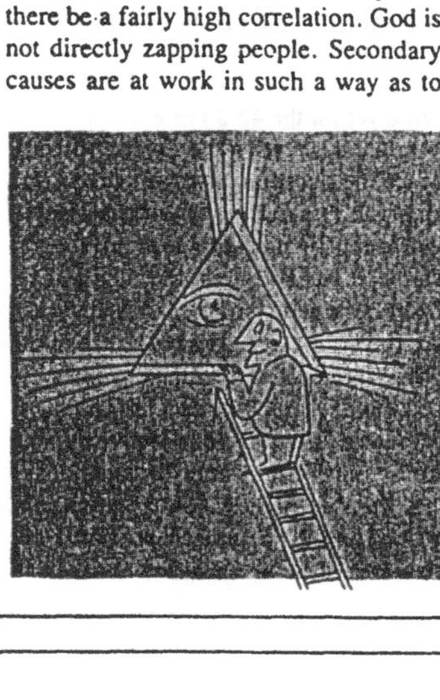

A New Age interpretation of AIDS, which is something of the flip side of Antonio and Mullor's positions, is claimed to have been "channeled" by Kevin Ryerson from John of Zebedee, who lived 2,000 years ago and was a follower of Christ (see *Psychoimmunity and the Healing Process*, Celestial Arts, 1986). To "channel" is to serve as a medium for a being from another spiritual plane or from another time. "John," the being who is channeled, envisions AIDS as a mirror reflection of the way that society has treated the high risk groups, homosexuals and drug abusers. In a separate channeling, a direct link is made between the collapse of the immune system and social disinvestment.

Like the positions of Antonio and Mullor, this New Age view presupposes a natural order that responds to moral outrages without the need for a special divine intervention. It is distinct from Mullor's position in that it locates the morally outrageous in society's *treatment* of high-risk groups rather than in *behaviors* of the high-risk groups themselves.

• *Discernment.* Believes that God is at work in the world in mysterious ways, without relying on a model of direct intervention. God somehow influences not only the consciousness of human beings, but also guides major historical events and shapes significant moments in the lives of individuals. Although the ways of God are difficult to discern, the ways in which things happen are surely more than coincidence.

Such an approach underlies the position taken by the gay activist writer John Fortunato in his book, *AIDS: The Spiritual Dilemma* (Harper and Row, 1987). Fortunato rejects the idea that AIDS is a divine punishment. He believes that we cannot know the ultimate reason for AIDS. And yet he still feels compelled to wrestle with the question of the meaning of AIDS in the divine scheme of things. Fortunato writes: "I do not know why God—whose ways I wish I could just give up trying to understand—initially chose gay men to comprise most of AIDS' victims." Fortunato is of the school of thought that there is a reason for everything. Ultimately God is writing straight with crooked lines.

Fortunato speculates about redeeming elements that might be uncovered in the AIDS epidemic. Although Fortunato emphasizes that it is all a great mystery, he offers what he labels the "non-rational" suggestion that AIDS will put sufferers in touch with a true spirituality of death, resurrection, hope, and compassion, and that perhaps it will be through AIDS that society's attitude toward gays, drug abusers, and other marginalized groups might be converted.

What is fascinating about Fortunato's position is that he combines a gay activist view with the notion that AIDS has meaning in the divine plan.

John Paul II, although his specific discernment differs from Fortunato's, seems to take a similar approach to the question of God's activity in the world. Last fall, on the night he arrived in Miami for his second U.S. tour, the pope was asked whether AIDS is a punishment from God. He replied, amid many T.V. cameras, that "the ways of God are very difficult to determine." He said further that "homosexuals are in the heart of the church." During his trip, he both reached out compassionately to persons with AIDS and reasserted the church's official stand against homosexual activity. The pope's approach is neither to deny nor to overinterpret the activity of God, but to model an appropriate response in the face of an epidemic that challenges our powers of discernment.

• *Intentional*. Believes that God works through our inner life. God is experienced as a tug on our subconscious toward truth, goodness, beauty, and love. God is involved in human affairs insofar as human beings respond to this inner call and give themselves over to it.

That Eileen Flynn takes such a position is reflected in the title of her book, *AIDS: A Catholic Call to Compassion* (Sheed and Ward, 1985). Flynn discerns in AIDS a call for human beings to exercise Christian love of neighbor. She emphasizes universal human dignity, the special claims of the needy and the suffering, the imperative not to judge, the taking up of one's cross, being steadfast in hope, and many other central Christian themes. Flynn is critical of official Catholic teaching about homosexual activity, and suggests that monogamous relationships be encouraged.

Flynn discusses in depth the place of God in the phenomenon of AIDS without ever bringing up the question of whether God causes AIDS. The immanence of God is God within the human heart; the transcendence of God is the divine call to growth in love. Flynn presents a God who acts not through any kind of direct intervention but rather as a forceful tug on human intentionality.

The U.S. Catholic bishops in "The Many Faces of AIDS" (*Origins* December 24, 1987) take a position on the question of divine activity that sounds very much like Flynn's. They say, "Jesus has revealed to us that God is compassionate, not vengeful"; and stress that "as with all other diseases, AIDS is a human illness." The bishops outline a compassionate response that respects official Catholic teaching on the meaning of human sexuality, and implicitly criticizes any position which discerns in AIDS a direct punishment from God. They call for Catholics to respond as Jesus would. They focus on revelation as the disclosure of the possibility of new life and the deeper meaning of divine love.

The position of the bishops is echoed in a pamphlet put out by the Catholic Health Association of the United States, "AIDS: Ethical Guidelines for Healthcare Providers" by Diana Bader and Elizabeth McMillan, 1987. These guidelines insist on the importance of correcting the belief that AIDS is a punishment from God: "Such an attitude, personally demeaning to the person with AIDS, has the further disastrous effect of isolating from the community the sick person most in need of its practical support. The Catholic voice needs to make these ethical points even more forcefully because some persons both inside and outside the church think that Catholic moral doctrine sanctions the punishment idea."

• *Process*. Believes that God's power is persuasive, not controlling. God created a universe with many risky possibilities. What God most offers human beings are choices. God does not foreknow the future, but rather struggles and suffers,

Advertisement deleted.

triumphs and rejoices along with us.

This approach informs the position of Earl E. Shelp and Ronald H. Sunderland in their book, *AIDS and the Church* (Westminster Press, 1987) These scholars interpret AIDS as one unfortunate actualization of the many possibilities of this free and diverse universe that God has created. They argue that "God does not 'send' AIDS for some retributive purpose (such a thought flies in the face of the New Testament witness to a loving God). Rather, God 'risked' creating a world in which HIV could develop."

Shelp and Sunderland are therefore not as concerned about the cause of AIDS as they are about the human response to AIDS. God offers humankind the choice between accepting and rejecting the role of caregiver i.e., risking possible sufferinto to lovingly respond to the afflicted.

• *Secular.* Believes that the causes of this-worldly happenings can be explained adequately without any reference to God. Secularists characterize the "religious" view as holding that AIDS is a divine punishment, and sharply criticize that view. Loretta Koppelman, writing in a collection of essays, *AIDS: Ethics and Public Policy* (ed. by Christine Pierce and Donald VanDeVeer, Wadsworth, 1988), uncovers the contradictions inherent in the "punishment concept of disease," both religious and secular, when applied to AIDS. Her overall thrust, however, dismisses the value of any discussion whatsoever about the morality of behaviors involved in the transmission of AIDS. Her conclusion suggests that any wrestling with an ultimate meaning for AIDS is senseless and self-serving.

Writing in the same volume, Judith Wilson Ross offers an incisive analysis of various metaphors used to talk about AIDS. Drawing upon the thought of Susan Sontag, Ross concludes, "AIDS has been permitted and encouraged to carry a moral meaning, but the morality is in our minds, not in the disease." In yet another essay in the same volume, Allan M. Brandt writes, "In some quarters the misapprehension persists: AIDS is caused by homosexuality rather than a retrovirus. In this confused logic, the answer to the problem is simple: Repress these behaviors. Implicit in this approach to the problem are powerful notions of culpability and guilt."

Common to these interpretations is the insistence that AIDS is caused by a virus, period. Any attempt to import a dramatic meaning from outside the strict medical model will result in a destructive distortion of reality.

The debate about the meaning of AIDS is inextricably mixed with the debate about the meaning of God. Positions taken on AIDS education, prevention, and research are grounded in presuppositions about the way in which God is at work—or not—in the world.

Thus, to challenge any of the positions I have outlined is to challenge not just an opinion about a disease but deeply held sets of presuppositions and beliefs. It is futile to argue against an interventionist that divine justice is not at work on the grounds that not every case fits a neat pattern. Nor is it effective to argue against an avowed secularist that the combination of factors involved is too uncanny to be mere coincidence.

Nor is this by any means a debate confined to interventionists and secularists. Most Catholics, for example, would find the secular view foreign to their consciousness. Yet a broad pluralism exists even among Catholics who may think in terms of the interventionist, discernment, intentional, or process model, or more likely some combination thereof.

The trouble with this variety of competing beliefs is that issues that should be central to society's response to the AIDS epidemic—such as care-giving, prevention, and societal values—are becoming exclusively associated with certain sets of presuppositions, hampering the debate about what is a proper public response. For example, those who see AIDS as the hand of God warning about social permissiveness seem inclined to permit "the sinners to suffer" the consequences of their misdeeds. In other circles, it is difficult to discuss the behaviors by which the disease has most often been transmitted in the U.S.; any mention of "morality" is taken, of itself, to be judgmental and reactionary. Among those who see in AIDS an opportunity to exercise Christian charity and healing, any general questioning of social permissiveness is viewed as inappropriate and irrelevant to the task at hand.

Can society distinguish between giving heartfelt material and spiritual help to the suffering and condoning, without hesitation, any lifestyle whatsoever? Can society distinguish between blaming AIDS victims for the outbreak and spread of the disease on the one hand, and discussing the morality and risk associated with those behaviors? The bishops' perspective in "The Many Faces of AIDS" is a striking example that we can. Although the bishops' moral objection to any homosexual activity is hotly contested within society at large, the bishops still manage to stress a loving response to persons with AIDS while upholding the church's guidelines for moral sexual behavior. □

British Journal of Psychiatry (1986), **148**, 421–425

Homosexuality in Monozygotic Twins Reared Apart

ELKE D. ECKERT, THOMAS J. BOUCHARD, JOSEPH BOHLEN and LEONARD L. HESTON

We describe six pairs of monozygotic twins, in which at least one member of five pairs were homosexual, and one of the remaining pair was bisexual, from a series of 55 pairs, reared apart from infancy; all the female pairs were discordant for homosexual behaviour. This and other evidence suggest that female homosexuality may be an acquired trait. One male pair was concordant for homosexuality, while the other was not clearly concordant or discordant; this suggests that male homosexuality may be associated with a complex interaction, in which genes play some part.

There have been a few reports of homosexuality in male twins ascertained as part of a series. Kallmann (1953) reported 100% concordance in 37 monozygotic (MZ) pairs, compared to 12% in 26 dizygotic (DZ) pairs, but came to regard that rate for MZ pairs as excessive, because the twins were recruited from the 'clandestine world' of New York City homosexuals of the 1940s, which might favour over-inclusion of concordant pairs. In a series of 14 MZ pairs ascertained because of criminality, Lange (1931) found homosexuals in one concordant and one discordant pair. Sanders (1934) located twins through homosexual probands, and found five of six MZ male pairs concordant. Habel (1950) started with five MZ and five DZ probands in German prisons; he found three of the MZ and none of the DZ co-twins to be homosexual. In an unselected series of 495 German twins, Koch (1965) found one pair of discordant DZ males, and one pair of discordant MZ females. Heston & Shields (1968) obtained proband twins from consecutive admissions to London psychiatric facilities. They described five MZ pairs, two definitely concordant, two definitely discordant, and one equivocal; among seven DZ pairs, one was concordant. In addition, they described a family with 14 siblings, including three sets of male MZ twins; all of the twin pairs were concordant—two for homosexuality, and one for heterosexuality. A family in which six out of ten siblings were homosexual was later described by Dank (1971). However, we know of no systematic studies of sexual orientation based on a series of twins, which included either female twins, or twins reared apart.

The use of twins to estimate the relative contribution of genetic and environmental factors to phenotypic traits is well known, and authoritative reviews are available (Hrubec & Robinette, 1984; Gottesman & Carey, 1983). Only one special problem of analysis will be discussed here—the search for specific environmental factors which might reasonably be associated with specific phenotypic dissimilarities between members of an MZ pair. Such dissimilarities, which are evident in all pairs examined, must be non-genetic, and should in principle, be traceable to environment. In typical studies, the heritability of behavioural traits has been estimated at about 0.5, leaving sufficient scope for environmental effects (Bouchard, 1984). Yet assiduous searches, albeit mainly retrospective, for specific environments which affected only one member of a pair, and which therefore might underlie discordance, have yielded few findings (Hrubec & Robinette, 1984; Pollin *et al*, 1965). In large part, this failure might be due to the special environments of twins reared together, which include the presence of a genetically identical individual. They may be so similar for each member of a pair that differences in environment possibly associated with phenotypic differences may be too fine to be caught in the crude nets provided by our instruments for assessing environments.

The study of twins reared apart from infancy removes the confounding effects of environmental similarity. Thus similar outcomes for MZ pairs reared apart may be more confidently associated with shared genes, and dissimilar outcomes may be more clearly associated with environmental factors, because the early environments are more likely to be definably different. Further, one major confounding environmental factor will be eliminated—the other identical twin.

Method

At the University of Minnesota, we have recruited twin pairs who had been reared apart, and have brought them to Minneapolis for a week of intensive psychological and

TABLE I
Clinical details of male pairs

Twin 1a
Examination
Age 25, weight 58.3 kg, height 180 cm.
Development
1st born, weight 2.67 kg, height 49.5 cm. Pubic hair, age 12; facial hair, age 14; masturbation, age 13; first aware of his homosexuality, age 13; limited heterosexual petting, age 14; no heterosexual dating.
Sex practice
No heterosexual intercourse; homosexual experience starting age 13. Less active sexually than twin; estimates he has had homosexual contact with 25–30 men. Homosexual partner to twin, age 24.
Other
Learning disability, hyperactive, speech impediment with lisp as child. Emotionally labile, subject to episodes of anxiety and depression.

Twin 1b
Examination
Age 25, weight 59.8 kg, height 175 cm.
Development
Second born, weight 2.56 kg, height 49.5 cm, pubic hair, age 12; facial hair, age 14; masturbation, age 12; some heterosexual petting and dating starting in late teens.
Sex practice
Several heterosexual contacts with intercourse starting age 19; homosexual experiences starting age 13. More sexually active than twin, estimates he had had homosexual contact with about 500 men. Homosexual partner to twin age 24.
Other
Learning disability, hyperactive, speech impediment with lisp as child. Emotionally labile and subject to episodes of anxiety and depression. Hospitalized three times for depression, anxiety, and anger outbursts.

Twin 2a
Examination
Age 35, weight 71.0 kg, height 175 cm.
Development
Birth order, wt, ht, unknown (but said to be larger than twin at birth). Pubic hair, age 14, facial hair, age 17; masturbation, age 13. Some heterosexual dating in high school, but no sexual contact.
Sex practice
First homosexual contact age 12. Two brief heterosexual contacts age 17–18. Regarded himself as bisexual until age 19 when he became exclusively homosexual. Has had homosexual contact with seven men; prolonged contact with one man. Feels sexually attracted to twin, but no sexual contact with him.
Other
Enuretic until his teens. Adopted into large family on east coast.

Twin 2b
Examination
Age 35, weight 76.2 kg, height 173.5 cm.
Development
Birth order, ht, unknown, weight 1.9 kg, pubic hair, age 15; facial hair, age 15; masturbation, age 15; some heterosexual dating and petting in high school.
Sexual practice
Homosexual affair with an older man between ages 15–18. First heterosexual experience, age 20, with future spouse. No heterosexual contact, except with spouse. Married age 20, four children. Regards himself as exclusively heterosexual. Sexual relations once or twice a month. Happy with his sexual adjustment.
Other
Adopted and reared by a family in a small southern farming community.

medical study. The procedure included standardised medical-psychiatric interviews and examinations, and questionnaires and interviews concerning current and past sexual practices. Zygosity was established through blood typing. A complete description of the recruiting and study methods was given by Bouchard *et al* (1981). Among the 55 pairs so far studied (counting two sets of triplets as three pairs each), members of five MZ pairs, two male and three female, described themselves as homosexual. A member of a sixth pair of MZ females has extensive homosexual experience, and is regarded as bisexual. The twin who first became known to our group was the homosexual member of a female pair in one case. In the other three female pairs, both members were approached at the same time, and were persuaded to participate in the study by one of the investigators (TJB); while both members of the concordant male pair agreed to participate after discussion with their parents. In the other male pair, contact was first made with the twin who regarded himself as exclusively heterosexual: these twins agreed between themselves to participate. The exclusively homosexual twin volunteered information about his homosexuality in his first telephone contact with one of the investigators (TJB). None of the 16 DZ pairs included a homosexual.

That the twins are highly selected cannot be doubted; they are not representative of twins or homosexuals. Nevertheless, study of them has yielded clues which warrant description. In the following descriptions, details have been changed in order to protect the twins identities.

Results

The male pairs

A male pair, seen by us shortly after their reunion at age 25, was the result of a normal pregnancy. After an unremarkable postnatal course, they were adopted by different families of similar middle-class status, who lived in different suburbs of a major western city. Neither twin

TABLE II
Clinical details of female pairs

Twin 1a
Examination
Age 35, weight 63.2 kg, height 164 cm
Development
Birth order, wt, ht unknown; tomboy before puberty; menarche age 12–13; breast budding, age 10; masturbation age 10; limited heterosexual petting, age 16; but no dating.
Sex practice
Age 19 had heterosexual intercourse, not pleasurable, and during same year, realised that she was homosexual. First organism, mid 20's. Has had affairs with five women, the last and current eight years in duration.
Other
Enuretic to age 12, probable addiction to sedative drugs age 25.

Twin 1b
Examination
Age 35, weight 62.2 kg, height, 158 cm
Development
Birth order, wt, ht, unknown; menarche age 10.5; breast budding, age 8; masturbation age 11; heterosexual dating and petting in teens.
Sex practice
Age 18, heterosexual intercourse. Age 25, only marriage, which has continued to date. No homosexual experience. Heterosexual intercourse two to three times weekly, enjoyed.

Twin 2a
Examination
Age 40, weight 82.1 kg, height 163 cm
Development
Birth order, first; birth wt, 3.38 kg; menarche age 14; breast budding and pubic hair age 13; masturbation, age 13.
Sex practice
Age 16 had heterosexual intercourse, then with several men through age 18; 'could take it or leave it' ... 'boring'; one induced abortion. By 18, knew self to be homosexual and has had affairs with several females.
Other
Alcohol problem in past—described loss of control drinking; also amphetamine abuse. Major depression after suicide of female lover.

Twin 2b
Examination
Age 40, weight 65.6 kg, 160 cm
Development
Second born; birth wt 2.0 kg; menarche age 11.0; breast budding and pubic hair, age 11; 'tomboy' before puberty; dating age 18; no masturbation.
Sex practice
First intercourse age 18, exclusively heterosexual. Marriage age 22, three children. Describes current sex as 'somewhat important'.

Other
Reared in small, geographically isolated community which, together with strict religious practice in home, limited opportunity for early dating. Age 16 suspended from school for fighting.

Twin 3a
Examination
Age 35, weight 55.6 kg, height, 163 cm
Development
Second born; weight 3.0 kg and length 45.25 cm. Menarche at age 13; age 10 breast budding and pubic hair; masturbation age 17; heterosexual dating through last one to two years of high school (age 17+); age 20, first heterosexual intercourse. Through age 24 to 25, heterosexual contact with about 12 males; never married or engaged. Age 27, first homosexual affair—'knew' she was homosexual.
Sex practice
Living with female sexual partner since age 28 toward whom she expresses deep emotional attachment.

Twin 3b
Examination
Age 35, weight 53.5 kg, height 162 cm.
Development
First born, 2.7 kg, 42 cm. Menarche age 11; pubic hair age 11; breast budding age 12; dated age 15; first intercourse age 17; married age 18, four children. No homosexual contacts or feelings.
Sex practice
'Very satisfied' with sex life in marriage.

Twin 4a
Examination
Age 48, 79.5 kg, 165 cm.
Development
First born; menarche age 10.3; breast budding and pubic hair age 9. No dating until age 21; heterosexual intercourse age 22; age 23, first marriage from which one child. Age 25, first homosexual contact; then three years with two successive female partners. Age 29, second heterosexual marriage, which has lasted to date with no homosexual contacts; second child.
Sex practice
Since age 29 regards herself as exclusively heterosexual with good heterosexual marriage and active sex life. At same time, feels sexually attracted to both males and females.

Twin 4b
Examination
Age 48; 92.5 kg, 164 cm.
Development
As child of 7, vagina was penetrated by adoptive brother, who was then age 9; menarche age 9.5; breast budding and pubic hair age 8; heterosexual intercourse, age 12; child at age 14; first orgasm and first marriage age 16. Divorced and remarried age 35.
Sex practice
Active heterosexual sex life, never homosexual contact. Was prostitute for one year between marriages.
Other
Significant depression after divorce.

knew that the other existed until one went into a bar frequented by homosexuals in a neighbouring city, and there was mistakenly identified as his brother. Their histories were strikingly similar. As children, both had been hyperactive, had learning disabilities, and had speech impediments, mainly lisps. Both were emotionally labile and subject to episodes of anxiety and depression. Both had been active homosexuals since age 13, starting with boys in their neighbourhoods. Although the second-born had had a few heterosexual contacts, both had been aware of being intensely attracted to males and indifferent to females since late childhood. After discovering each other, they became sexual partners.

The second pair, tested four years after their reunion at age 35, was also the product of a normal pregnancy and delivery. One twin weighed 1.9 kg; his co-twin was said to be larger at birth and was 2 cm taller as an adult. The larger twin was adopted by a family living in a large city on the US east coast. He had homosexual relationships starting about age 12; at age 17–18, he had two brief heterosexual contacts which led him to regard himself as bisexual until age 19, when he became exclusively homosexual. He felt sexually attracted to his co-twin, who had been adopted and reared by a family living in a small southern farming community. He had married, had four children, and regarded himself as exclusively heterosexual. However, between ages 15–18, he had had a homosexual affair with an older man who lived in the same town. His only female partner has been his wife and, although intercourse is infrequent, he described his current sexual adjustment as a happy one. Table I contains further details.

The female pairs

Table II presents the major features of the four female pairs. Without reservation, three of the four pairs were discordant for sexual preference. One member of pair 4 had had a homosexual affair, which was intense and prolonged, so that we regard her as bisexual, although she describes herself as exclusively heterosexual since her second marriage in her late twenties. Her co-twin, like the other three co-twins, denied any homosexual experiences, and described herself as enthusiastically heterosexual.

All four pairs were adopted by ordinary families which did not have especially notable features. All were reared in medium-sized cities or suburbs, except for twin 2b, who was reared in a small town that was exceptional for its geographical and cultural isolation. In every pair, the homosexual member was the larger throughout life, but had experienced menarche later than her co-twin. The homosexual twin also lagged behind her co-twin in the development of secondary sex characteristics and in the age at which sexual experiences commenced. After menarche, the menstrual history of the two pairs for whom adequate information was available did not distinguish the homosexual from the heterosexual twin.

Discussion

The male pairs are typical of others which have been described, with the single main difference that they were reared apart in different environments. One pair was clearly concordant for homosexuality. Whether to count the other pair concordant or discordant, or partially one or the other, is problematic; analogous problems of classification often occur in twin studies. It is notable that the male homosexuals said that they were attracted sexually by their co-twins. Twins reared together strongly deny such feelings according to Kallmann's experience, and ours (Heston & Shields, 1968), although exceptions have been reported (Meyers, 1982).

Overall, the male pairs tend to confirm earlier studies of twins and twin families: the concordance rate for sexual orientation among MZ pairs is consistently above that of DZ pairs, and despite all problems of ascertainment and diagnosis, it is hard to deny genetic factors an aetiological role.

The female pairs yield evidence leading in an opposite direction. Either three or all four of our female pairs were discordant, depending on how one classifies twin 4a. This evidence suggests that in the women, environmental factors were decisive. Moreover, in each pair, the homosexual twin was taller and heavier, but achieved menarche later. In our four pairs, the mean difference in age at menarche was two years, whereas in normative series, the mean difference is about 0.3 year (Fischbein, 1977; Stern, 1973 and Gedda & Brenci, 1975). In our series, the 15 heterosexual female MZ pairs averaged 0.9 years difference in age at menarche, or 1.1 years less than the homosexual twins. In the homosexual pairs, the interval between the menarche of the first and the second twin, was significantly greater than the comparable interval observed in either the normative series, or in our reared-apart heterosexual twins ($P<0.05$, Mann-Whitney U statistic).

The difference of 0.6 years between members of our heterosexual pairs and normative pairs may well be associated with the separate rearing of our pairs. Shared rearing environments, or a tendency for twins reared together to compare notes when asked about developmental milestones, could logically explain the small difference in reported age at menarche between our heterosexual reared-apart twins and reared-together twins.

This pattern of findings suggests that female homosexuality is a trait acquired after conception, most likely after birth, but before menarche. It may be associated with delayed puberty and just possibly with larger physique. With this possibility in mind, we reviewed the medical history of the twins, but found no episodes of illness or other events which differentially affected the homosexuals.

These findings are descriptive only, and should be

regarded as clues upon which to base hypotheses; e.g. do lesbian women tend to have menarche at later ages than their heterosexual female siblings? If so, this would support our findings, and it would seem to warrant search for an acquired cause, perhaps an endocrinopathy. Neuroendocrine differences may be associated with male homosexuality (Gladue *et al*, 1984). Our evidence, though based on a small sample, implicates environmental factors as the major determinant of female homosexuality. If this remains a constant finding, it will, apart from general features of a culture such as language, be the strongest evidence known to us which attributes a major behavioural complex exclusively to environmental factors.

References

BOUCHARD, T. J. (1984) Twins reared together and apart: What they tell us about human diversity. In *Individuality and Determinism* (ed. S. W. Fox). New York: Plenum Press.

—— HESTON, L. L., ECKERT, E., KEYES, M. & RESNICK, S. (1981) The Minnesota study of twins reared apart: Project description and sample results in the developmental domain. In *Twin Research 3, Intelligence, Personality and Development* (eds. L. Gedda, P. Parisi, W. E. Nance), pp. 227–233. New York: Alan R. Liss.

DANK, B. M. (1971) Six homosexual siblings. *Archives of Sexual Behavior*, **1**, 193–204.

FISCHBEIN, S. (1977) Onset of puberty in MZ and DZ twins. *Acta Geneticae Medicae et Gemellogiae*, **27**, 151–158.

GEDDA, L. & BRENCI, G. (1975) Twins as a natural test of chronogenetics. *Acta Geneticae Medicae et Gemellogiae*, **24**, 15–30.

GLADUE, B. A., GREEN, R. & HELLMAN, R. E. (1984) Neuroendocrine response to estrogen and sexual orientation. *Science*, **225**, 1496–1499.

GOTTESMAN, I. & CAREY, G. (1983) Extracting meaning and information from twin data. *Psychiatric Developments*, **1**, 35–50.

HABEL, H. (1950) Zwillingsuntersuchungen an Homosexuellen. *Zeitschrift für Sexualforschung*, **1**, 161–180.

HESTON, L. L. & SHIELDS, J. (1968) Homosexuality in twins: A family study and a registry study. *Archives of General Psychiatry*, **18**, 149–160.

HRUBEC, Z. & ROBINETTE, C. D. (1984) The study of human twins in medical research. *New England Journal of Medicine*, **310**, 435–441.

KALLMANN, F. J. (1953) *Heredity in Health and Mental Disorder*. New York: Norton.

KOCH, G. (1965) Die Bedeutung genetischer Faktoren für das menschliche Verhalten. *Arzliche Praxis* **17**, 823 and 839–846.

LANGE, J. (1931) *Crime as Destiny* (translated by C. Haldane). London: Allen & Unwin.

MYERS, M. F. (1982) Homosexuality, sexual dysfunction, and incest in male identical twins. *Canadian Journal of Psychiatry*, **27**, 144–147.

POLLIN, W., STABENAU, J. R. & TUPIN, J. (1965) Family studies with identical twins discordant for schizophrenia. *Psychiatry*, **28**, 60–78.

SANDERS, J. (1934) Homosexueele tweelingen. *Nederl Geneesk*, **78**, 3346–3352 (from an abstract in English prepared by E. Slater).

STERN, C. (1973) *Principles of Human Genetics*, 3rd ed. San Francisco: W. H. Freeman.

Elke D. Eckert, MD, *Associate Professor of Psychiatry, University of Minnesota,*

Thomas J. Bouchard, PhD, *Professor of Psychology, University of Minnesota,*

Joseph Bohlen, MD, PhD, *Psychiatric Resident at Southern Illinois University School of Medicine,*

*Leonard L. Heston, MD *Professor of Psychiatry, University of Minnesota, Box 393, Mayo Building, Minneapolis, Minnesota, 55455, USA.*

*Correspondence

(Accepted 27 March 1985)

The conservative movement and the AIDS virus.

THE POLITICAL USES OF AN EPIDEMIC

BY MICHAEL J. FUMENTO

IN THE TRAGEDY of AIDS, some conservatives believe they have found a shiny weapon with which to restore traditional sexual morality. They wish to recapture their vision of a better world—one where homosexuality is pushed back into the closet (or further), where chastity, monogamy, and sexual morality are revered, and where sexual behavior is once again within the domain of law.

Michael J. Fumento is the author of *The Myth of Heterosexual AIDS*, to be published by New Republic Books, an imprint of Basic Books.

But in order to do so, they have been forced to distort the true nature of the epidemic. They will find, however, that the epidemic will not change to fit their wishes. Whatever short-term gains they make through disinformation will eventually disappear and leave their causes worse off than before. They have already victimized the sufferers of the disease. Another victim may be American conservatism itself.

At the root of conservative confusion over AIDS policy is confusion over the AIDS virus itself. There are essentially three theories of transmissibility. Theory One assumes that in addition to being blood-borne, the contagion can be transmitted casually, that it can be passed through mere close proximity as well as sexual intercourse. Theory Two assumes that HIV (the AIDS virus) is transmitted efficiently through both homosexual and heterosexual sex. Theory Three is that because HIV is blood-borne, it will continue to plague those who exchange fluids through anal sex and needles, but will pose far less of a threat to the general heterosexual population.

As a matter of logic, all three of these theories can't be right. Either AIDS is a "gay plague" or it's not. Either it is just a fluke that AIDS emerged in the gay community first or it is confined primarily to homosexuals (and drug users) by its very nature. Similarly, either AIDS is casually transmitted and hence no more a behavioral contagion than tuberculosis or influenza, or it's not. Yet conservatives frequently combine all three models depending on their state of confusion—and depending on their agenda.

THEORY THREE is correct. Ten years after the first heterosexual AIDS cases began showing up in New York City, AIDS remains confined almost exclusively to homosexuals, intravenous (i.v.) drug abusers, recipients of blood products prior to 1986, and their steady sexual partners. Only about two percent of all diagnosed AIDS cases in this country have been attributed to heterosexual transmission in native-born Americans, a figure that has held steady for several years now. In New York City only eight males have been identified as having gotten AIDS from heterosexual sex. If other health departments interviewed patients as carefully as New York and could thus screen out those who claim sex with women as their only risk when in fact they've had sex with men or shared needles, it's quite possible that they'd find fewer than a score of such heterosexual men in the country. Blood tests for HIV infection among military applicants, blood donors, and hospital patients also indicate that the problem remains tightly confined to a few groups.

Most conservative leaders and writers have remained impervious to these facts. While writers such as George Will and Norman Podhoretz have insisted on Theory Three (the correct one), Theory Two (easy heterosexual transmission) holds sway with the Reagan administration. Secretary of Education William Bennett and White House Director of Policy Development Gary Bauer have thrown in their lot with Theory Two, as to some extent has President Reagan, who has declared that "AIDS is surreptitiously spreading throughout our population."

The president is advised in these matters by Bauer and assistant for domestic policy Kenneth Cribb. These conservatives, advised often by the kookiest of scientists, have used the theory to push programs from mandatory premarital testing to chastity-based sex education in schools, all to combat a virus that, according to the theory, spreads about as efficiently as syphilis. In fact, syphilis is so infectious that you can get it on the back of your hand. The infection rate of this microbe during coitus is about 20 percent to 50 percent, depending on which sex it is being transmitted to (sexually transmitted diseases are transmitted more easily from male to female). HIV has an infection rate estimated by Centers for Disease Control epidemiologist Dr. Thomas Peterman at less than 0.1 percent going from male to female and less than 0.05 percent going from female to male. Thus, for males syphilis appears to be 400 times more infectious than AIDS; for females 500 times. Yet syphilis is the Reagan administration's favored analogy.

Republican presidential candidates Jack Kemp, Pierre du Pont, Alexander Haig, and Pat Robertson all supported mandatory premarital testing, on the syphilis prevention model. Two states have complied, and many others have such legislation pending. Senator Jesse Helms and Representative William Dannemeyer, both normally fierce champions of federalism, have introduced legislation to penalize states that refuse to mandate premarital testing. (Dannemeyer has deluged Congress with AIDS legislation, all of which remains bottled up in committee.)

We now have some evidence of how such strategies work. Couples preparing for marriage, by virtue of that fact, are in an extremely low-risk group for HIV infection. Some may be drug abusers or bisexuals, but few will be homosexuals. Thus in Illinois, by the end of May, of an estimated 60,000 tested marriage applicants, only six were HIV-positive. The price of these tests vary, but they average over $100 for each individual. Thus it costs an average of more than $1 million per AIDS case detected. Testing clinics are doing handsomely, but it's hard to see what benefit accrues to the people of Illinois. Detecting cases doesn't necessarily prevent even one case of AIDS. Testing premaritals simply because they have to get a licence is like the drunk who looked for his lost keys under the street lamp because the light was better there.

THE EDUCATION DEPARTMENT, under Bennett, distributes AIDS information materials to government and private institutions; included is a thick package detailing the syphilis control measures instituted under President Franklin D. Roosevelt. The department urges that similar measures be taken against AIDS. Bennett, the administration member most active in promoting monogamy and abstinence as a method of preventing AIDS, has also predictably taken the lead in criticizing the use of condoms. He publicized the term "condomania." Disguising moral indignation behind the shield of practicality, Bennett has tried to impeach the value of condoms in preventing AIDS. Studies have been dragged out demonstrating condom usage failure rates. Most frequently cited are the Planned Parenthood survey showing a ten percent failure rate for condoms as contraceptives and a University of Miami study showing a 17 percent failure rate in preventing transmission of the virus in partners of men infected with HIV.

A booklet circulated by Education Department staffers warns in all capitals: "DON'T ENGAGE IN INTIMATE CONTACT AT ALL. IF YOU HAVE HAD THAT KIND OF CONTACT IN THE PAST, STOP NOW. THAT IS THE ONLY 'SAFE SEX.' IF YOU ENGAGE IN CLOSE SEXUAL CONDUCT, YOU ARE PLAYING RUSSIAN ROULETTE WITH YOUR LIFE." The book also declares: "The Black

Plague was a disease that during the 14th century killed one-third or more of the people who live in Europe. . . . [Unlike AIDS] the plague killed only one out of every four people who caught it." Apart from the fatuousness of comparing an insect-borne disease with a blood-borne one, the mathematics are impossible.

Bennett and his allies replace "safe sex" with the phrase "safer sex," because, after all, one can never be 100 percent sure that one's partner is uninfected, nor 100 percent sure that a condom will be an effective barrier. Bennett et al. favor the term "Russian roulette." The only truly safe behavior is described as chastity until marriage, and then monogamy. One difficulty is immediately apparent. Urging homosexuals to remain chaste until marriage is obviously problematic. Because heterosexual transmission of AIDS is so rare, emphasizing chastity and monogamy as AIDS preventatives is clearly misfocused.

EVEN FOR that two percent who get AIDS heterosexually, Bennett's advice is problematic. First, since most of these two percent are female partners of drug users and probably tend to share the addicts' penchant for instant gratification, the chastity message is unlikely to affect them. Second, strange as it may seem in light of the campaign against promiscuity, the overwhelming number of heterosexually transmitted AIDS cases occur not in people engaging in "casual sex" but as a result of monogamous or near-monogamous relationships with i.v. drug users or, much less commonly, with bisexuals. This is because in a population with a low percentage of infected individuals and where transmission is highly difficult, only a regular relationship can expose one frequently to infection.

It follows that the same arguments conservative moralists use against condoms also apply to monogamy. There is no such thing as "safe" monogamy, because there is no way to know for certain that one's partner is neither cheating nor shooting up. Studies done in recent decades estimate extramarital infidelity rates upward from 21 percent for females and 26 percent for males. Those who tell us not to place our faith in "one thin sheet of latex" might better trust latex than a spouse.

Monogamy may be no more effective than condoms in preventing AIDS among heterosexuals. Both have their place, and that place is limited. Jack Kemp pointed out in an address that there's no need, moral concerns aside, for condom education for third-graders. But there's also no need, moral concerns aside, for impressing upon third-graders the importance of chastity, at least in order to prevent AIDS, for the same reason: AIDS is not being transmitted between third-graders. When engaged in properly, both condom usage and monogamy can reduce what is for most heterosexuals virtually no risk to absolutely no risk.

The director of a company that produces chastity-urging videos for schools (which don't even mention homosexuality but do warn against the terrors of deep kissing) is undaunted by the astronomical odds against acquiring HIV through intercourse with other drug-free heterosexuals. "If there is one chance in ten million that a kid will catch AIDS, he shouldn't take it." Of course, to avoid such odds with everything that could kill us would end life as we know it. This year, more than one in 5,000 Americans will die in automobile accidents, or about 2,000 in ten million. About 500 in ten million will die in accidental falls, while over 200 in ten million will die from accidental drowning. Are we thus to conclude that there is no such thing as "safe driving" or "safe walking" or "safe swimming," or even "safer driving" or "safer walking" or "safer swimming"?

What the video producer is saying is that, to him, extramarital sex has zero utility. Unfortunately, he doesn't have the honesty to come out and say so. It is dishonesty that underlies the entire moralistic scheme to exaggerate the heterosexual AIDS problem. Frustrated with the failure of the message "Sex will cost you your soul," the moralists have cynically replaced it with "Sex will cost you your life." Moral suasion is replaced by mortal terror.

One prominent conservative columnist, while acknowledging the low risk of AIDS to heterosexuals, nevertheless confided to me that he saw nothing wrong with the "chastity or death" message. He saw the end as being so important as to justify a "whatever works" approach. Yet such an approach is fraught with danger. At some point, sexually active heterosexuals are going to wake up and find they're still alive. Their chaste-out-of-fear brethren will see the same. What then? If the moral position is abandoned for a pragmatic one, how can the moral one be reclaimed once the reason for pragmatism is gone?

CONSERVATIVES HAVE to a great extent ignored the i.v.-drug aspect of AIDS, presumably because i.v.-drug use has nothing to do with syphilis or chastity. Given the overemphasis on heterosexual AIDS cases, this is rather amazing. Almost 60 percent of i.v.-drug abusers with AIDS are exclusively heterosexual. Even in heterosexuals who acquired the disease through intercourse rather than through needle-sharing, drug use is the overwhelming cause. About 85 percent of heterosexually transmitted cases occur in the partners of i.v.-drug abusers. Virtually 100 percent of males infected through heterosexual intercourse were the partners of i.v.-drug abusers. Yet no conservative member of Congress has introduced legislation dealing directly with the AIDS/i.v.-drug connection, and none has signed on to the bill introduced by Representative Charles Rangel that does deal with it.

Mention of the AIDS/i.v.-drug abuse connection is almost absent from the speeches of Bennett and Bauer. Bennett's booklet, "AIDS and the Education of Our Children," was put out last October. Almost two million copies have been printed. In this booklet, 15 sentences concern drugs only, 13 concern both sex and drugs, three sentences concern exclusively homosexual intercourse, and two exclusively heterosexual intercourse. By contrast, a whopping 79 sentences make reference to sex in general, without mentioning drugs and without differentiating between homosexual and heterosexual sex. (Of these, 18 are devoted to disparaging condom usage.) Nowhere is anal sex mentioned. What can be said of a man who complains bitterly that the surgeon general's report was incomplete because it did not mention condom failure when his report fails to mention that over 95 percent of sexually transmitted AIDS cases occur from anal sex? Nowhere is the reader told that AIDS is virtually nonexistent in heterosexual men whose partners do not inject drugs. The silence is all the more amazing given the Reagan administration's usual habit of using any evidence to inveigh against the "epidemic" of drug use in the United States.

According to *Chicago Tribune* reporter John Crewdson, at an October meeting at which White House officials and officials from CDC were present, Bennett confronted CDC Director James Mason. Bennett said, "You mean this thing is not exploding into the heterosexual community?" Dr. Mason replied, "No, it's not." Whereupon Bennett said, "Well, why have you been telling everybody that it is?" Why indeed? But why did Bennett then proceed with the mailing of his booklet, with a reprinting several months later?

AS UNFOUNDED as the syphilis theory is, the casual contact theory is nothing short of bizarre. And unlike the syphilis theory, it appears to be almost the sole domain of the right. Because responsible public officials and reporters will not credit the casual contagion model, its proponents are prone to conspiracy theories. The guru of the casual contagion theory is John Seale. Although he is a medical doctor, he gains most respectability from being a member of Britain's Parliament. He has testified before a committee of the California General Assembly at the behest of conservative Republican legislators, and also elsewhere at the behest of New York Governor Mario Cuomo.

Seale submitted a report to the House of Commons in May 1987, in which he admitted—indeed, trumpeted—that the material therein was completely in conflict with the reports in British and American medical journals. Among Seale's claims was that "male homosexual contact of the finger, penis, or tongue with the rectal wall of another man transmits the virus very easily. . . . Moderately efficient means of transmission include mouth-to-mouth and genital contact [and] oral salivary contact between small children."

Such a kook would be only amusing if he weren't taken so seriously on the mainstream American right. His influence extends beyond fringe publications such as Reed Irvine's "Accuracy in Media" newsletter and the *Washington Inquirer*, which have made much play of Seale. Wayne Lutton, writing a scathing critique of "The Surgeon General's Report on AIDS" in *National Review*, quoted Seale as saying that "the genetic information contained in [AIDS'] tiny strip of RNA has all that is needed to render the human race extinct within 50 years." He mentioned none of Seale's quirks. Lutton reprinted Seale's California testimony in a book he co-authored on AIDS, again without disclaimer. Last December presidential candidate Pat Robertson, in an interview with New Hampshire's *Concord Monitor*, declared that "if say, we're in a room with 25 people with AIDS and they're breathing various things into the atmosphere, the chance of somebody catching it has become quite strong." Robertson's source, according to a spokesman, was Dr. John Seale.

Other conservatives, such as nationally syndicated columnist Gregory Fossedal, don't even feel the need to cite a physician or theorist like Seale to push the casual transmission line. Fossedal wrote in one column:

> Polls show that a majority of Americans think they are being lied to about the disease, and they're right, as the provocative book *The AIDS Cover-up?* suggests. They can tell that doctors are telling the truth but not the whole truth when they say there's no evidence AIDS can be spread through casual contact. (There's nothing proving it can't, and common sense suggests erring on caution's side.)

Fossedal merely states the logical proposition that one can't prove a negative. That AIDS is not casually transmitted is demonstrated in the same way as so many other negatives we accept are, by lack of evidence on the other side. AIDS has been recognized as an epidemic for seven years now. During that time there has yet to be identified a single case of casual transmission.

THE BOOK cited by Fossedal, *The AIDS Cover-up?*, was written by Gene Antonio, a heretofore unknown former minister, and published by the Catholic Ignatius Press. It has become a cult classic, with over 200,000 copies sold. It makes no bones about its purpose being to terrify, and it succeeds. "I got a copy of it from my dentist," related a friend of mine. After which she, a virgin until her marriage a year earlier, promptly got an HIV test. *The AIDS Cover-up?* has been offered as a selection of the Conservative Book Club, a popular book-of-the-month organization for conservatives. Copies of the text are displayed prominently on conservatives' bookshelves and desks throughout Washington. If you are a conservative journalist who writes about AIDS, like me, you are constantly plagued with the question: "Have you read Gene Antonio's book?" Antonio has written updates that are circulated by the Department of Education. He has spoken at meetings of Phyllis Schlafly's Eagle Forum. His agenda is also stridently anti-homosexual, portraying gay people as agents of human destruction.

The AIDS Cover-up? cites Seale 13 times. But Antonio is fully capable of apocalyptics himself. He uses the average doubling time of AIDS cases (12 months at that time, now thought to be at least 15) and extrapolates that as many as eight million Americans would be infected by the end of 1987 and 64 million by the end of 1990. Antonio appears ignorant of the standard epidemiological curve, which indicates that as a new infection spreads, it slows down as the most vulnerable potential victims are struck and only harder targets are left. Eventually the rate peaks, drops, and levels off, as with syphilis or gonorrhea, or drops almost to a point of nonexistence, as with bubonic plague and influenza epidemics. (In the most AIDS-afflicted city in the United States, New York, the rate of new cases among homosexuals has already leveled off.) Antonio has also peddled an absurd comparison between AIDS and a completely unrelated lentivirus in sheep that can be transmitted through coughing.

One source quoted in *The AIDS Cover-Up?* probably constitutes the most egregious AIDS scare article printed in the mainstream conservative press. The March 1986 *American Spectator* featured an article claiming that 30 percent of all men patronize prostitutes, that cow's milk could transmit the virus (even were this true, the heat of pasteurization would kill HIV), and that AIDS can be transmitted by coughing. After summarizing the various categories of persons at risk, the article concludes ominously, "Who will be left?" To which the apparent answer is "nobody." Later, the *Spectator* ran an article by a former special adviser to Margaret Thatcher calling for compulsory universal testing with enforced isolation for the infected. A half year later, though, when the authors proposed a follow-up, the magazine was more wary. "I was beginning to notice no one was dying," managing editor Wladyslaw Pleszczynski told me.

THE *Wall Street Journal*, with the most prestigious conservative op-ed page in the country, has run two pieces advocating the heterosexual AIDS breakout theme. One was an anti-prostitution article in which the author, asserting that prostitution was no longer "victimless," claimed without citing any source that "between 1,000 and 10,000 men will become infected with the AIDS virus this year by having sex with female prostitutes." A year later in New York City, which has more heterosexual AIDS cases and probably more prostitutes than any city in the country, a total of eight men have been identified as having acquired AIDS sexually from women, prostitutes or otherwise. Another *Journal* op-ed was written by Katie Leishman, pushing the theory that AIDS is really syphilis. In an editorial just last year, the *Journal* also stated, "An African-style epidemic is certainly possible, especially with a mutation of the virus." (In fact, no virus known has ever mutated so greatly as to change its mode of transmission.) The *Journal*'s op-ed page has yet to publish a piece challenging the heterosexual epidemic myth.

The mainstream journal *Conservative Digest* is also not above using fanciful statistics. It reported that 1.5 million homosexual and bisexual men in the United States were infected with HIV and that 20 percent of these men were married and had passed the virus on to their wives. In fact, the official CDC estimate released nine months later indicated 625,000 to 1.1 million homosexual and bisexual men infected, a figure that many believe to be too high. As to their 300,000 infected wives, while CDC has no estimate of this, as of July only 1,500 full-blown AIDS cases were reported to have been infected through heterosexual intercourse. Of those, about 15 percent, or 225, appeared to have been infected by a bisexual.

The Rev. Jerry Falwell has employed all three AIDS transmission theories, calling for "immediate action [or] AIDS will prove to be the final epidemic—with millions dying each year—including your loved ones." Falwell makes no bones that the virus is being spread by evil practices of perverted sodomites. So is he saying that our loved ones are homosexuals? Or is he adopting Theory Two, in which case he must be saying our loved ones are humping like bunnies—not a very nice thing to say to someone on the Moral Majority direct mail list. Or is he saying the virus is casually transmitted, in which case why is the solution abstinence and monogamous marriages?

The honorary national chairman of the AIDS Prevention Institute, a chastity-pushing organization, is singer Pat Boone. The newsletter contains such admonitions as: "Save sex for marriage! You owe it to your future children!" Authorities such as Miss America 1988 are cited as calling for mandatory testing. A story in the newsletter tells the story of a heterosexually promiscuous young man whose glands remain swollen for more than a week. He sweats through an AIDS test that after an agonizing wait comes back negative. "Never again!" proclaims the prodigal youth. The newsletter terrifies heterosexuals into thinking they may be infected, then uses accounts of those needlessly terrified heterosexuals to needlessly terrify more heterosexuals.

CONSERVATIVES are not alone in exaggerating the terrors of the AIDS epidemic. Liberals have pushed the AIDS-doesn't-discriminate line in order to advance their pre-epidemic causes, such as sex education in schools, and to generate more research funds and reduce the stigma of homosexuals. The difference is that liberals are winning, and conservatives will lose. And ironically, conservatives will lose because they've failed to act like conservatives. The AIDS crisis called for what used to be thought of as conservative virtues: caution before all the evidence is in and dispassion when weighing public policy. Instead, conservatives have reacted as hysterically as their radical adversaries. In the process, they also lost two old battles. They conceded that sex education in schools was necessary in order to promote their own moral agenda. (They will have trouble now arguing that it should not occur at all.) And by ignoring the drug connection while grossly overemphasizing heterosexual sex, they also passed up a key opportunity to talk about the immorality of drug abuse.

When the *American Spectator* ran its first hysterical AIDS story, assistant managing editor Andrew Ferguson wrote this dissent. It stands in stark contrast with the attitude of the American conservative leadership:

> This grotesque but recently voguish hysteria is ludicrous on its face, or anyway it should seem so to someone who prizes the principles on which [conservatism] is supposed to be based—limited government, prudence, and individual responsibility, to name a few. It is simply the latest version of the totalitarian flimflam that is forever drawing believers from the ranks of the weak-minded and the perpetually alarmed.

The conservatism of which he writes is that not of a Bennett or a Bauer, but of a Burke.

Some of today's conservatives seem to have forgotten that it is a liberal precept that "in the long run, we shall all be dead." After the long run of AIDS, the vast majority of us will still be alive. What short-term victories could the conservatives gain that, come the morning after, could possibly be worth what they will lose? □

Acta Sociologica 1987 (30), 1:53–66

Power, Prestige, Profit: AIDS and the Oppression of Homosexual People

Martti Grönfors and Olli Stålström
Department of Sociology of Law, University of Helsinki

Scientific discussion about homosexuality is often a mixture of science, myth, religion, politics and emotion. Homosexual behaviour has been variously defined as sick, criminally deviant and heathen, its participants in need of punishment, cure and control. In the 1980s, with the appearance of the deadly AIDS virus, this overt and covert hostility has gained new impetus. Not only are gays a threat to a multitude of 'decent' values in society, they are also a *threat* to the 'decent' members of society. Alongside control-talk, the new virus has provided a challenge to the medical profession. Careers and monetary gain can be made out of AIDS. The news media received its cut by exploiting public curiosity and fear and by satisfying the need for villains and heros, entering and feeding the general rush for emotion, using and being used, all for profit. Struggle for expertise means defining out the perceived competition and alternative viewpoints. An attempt by the medical profession to define the AIDS issue as a medical problem has, above all, to do with power, prestige and especially profit. In the middle of all these secondary issues, those suffering from AIDS or fearing it, tend to be forgotten.

Until the 1960s there was a blanket of silence over homosexuality. The topic became acceptable in public discussion in the general climate of the liberal ideas of the 1960s. Coming to the 1970s homosexual people had acquired a certain optimism about their acceptance in society. These hopes were quickly shattered in the early 1980s, however, when AIDS drowned the budding optimism. Once again homosexuality and homosexual people were being thought of primarily in negative terms, control policies again dominating the discussion in such volume and ferocity as never before. Homosexual people were now not only deviant in their sexual habits, but a threat to the whole humankind. Homosexual behaviour is as old as human history, so is its control. Only the rationale and the source of control appear to change according to the perception of gains it offers to various interest groups at any particular moment of time.

The relativity of sex roles and attitudes toward sexual preferences have been pointed out by, among others, Edward Westermarck and Margaret Mead. Even today, within contemporary Scandinavia, there are subcultures whose views on sex roles differ remarkably from those of the dominant cultures. Among Finnish gypsies it is the men who are expected to be emotional – even irrationally so. It is the women who, in the end, are supposed to carry the responsibilities of livelihood, including that of their men, while the men legitimately use their resources for their own, often secondary and even frivolous, purposes (Grönfors 1977 and 1979).

Among many African peoples homosexual activity is both generally condoned and has a specific role in social relations between men. It has been observed that

> Homosexuality is especially common among the Dahomey, Ila, Lango, Siwa, Thonga, Wolof and Zande. Homosexuality is obligatory in the Siwa Oasis, where persons of social distinction exchange their sons. A man who is not a dedicated homosexual is considered odd (Rachewiltz 1964:63 and 280).

According to a review of available data on cultures outside our Western culture, homosexual relationships are considered normal or socially acceptable for either some or all members of society (Ford & Beach 1952). It is quite evident that the various definitions and prescriptions of sexuality are cultural, as are those of procreation and parenthood, all of which can be and, indeed, have also in practice been defined independently of one another. The entire concept of sexuality and issues related to it should be viewed not as static, but in relative terms of time, place, culture and history (see Foucault 1979). The fascination of sexuality as an object of scientific inquiry as well as an ideological issue rests in this.

Our society's attitudes, social and legal prescriptions and proscriptions, as they are today, have not always been the same; nor are they 'god-given' and immutable. They evolve as the other cultural spheres evolve and, above all, change to meet the ideals of equality, democracy and social justice.

All available research shows clearly that homosexual persons do *not* constitute a uniform cultural or social minority with a common culture or lifestyle, not even within one country (see Weinberg & Williams 1974; Bell & Weinberg 1978; Hart & Richardson 1981). Sexual preference in itself – whether heterosexual or homosexual – does not entail common group characteristics. Individuals choose their frame of reference on an entirely different basis, whether it be political belief, religious conviction, social background or whatever. However, homosexuality, which is often feared, hated and felt to be wickedly attractive, induces stereotypes which disguise reality. These stereotypes are of paramount importance for the legitimation of social control.

Social control of sexuality

Manipulation of the means and resources for satisfying the basic needs of human beings is a particularly powerful tool in social control. Direct control of food and shelter have a direct impact on people's welfare. Control of sexuality and sexual behaviour, while also having a more or less direct impact, is more often hidden behind other issues, given other names, etc., until it is difficult sometimes even to discover that what is being controlled is sexual behaviour. Wilhelm Reich, for example, says that when society limits access to the satisfaction of basic needs, it is done on purpose. Monogamy and the patriarchal family reflect authoritarian and unegalitarian society, where those who have power govern those who do not. In such a society, rigid sexual norms are necessary for this hierarchical system to be upheld (Reich 1972:145–161).

In other words, examination of a society's sexual norms and attitudes towards sex-related issues effectively reveals something essential about that society, its structures and power relationships. When attitudes towards and attempts to control homosexuality are examined, these general points about social control via sexuality become apparent.

One main branch in Western attitudes towards homosexuality is the Judeo-Christian heritage of our culture. The patriarchalism of the traditional Jewish culture which became sanctified in the Old Testament has affected the laws, general culture and attitudes of Western peoples. In contrasting the Jewish and Jewish-based legal system with that of the Japanese, Ben-Dasan puts the difference very succinctly:

> The Jews . . . regard obedience to divine law as the inevitable outcome of the God–men relation; the Japanese, on the other hand, believe in a law that transcends all codified law, and one that demands flexibility of attitude and adaptability to the human circumstances of the moment rather than unquestioning obedience to some abstract principle (Ben-Dasan 1976:292).

In countries such as Finland, where the Judeo-Christian belief system has reigned for a long time, laws have a rationale of their own, separate from people's everyday lives. In Japan, the people and their relationships form the dynamics of the law, so it is not surprising that, for example, homosexual activity has never been against the law there.

The development of laws even in the West has not, however, been quite linear. When, for example, the power of the Church declined, as it did during the so-called Enlightenment in the eighteenth century in France, the attitude towards homosexuality also changed, and for a period it was decriminalized in the Napoleonic Code. Similarly, the overwhelmingly secular Russian Revolution in the early 1900s initially decriminalized homosexuality, together with many other so-called moral offences.

It appears to be a recurrent characteristic that when social control of sexuality and sexual morality as a tool for furthering the interests of the prevailing power groups is reduced or removed, attitudes towards matters related to sexual behaviour relax for a time, *only* until a new interest group discovers the potential for its own power-pursuits. This aspect can be highlighted in examining attitudes towards homosexuality.

The period of Enlightenment with respect to homosexuality continued in several European countries from the early 1800s until the advent of industrialization in the mid- and late 1800s, when capitalism saw the control of sexuality as one tool for supporting its needs (see e.g. Weeks 1977:23). Labour-intensive production, characterstic of capitalism, required a ready and continual supply of reasonably amenable and cheap labour. Not only did it require large numbers of people moving from the countryside into industrial towns, but at the same time it was necessary that the conglomerations of people in these towns become productive units in providing a continuous supply of new workers.

An ideology and a system to support and legitimate this was necessary. Men were expected to put all their energies to the service of industry, and were enabled to do so by the unpaid labour of women in the home, who serviced the men while at the same time producing and raising the next generation of labour. In this system, male supremacy was ensured, and a sharp distinction between the workplace and the home was made. Anything which was thought to undermine this structure or to be a hindrance to the system of capitalistic production was proscribed.

Against this background it is easy to see why homosexuality fitted rather poorly into the early labour-intensive capitalistic scheme of things. Homosexual relations were naturally considered non-productive, standing in sharp contrast to the idea of sexual production; hence they had to be controlled. In the Soviet Union, the rise of general authoritarianism during the Stalinist period in the 1930s saw the re-introduction of most of the repressive sexual laws, including a law in 1934 recriminalizing homosexuality. Freedom in the sexual sphere, while considered a threat to the basis of production under capitalism, is seen as anti-authoritarianism under socialism. The rationale is remarkably similar in both (see Reich 1972 passim; Weeks 1977:141).

In early Scandinavian laws there were references to 'sodomitic activity', which was extended to various types of unacceptable sexual practices and not just to homosexual relations. The latter were not specifically mentioned or defined – sometimes for fear that describing them in the law might encourage them (as was argued in the preparatory work for the 1734 law in Sweden–Finland). The prevailing attitude towards sexuality in the mid-1800s was the so-called 'absolute sexual morality', which condemned all sexual activity outside marriage. The laws enacted in this period (Norway 1842, Sweden 1864, Denmark 1866, Finland 1889) – while using terms such as 'unnatural behaviour' or 'indecent behaviour' – were now for the first time being applied only to homosexual acts and for the first time the laws specifically defined sexual acts between members of the same sex (see Månsson 1984).

Homosexual activity between consenting adults in private has, in the main, been decriminalized in Western countries (e.g. Denmark 1930, Sweden 1940, Britain 1967, Finland 1971 and Norway 1972). It might be of interest to mention that although Norway was relatively late in decriminalization, it put homosexuality on a par with heterosexuality at the same time (unlike most other countries) by making the age of consent the same for both. In 1981 Norway also passed the first law which actively prohibits discrimination on the basis of sexual preference.

A thorough analysis remains to be done of the reasons why the decriminalization of homosexuality took place when it did in the West. On the basis of what is known about earlier criminalization and decriminalization, certain assumptions can be made. Firstly, it would be logical that some basic changes occurred in the structure of societies, which then affected attitudes towards sexual behaviour as well. It may not be too far-fetched to imagine that the state of industrialization in the Western world had progressed to a stage where reliance on labour was no longer paramount. Hence, the ground was more ready than earlier for the relaxation of certain laws connected with sexuality, including homosexuality. In the same way, attitudes towards birth control became much more liberal than earlier, and the reasons were probably very much the same. It is interesting that attitudes towards the control of women through birth control and abortion have always closely followed the attitude towards homosexuality.

However, the control of homosexuality was vacated for those interest groups who found it useful for gaining and maintaining power. One such group was the medical profession, which needed 'pathological' individuals to be 'treated'. Thus the medical model changed the conceptualization of homosexuality from specific *acts* to specific *people* committing these acts. The effect was the creation of a special category of people – 'homosexuals', as the term which was coined by psychiatrists as late as in the 1860s.

It is quite evident that certain professions, in this age of professionalism, have discovered now more than perhaps ever before the power of sexuality in promoting their own concerns. This applies in particular to sections of the medical profession which have been the guardians of ideologies on sexual normality, such as psychoanalysts in earlier years and venereologists more recently.

As a concrete example of this, we shall take a look at the way in which some of the medical profession are currently attempting to control the definitions of sexual norms, making value judgments not traditionally belonging within their competence and attempting to subordinate other interest groups in the discussion and decision-making. This is most evident in the issues surrounding the AIDS panic.

History of the AIDS panic

During 1983, the acquired immunodeficiency syndrome (AIDS) caused an unprecedented wave of panic and a sharp increase in discrimination and violence against gay men in some Western countries, most notably in the US (and also in Finland). The panic took such dangerous forms in the US that a congressional committee was set up to study the causes of the situation. The committee's report, issued at the end of 1983, provides startling insights into how the US Federal Government conducted – and did not conduct – its campaign against the outbreak of AIDS (*Federal Response to AIDS* 1983).

An unusual outbreak of Kaposi's sarcoma and *Pneumocystis carinii* pneumonia was first reported to the Centers for Disease Control (CDC) in the spring of 1981. Within a few months, physicians and scientists realized – according to the congressional report – that the nation was facing a frightening and deadly disorder of epidemic proportions. Although the medical experts at the CDC sounded the alarm and demanded immediate resources, the US Department of Health and Human Services (HHS) and other Federal agencies refused to give any funds for the research. Although, as the report points out, the funding system for health research is slow and complicated in the States, it is clear that the Federal resistance was active and deliberate. An appropriation for research funds was vetoed by President Reagan himself. The report also points out that government officials told untruths to the public. The HHS Secretary told the press that she 'would leave no stone unturned to pursue an answer to AIDS' at the very time that the existing small funds were actually being reduced.

As a result, according to the congressional report, the medical experts of the CDC had funds to conduct nothing more than 'passive surveillance' for 18 months from the first alarm. Up to the beginning of 1983, all they could really do was to count bodies. When the CDC finally got sufficient funds to start research in the summer of 1983, the number of reported AIDS cases was over 2000, with around 800 deaths.

According to the congressional report, the Public Health Department did not design, plan or coordinate a strategy for systematic dissemination of information until June 1983, at which point the growing myths and misconceptions about the disease had caused an 'epidemic of fear'. The chairperson of the Committee concluded that the congressional findings 'document inexcusable and unconscionable gaps in the Federal effort to resolve this crisis' (*Federal Response to AIDS*, 1983).

The initial response of the state bureaucracy and the medical experts is poignantly illustrated e.g. by Cahill (1984:2):

> But even as the disaster escalated, the organized medical community was strangely absent. When a fatal infection had struck down veterans attending an American Legion convention, health professionals across the country joined in the search for a solution. When women using tampons became ill with toxic shock syndrome, medical societies and research centers immediately focused their enormous talents on that problem.[1] But when the victims were drug addicts and poor Haitian refugees and homosexual men, their plight did not, somehow, seem as significant to those expected to speak for the health professions. No major research programs were announced, and until it became clear that the disease could spread to the general population through blood transfusions, organized medicine seemed part of the curious conspiracy of silence.

The disease appeared at the right time for the Moral Majority, Reaganism and the present conservative atmosphere in the US. The committee report also indicates that part of the panic had to be created by the gay liberation movement itself in a desperate effort to make the Federal Government do something to stop the rapidly mounting death figures. American public opinion was electrified when the distorted face of a young man dying of AIDS was shown in the news media. This unleashed a feverish panic in the States – but also brought pressure on the Federal Government.

The history of AIDS has shown that there is a strong view that some people are worthier of being kept alive than others. Although the main resistance has come from the US State bureaucracy, some medical researchers do not hide their racist or otherwise prejudiced views. In an interview in Finland in 1984, Dr. Robert Gallo, who claims to have discovered the virus causing AIDS, stated that the virus had been present 'heaven knows how long' in Central Africa and in homosexual men for a number of years. He commented that 'it is *most disturbing* now that the disease has been discovered in new population groups, such as women and children' (emphasis added) (Gallo 1984). Similar attitudes have been expressed by several medical experts in Finland.

A Finnish professor of virology recently suggested (in the *Finnish Journal of Medicine*) police action against suspected HIV carriers and their internment in an old leper hospital on a remote island. He compared the sexual equality movement with a hypothetical 'equality movement for syphilitics' and added that when AIDS was thought to be only a homosexual disease, it had only 'limited curiosity value among physicians', but when it was found in heterosexuals, it became 'a problem touching every physician' (Halonen 1985).

It should be kept in mind that AIDS is not a mystical 'gay disease'. It is transmitted via sperm or blood (not through social contact) by a virus. Any research on AIDS will therefore produce important information on the immunological system of the body. Had AIDS been taken seriously right from the beginning and not been dismissed as merely a 'gay plague', the virus could have been identified earlier.

As research into such a taboo-laden area can be done more or less responsibly, we shall compare the methodological and ethical aspects of the Dutch AIDS research programme and the Academy of Finland AIDS research programme.

AIDS research strategies in the Netherlands[2]

In the Netherlands there were few problems of funding and attitudes were not as negative. In part this reflects the difference between the health policies of the US and continental Europe, and in part the more enlightened attitudes of Dutch medical and government personnel. From the beginning, the AIDS problem was perceived as something wider than just a medical or panic issue. A national AIDS research team was set up, consisting of representatives of medicine, sociology, health administration and the gay liberation movement (COC). In 1984 a comprehensive study began of 3 000 gay men with various lifestyles, the Dutch government footing the bill of over four million Dutch guilders.

Extreme care is being taken to prevent premature or false information being given to the media, to prevent the use of any information being used in a sensational manner and to coordinate the dissemination of information with all groups involved. A research contract setting forth ethical principles was signed between the state and members of the research team. There is also a research contract between the research team and each individual person to be studied, guaranteeing total anonymity, among other things (see e.g. Tielman 1985a and 1985b).

Most importantly, the project has a special person responsible for publicity preparing information bulletins in cooperation with all parties involved in the research. These bulletins are circulated among selected representatives of the mainstream news media. The researchers have not appeared in or provided information to the sensational, pornographic or tabloid press. Individual events, such as new cases or deaths, are generally not reported as sensational news; only the general situation is given, in a statistical form. A special project ombudsman has been appointed for the efficient handling of any complaints concerning violations of medical ethics.

The research programme consists of a thorough blood analysis coupled with a sociological in-depth interview of the subjects, covering their medical, social, mental and practical circumstances. Special emphasis is placed on emotional support, as it has been suggested that the severity and course of the disease may be connected with the mental and physical condition and anxiety felt by the virus carriers about the negative publicity given to AIDS and people affected by it.

In addition to being multidisciplinary and representing all parties whose interests are involved, the research team includes both gay and straight people, guaranteeing a more accurate understanding of different lifestyles. As a result, no great panic ever occurred in the Netherlands.

AIDS research in Finland[3]

In 1982 the Finnish Gay Liberation Movement (SETA) started asking the Helsinki

City VD clinic to prepare for a potential AIDS crisis, even though no case had been found at that time in Finland. One reason for this was the sensational overseas news items about the 'gay plague' that were spreading in the Finnish news media. No serious attention was paid to the requests. On the contrary, leading venerologists fuelled the panic with press comments such as 'the spread of the disease is connected to homosexual rituals' and 'homosexuals have a terrible number of different infections'. Delegations from SETA continued pleading with the venerologists up to the end of April 1983. The approaches were met with aggressive responses that taking care of press coverage and considering the rights of gay people were of 'secondary importance'.

In April 1983 a venerologist from another clinic began collecting data on the clinical side of AIDS for an M.D. thesis. The potential medical points to be scored from AIDS had now been discovered in Finland. In contrast to the situation in the Netherlands, ethical principles were not adequately safeguarded in the Finnish research project, not even those usually associated with research practices in Finland. Participation by sociologist and gay liberation representatives was strongly opposed. The anonymity of the subjects, which was guaranteed in writing to the Academy of Finland, was violated from the beginning. In reply to complaints to the Ethics Committee of the Academy of Finland, the Committee urged stricter adherence to the stated ethical principles. However, full anonymity was never maintained in spite of the promises made to the Academy and to SETA, who recruited the subjects for the study.

The news media, especially the tabloid press, managed to get detailed information about individual cases and events. Thus the research programme in fact fuelled the panic in Finland in the summer of 1983 when the first AIDS cases were found.

In spite of the promise made by the Minister of Social Affairs in 1983 to establish a broad-based committee, the matter dragged on for about a year until the first working group – consisting solely of medical experts – was set up in 1984. Its brief was formally to study the incidence and prevention of AIDS, but in reality the work of the group was limited to planning treatment for those individuals who had been discovered to have HIV antibodies.

By delineating the problem as purely a medical one, the medical profession enhances its own status. Examining other problems created by AIDS would have meant sharing responsibility and hence sharing status and expertise. Thus sociologists, psychologists, gay liberationists and especially gay people themselves, had to be kept out of the proceedings.

The powerful position of medical doctors in society meant that the interests of the medical profession were given priority over ethical considerations in information production and dissemination on AIDS. What would have happened had they taken into account right from the beginning the societal and emotional aspects of AIDS and had included in the working groups representatives of all concerned parties? Instead of limiting the issue to individual medical problems, the working group would have been forced to look at the situation of gays in the wider societal context as a discriminated and stigmatized minority, a subject which would have been rather more complicated and uncomfortable for the state and the medical profession. It was more expedient to keep the matter a purely clinical problem. This is not to say that all medical people involved shared that view, but no alternative medical voices were given publicity.

Persistent pressure from SETA finally resulted in the formation of a multidisciplinary AIDS committee in March 1985. The committee consists of, among others, representatives of clinical AIDS research, medical ethics, the Institute of Public Health, the Finnish Red Cross and SETA. The brief of the committee is to coordinate treatment and testing and preventive information (Krohn et al. 1985).

Tactics in status pursuit

Subterranean conscious or semi-conscious tactics to maintain and increase the power and influence of an interest group, such as the medical profession in the AIDS case, can include the following: secrecy, telling half-truths or outright lies, telling truths out of context or without context, withdrawal or release of information especially at strategic moments, giving false hopes, taking away hope, demeaning and attacking the opposition, excluding the subjects involved, appealing to expertise, mystifying the role of the experts, and appealing to even higher authorities (religion, morality, etc.).

Examination of the details of the developments around AIDS in Finland supports the interest-base analysis. Secrecy has surrounded the methodology of the research project. Publicity used instrumentally with selected information, and tactically selected AIDS-patients, has resulted in a new stereotype that all or most homosexuals are infested with huge numbers of sexually transmitted diseases and have hundreds of partners. Tactically, the most promiscuous subjects are presented to the news media as examples of homosexuals. The researchers, however, have steadfastly refused to make sufficiently clear that their speculations are made from clinical samples heavily based towards self-selected high-risk groups of men whose lifestyle incorporates a multi-partner, special-sexual-practices identity. The bias is further increased by the fact that participation in the Academy of Finland project was for a long time the only way of getting a medical test for those who had, or who suspected, symptoms, of the disease.

The death of the first Finnish AIDS patient was reported in the press in July 1984. Because of the lack of controls on publicity, the wrong man was described as dead! In the same articles, clinicians bemoaned the fact that there were no finances left for AIDS research to continue. This was strategically good timing to complain about the lack of money for research. What was not told, however, was that finance had been temporarily suspended because of the complaint lodged with the Academy of Finland concerning violations of research ethics, anonymity, publicity, etc.

Many 'cures' for AIDS have appeared in the news media, in spite of the knowledge that they are either pure speculation or at most experimental symptomatic treatment. These are initiated by speculations and hypotheses by clinicians in various countries. Many causes of AIDS have been suggested in the press, ranging from swine flu and fungi to viruses, supported by comments from medical experts, each promoting their pet theories. Speculative 'causes' mean speculative 'cures' and false hopes for patients. Other reports emphasize the highly contagious nature of AIDS (which is not supported by empirical facts). Frequent speculations appear as to how many people are at risk, ultimately the majority of humankind.

It has been suggested that the patient's level of anxiety might be related to the progress of the disease. All unfounded speculations and devaluation of the life of gays only serve to increase the anxiety of those affected, those at risk – and those not at risk.

The gay liberation movement has been the main target of attacks from some clinicians. This has happened in a variety of ways: initial efforts aimed at influencing the manner in which the research was conducted were systematically dismissed, as were attempts to make the researchers adhere to basic ethical and methodological principles. Some subjects in the Academy of Finland AIDS project report having received long lectures against the gay liberation movement. One example of this adverse propaganda appeared in a Finnish popular scientific journal in January 1984, where AIDS was linked to the gay liberation movement, which was blamed for promoting conditions helping its development and spread (Valle 1984). This is a very common tactic used against groups fighting for minority rights, an attempt to discredit them by appealing to common prejudice and making the victim the guilty party.

When the clinicians responsible for the AIDS research were initially approached about the violations of ethical principles, the usual retort was that such pleas were attempts to hide the truth for political aims. This is another common experience of those defending minority rights. The 'experts' may say that the two sides are talking in different languages, the clinicians with a 'scientific' one and their critics with an 'emotional' one.

Apart from attempts to silence the critical voice, there was a systematic refusal to cooperate with the subjects and their representatives. It was openly stated that the concerns the subjects had about the research only confused it. Written promises about research ethics made at the outset were not honoured. For example, details about subjects participating in the research, including their real names, were passed on to numerous clinics, and a person giving a sample in any of the clinics which take samples for the research is immediately identified as an AIDS research subject. All this has caused embarrassment to those who volunteered in the research, shows disregard for their personal dignity and is a violation of the ethical promise the researchers gave in order to secure the subjects' cooperation.

The entrenched authority of the clinicians carrying out the Finnish AIDS research has meant that few arguments which contradict or counter those put forward by the medical experts are heard. The status of a medical doctor gives the required justification. The mystification of the profession supports the maintenance of this power. Christian-based morality, which favours heterosexual chastity, and where 'immoral' – homosexual – encounters are punished by dreadful diseases, such as AIDS, is reflected in doctors' statements. One of the AIDS researchers said explicitly in a radio interview that *neomoralism* is the recommended prevention. It would be hard to imagine many other 'scientific' studies which conclude that Old Testament prohibitions against homosexuality may have been medically justified (Vaheri 1985).

News media in information manipulation

In the commercial news media, the selection of material takes place not on the basis of its inherent value as discoveries, events or analyses, but on its ability to attract an audience or sell more copies. This offers a great tool to those groups or individuals who want to further their particular interests or positions of power. Here the interests of power-wielding groups and the news media coincide. Both get what they want.

AIDS is a fruitful topic for the news media, in that it combines some basic elements of human drama: sexuality, immorality, terminal disease and death. Billions are made annually on those topics, and recently a goodly proportion via AIDS. So many taboos culminate in AIDS that almost any story which can include AIDS becomes profitable. Even a piece of non-news, when linked with the disease, sells. Several local papers in small Finnish towns reported with large headlines that AIDS had not reached the town yet. Any new 'discovery' is reported, similarly its correction.

Although the media are keen to tackle anything to do with AIDS, there are issues which are not handled despite being very relevant to the topic. The reason for the silence on these is that they remove the drama, making AIDS an 'ordinary' disease, and therefore reducing its market value. Facts such as that the majority of gay men are as healthy as anybody else, and in no danger of contracting AIDS, are not as interesting as telling the readers about the 'homo virus'. It is financially more rewarding to write that homosexuals contract AIDS. It is 'horrifying' to report that the HIV virus spreads through the air, but 'comforting' to report that the airborne spread is limited to homosexuals only. Normal people are safe.

Much of the onus of distorted reporting falls on Finland's afternoon tabloids and soft-porn men's magazines. Their sales figures rest heavily on captivating headlines and billboards. When a page is decorated with a skull and crossbones, the story to which it refers is almost irrelevant. When the front page promises 'good stuff', one has to buy the paper in order to get the story inside; never mind if that story bears little resemblance to the enticing headlines.

To tell readers that a despised group of people are having it rough entertains some, disgusts others, creates pity in a few, but interests most. To speculate that thousands might die titillates people's sense of morbidity, and to suggest that thousands of gays may die might satisfy those who think that to be gay is worse than to be dead anyway. To report the 'discovery' of a vaccine for AIDS extols human ingenuity and inventiveness, be it true or not. To give space for medical experts to air their theories about the 'causes' and 'cures' for AIDS satisfies the human desire for heroes. To hint at the 'lurid sexual practices' of gay men allows ordinary people into bedrooms which they would never otherwise have entered.

In short, the news media know their readers, make use of them and create the news which is wanted. In so doing, and in addition to making money on AIDS, the media also act in collaboration with other interest groups, such as the medical profession. Each needs the other, one for money, the other for power and publicity. This closed-circuit relationship is so tight that it is almost impossible for anything which does not support either group or their interests to penetrate it. In the web of this vicious relationship are caught those people who form the subject matter, in this case homosexual people.

The medical profession and the press in close cooperation generated close to 1 000 articles on the first two cases of AIDS in Finland (at the time of writing, a total of 17 cases have been found). Many of the articles have been distorted, negative or hostile. As a result of the panic created by the press, the Finnish gay liberation movement (SETA), for example, lost the disco which was the source of 90% of its income, resulting in the loss of most of its paid social workers and a state of de facto bankruptcy, now that the need for support and information is at its greatest. The near destruction of the gay liberation movement and the remedicalization of homosexuality in the public mind shows the tremendous potential and real power of the medical profession.

Who next?

If our analysis is correct, then it should be reasonable to assume that the vehemently negative attitudes towards homosexuality which were produced by religious interests and the interests of capitalist industrial production may diminish in the future, after the AIDS crisis is over. Some signs already in sight of a new interest group, the importance of which might be most significant in the future, include the 'gay lifestyle' as commodity. In some American cities with visible 'gay ghettos', commercial interests in gay life are already quite apparent. The entertainment industry is now freer to make gay topics more respectable, even desirable. The lack of information and an acceptable social milieu, caused by decades of repression, is rapidly being met by private business interests which thus, in fact, are acquiring control of the public image of homosexuality by promoting a particular gay lifestyle. However trend-setting the new visible gay subculture may be, the underlying problem is that most of it is motivated by private commercial interests rather than by genuine emancipatory ideals.

In a historical perspective we may perceive a progression of changing sources of control: the oppression of gays by the Church in pursuit of worldly power was replaced by the exploitation of gays by the medical profession in pursuit of prestige and social control, and that is being replaced by the exploitation of gays by private commercial interests in the pursuit of profit.

The future will become even bleaker if some newly-suggested forms of control take effect. For example, there have been suggestions in the Swedish press that it be made a criminal offence for anyone with HIV antibodies to have sex. A law has been enacted in Australia to criminalize gay blood donors if they do not reveal their sexual preference. The Finnish National Board of Health has started to register everybody with HTLV-III antibodies. The Helsinki University VD clinic has been marking the patient cards of all known homosexual clients since 1984 with a yellow triangle (why not pink, as the Nazis did?). There is recent evidence that suspected homosexuals are being tested for HIV without their knowledge or consent.

Quite apart from the discriminatory nature of such proposals, a more serious problem would be the effect of such forms of control on the health and civil rights of gay people. Repressive measures, criminalization and threat of internment would only drive homosexuality underground. The increase in secrecy and fear of medical treatment would most probably actually increase the risk of all sexually transmitted diseases. This situation would violate the basic principles of medical ethics and public health.

AIDS is a very serious medical problem. However, it is more than merely a medical problem, it is first and foremost a *social and psychological* one which has serious consequences both at the level of individual suffering and at the wider societal level of *human rights, equality as well as the quality and value of human life*, all of which are under threat at present. Consequently, any action to combat the spread of the disease and helping those affected by it must include more than medical considerations alone. In every public health campaign (e.g. anti-smoking) it is discovered that scare-tactics are not generally affective. What does work, seems to be related to the availability of factual and balanced information, and to the credibility and familiarity of the source of the information. For example, the Dutch National Board of Health has explicitly stated that the basic condition for the effective prevention of the spread of AIDS is complete trust between the medical profession and homosexual people. Non-moralizing preventive information in the long run will be a cheaper and more effective way of curbing the spread of AIDS than testing and treatment.

This grave human, social and medical crisis, threatening the well-being and human rights of many more people than are at a risk of contracting AIDS, requiring urgent, open, honest and trusting co-operation between all those parties who have the capacities, resources and responsibility to contain the crisis and reduce suffering.

Notes

1 A reading of feminist material raises queries as to whether it is true that toxic shock syndrome received immediate and massive medical attention.

2 Information on the Dutch programme is based on personal interviews with Dr. Rob Tielman (Utrecht University), Dr. Jan van Wijngaarden (Academic Medical Centre, Amsterdam) and Dr. Hans Moerkerk (Amsterdam City Bureau of Health Information and Education), January, April and August 1984 and January and July 1985 as well as *De AIDS factor*. Amsterdam: Radio STAT/COC, 1984. See also Tielman 1985a and 1985b.

3 Information on the Finnish programme is based on Finnish press analyses and the participant observation by Olli Stålström of the production and dissemination of information on AIDS and the negotiations between the gay liberation movement (SETA) and the Finnish AIDS researchers from December 1982 to August 1985.

See also the methodological and ethical statements in Pönkä, A., Valle, S-L., Ranki-Häyry, A-M. & Dowiatt, H. *The occurrence of predisposing factors for AIDS and changes in T cell subpopulations*. Helsinki, May 1983 (original research plan for the Academy of Finland) and Krohn, K., Vaheri, A., Ranki, A. & Weckström, P. *AIDS-asiantuntijaryhmän mietintö*. Helsinki, 1985. (The report of the expert working group on AIDS.)

References

Bell, A. P. & Weinberg, M. S. 1978. *Homosexualities: a Study of Diversity Among Men and Women*. New York: Simon & Schuster.

Ben-Dasan, I. 1976. The Japanese and the Jews. In H. Tanaka (ed.), *The Japanese Legal System*. Tokyo: University of Tokyo Press.

Cahill, K. M. 1984. Preface: the Evolution of an Epidemic. In K. M. Cahill (ed.), *The AIDS Epidemic*. London: Hutchinson.

Federal Response to AIDS. 1983. Twenty-ninth Report by the Committee on Government Operations. Washington, D.C.: US Government Printing Office.

Ford, C. S. & Beach, F. A. 1952. *Patterns of Sexual Behavior*. London: Eyre & Spottiswoode.

Foucault, M. 1981. *The History of Sexuality*. Vol. I, an introduction. Harmondsworth: Penguin.

Gallo 1984: Näin löytyi AIDS-virus (This is how the AIDS virus was found; an interview with Dr. David Gallo). *Suomen Kuvalehti*, 1984, *23*, 28–29.

Grönfors, M. 1977. *Blood Feuding Among Finnish Gypsies*. Helsinki: University of Helsinki, Institute of Sociology Research Reports, No. 213.
Grönfors, M. 1979. *Ethnic Minorities and Deviance: the Relationship Between Finnish Gypsies and the Police*. Helsinki: University of Helsinki, Sociology of Law Series, No. 1.
Grönfors, M. & Stålström, O. 1985. Ethical Aspects of the Production and Dissemination of Information on AIDS. In *European Group for the Study of Deviance and Social Control Working Papers in Criminology*, No. 6.
Halonen, P. 1985. AIDS – tasa-arvoako? (AIDS – equality?). *Suomen lääkärilehti 7*, 599–600. (Finnish Journal of Medicine.)
Hart, J. & Richardson, D. 1981. *The Theory and Practice of Homosexuality*. London: Routledge & Kegan Paul.
Krohn, K., Vaheri, A., Ranki, A. & Weckström, P. 1985. *AIDS-asiantuntijaryhmän mietintö*. Helsinki. (The report of the expert working group on AIDS.)
Månsson, U. 1984. Synti, rikos, ihmisoikeus – oikeustaistelun historiaa ja nykypäivää (Sin, crime, human rights – history and present-day of the struggle for human rights for gays). In K. Sievers & O. Stålström (eds.), *Rakkauden monet kasvot* (The many faces of love). Espoo: Weiling + Göös.
Pönkä, A., Valle, S-L., Ranki-Häyry, A-M. & Dowiatt, H. 1983. *The Occurrence of Predisposing Factors for AIDS and Changes in T Cell Subpopulations*. Helsinki, May (Original research plan for the Academy of Finland).
Rachewiltz, B. de. 1964. *Black Eros. The Sexual Customs of Africa from Prehistoric Times to the Present Day*. London: Allen & Unwin.
Reich, W. 1972. *The Invasion of Compulsory Sex-Morality*. London: Souvenir Press.
Rosen, W. von. 1982. Den homosexuella historiska traditionen (The homosexual historical tradition). In J. Hansson (ed.) *Homosexuella och omvärlden* (Homosexuals and society). Stockholm: LiberFörlag.
Tielman, R. 1985a. Het Grote AIDS onderzoek. In *De AIDS factor 2*. Amsterdam: COC-Magazijn, 11–12.
Tielman, R. (ed.) 1985b. *Meerjarenplan 1985–1990*. Utrecht: Rijksuniversiteit Utrecht, Interfacultaire werkgroep homostudies, 1985. For an English summary see R. Tielman, Outline of the Dutch Psycho-social AIDS-Project. Unpublished research plan. Utrecht: Rijksuniversiteit Utrecht, May 5.
Vaheri 1985: Interview with Professor Antti Vaheri in *Helsingin Sanomat*, January 6, 1985.
Valle, S-L. 1984. AIDS – mistä on kysymys (AIDS – what is it about?). *Tiede 2000*, (Science 2000), *1*, 47–50.
Weeks, J. 1977. *Coming Out: Homosexual Politics in Britain, from the Nineteenth Century to the Present*. London: Quartet Books.
Weinberg, M. S. & Williams, C. J. 1974. *Male Homosexuals: their Problems and Adaptations*. New York: Oxford University Press.

COMMUNITY

Gett to Ser

Do addiction programs sap our political vitality?

[redacted]

ANYONE WHO CARES to go looking can find serenity. It leaves tracks: neat rows of folding chairs lined up in musty church basements; the dull buzz of fluorescent lights in hospital lecture halls; schoolrooms where half-erased algebra problems remain on green blackboards. Literally hundreds of thousands of people across the country and around the world make regular trips to such places—as often as once each day. They are members of 12-step and other "recovery" programs.

Alcoholics Anonymous (AA) is the oldest and best known of these self-help programs, and its structure and philosophy have served as models for others: Narcotics Anonymous (NA); Overeaters Anonymous (OA); Incest Survivors Anonymous (ISA); Emotional Health Anonymous (EHA); Emotions Anonymous (EA) Gamblers Anonymous (GA); Al-Anon and Alateen (programs for family members and friends of alcoholics); and most recently, Sex and Love Addicts Anonymous (SLAA).[1] The only requirement for membership in any of them is a desire to stop substance abuse or change a compulsive behavior.

There is strong impressionistic evidence that, in the past few years, these programs have become so popular within the gay and feminist communities that they virtually constitute a 12-step "movement." Although many people know, through personal contact, that 12-step programs, especially AA, have literally been lifesavers, the programs sometimes have the look and feel of modern-day cults. They describe themselves in universal terms, pride themselves on excluding no one, suggest that their "fellowships" are supportive without ever being critical, and claim to offer a philosophy of spiritual enlightenment without any religious trappings. To the uninitiated, this description might sound like old-style evangelical religion or even like New Age pop psychology with a do-you-believe-in-magic touch thrown in for good measure.

I have never been a member of a 12-step program. In order to write this article, I attended a lot of meetings and talked to many people. Some of what I learned surprised me; all of it involved me. I have asked certain key

ing enity

by Ellen Herman

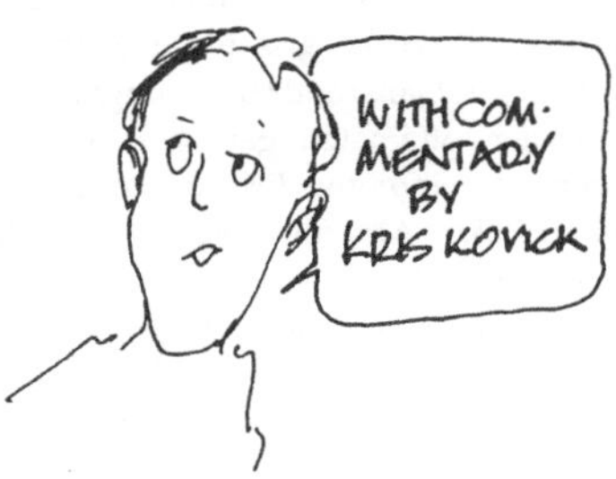

Ellen Herman works at South End Press in Boston, Massachusetts. She has written for Gay Community News, New Directions for Women, Sojourner, Women's Review of Books, *and* Zeta.

questions about the nature of addiction and the methods these programs offer for recovery: whether all the problems addressed by a variety of 12-step programs are fundamentally the same; what resources and analyses feminism and gay liberation have developed in response to addiction and other personal life crises; whether 12-step philosophy has anything to say about politics; what needs these programs are addressing that could or should have been met by political movements; and how living in a "just say no" culture can change the meaning of all of the above.

The Recipe for Recovery

The "steps" (see p. 13) are the heart of Alcoholics Anonymous and all the programs based on the AA model. They are twelve specific actions that the programs urge individuals to take and then repeat. They are the programs' official recipe for recovery, the ingredients of an addiction-free life. Their purpose is "to relieve pain and suffering, fill our emptiness, help us find the missing something, help us discover ourselves and the God within us, and release great quantities of the energy, love, and joy dammed up inside ourselves"[2]—all with a minimum of discomfort and a maximum of self-awareness.

Addiction has always been a dead-serious reality, and the fact that I.V. drug use and sexual behaviors favored by many gay men put people at high risk for AIDS has made the lethal consequences of addiction even clearer. The currently accepted estimate is that the rate of alcoholism and drug addiction among gay men and lesbians is about three times the rate in the general population—about one in three compared to one in ten.[3]

Unlike medical professionals, therapists, or some political activists, 12-step programs do not dwell on the "whys" of addiction. It is simply understood that anyone who uses substances or activities in a way that interferes with living has an addiction problem.

Accordingly, programs offer very simple explanations and a decidedly behavioral approach, two important reasons why they seem to work for so many people. They pay serious

Feminist and gay 12-step program members complain that their political movements did not make good on promises to create supportive spaces where people could go to air and heal the traumas of daily living.

attention to ordinary pain by requiring people to pay attention to it themselves: taking inventories (steps four and ten); admitting wrongdoing (steps five and ten); making direct amends (steps eight and nine); praying and meditating (step eleven); and carrying the message of spiritual awakening (step twelve). "Working the steps" one by one, and then repeating them indefinitely, gives people at least two things that neither science nor politics seems to trust people with consistently: a largely self-determined behavioral routine and permission to understand our problems differently at different stages in our lives, in ways that make sense to us even if they don't to anyone else.

Day to day, what programs offer members are handy directories of meeting times and places, "approved" literature on a range of topics, and slogans to live by, like "one day at a time" and "let go and let God." A set of 12 "traditions" governs program structure. Members are strongly urged to attend meetings frequently, although meetings are completely voluntary. Still, it is not unusual for individuals to participate in four or five each week for many years running. Meetings roughly follow a standard format: an opening statement, a speaker who comes prepared to tell his or her story, time for spontaneous sharing by those present, and a closing statement. When people speak, they do so for as long as they like without interruption. No one responds directly to anything that is said. There are slight variations on this format, and a meeting in rural Nebraska would certainly feel different than one on Castro Street in San Francisco, but a 12-step meeting anywhere would be easily recognizable to anyone who had ever attended one before. Predictability is the point.

Programs encourage a "sponsorship" system, where individuals who have been in the program for a while act as "buddies" for newcomers, orienting them to program philosophy and structure. In addition to their sponsors, members have no trouble finding willing ears outside meetings. Telephone numbers are exchanged and used, at all hours of the day and night, when people need help or support, or just want the comfort that comes from making contact with other human beings who care.

The Gay/Feminist Flood

Pick up almost any gay newspaper or resource guide and you will find listings for gay meetings, ads for "co-dependency therapy," and notices like this one: "SOBER, PROUD AND FREE, Friendly 12-stepping woman, 31, needs home..." Feminist publications from *Ms.* to *off our backs* also routinely publish letters by readers who identify themselves as "ACOA" (adult child of an alcoholic). Many women's centers that operate as crucial information clearinghouses and gathering places for feminists also offer a wide and growing variety of 12-step meetings for anyone interested.[4] During the past five years, organizers of women's music festivals and other such events around the country have started providing "alcohol and chem-free" spaces as a routine part of expressing their commitment to a feminist culture of inclusion. Women's bookstores have done a booming and steady business in recovery books and cards ("Expect Miracles—They are only 12 steps away!") during the past few years. Workers at New Words, in Cambridge, Massachusetts, have even created a new category in the store's accounting system to keep track of what they say are literally hundreds of sales.

The number of "official" gay and women's meetings offered by the programs is astonishingly large. In the Boston area, for example, AA lists 20 weekly gay meetings (one specifically for lesbians) and 60 meetings for women. Al-Anon offers ten gay, two lesbian, two women's, and one bisexual meeting, with names like "Amazon Lesbians" and "Glitter and Be Gay."

There are few ways to document accurately the number of gay or feminist (or any other kind of) members of 12-step programs, since one of the 12 traditions specifies "anonymity at the level of press, radio, and films." The overwhelming consensus though, among the 12-step members and social service professionals I interviewed is that gays and feminists have flooded the programs in recent years, and that the vast majority of predominantly gay meetings are "unofficial" (not designated by a "G" in program directories). People spoke repeatedly about the "phenomenal" growth of the programs, about "constantly overflowing" meetings, and about a 12-step consciousness among gays and feminists that has "spread," "mushroomed," and "gone wild."

Although feminism and gay liberation both tried to mend the personal/political split that seemed to be just a fact of life in progressive social movements, feminist and gay 12-step program members complain that their political movements did not make good on promises to create supportive spaces where people could go to air and heal the traumas of daily living, including addiction. One AA member described her experience this way.

> I was very politically active up until the point when I entered the program, and ever since then I've thought maybe I'd get myself back into politics, but there is something connected for me in being sober and being afraid of political activism, being afraid of how I felt when I did it, like using drugs and feeling out of control. [In my political organization] I felt like I had to be such a together person, do a lot of work, take a lot of responsibility. People saw me as a very reliable person, but I felt that the people around me didn't realize I was falling apart inside.... What I think now is that it was more important for me to get my personal shit together than to do the political work I was doing because I couldn't do good political work while I was such a mess.

It is ironic that many feminists and gay people felt, and continue to feel, that pressing personal concerns—like addiction—are often invisible within the movements that offered slogans like "the personal is political."

There are other important differences between belonging to a political movement and being a member of a 12-step program. Progressive organizations typically require people who may or may not like one another to get together often and for interminably long periods of time, to plan events or campaigns, divide chores, assign responsibilities, and periodically check in on the progress of their projects. When it's all over and everyone is completely exhausted, it's time to meet again for a humorless evaluation, a less-than-sincere session of criticism/self-criticism, or both.

Twelve-step programs literally require nothing. Meetings are always short and always start and end exactly on time. You can show up if you feel like it or skip it if you don't. If you do go, the format will be familiar no matter where you are. You listen. You might choose to share your story or socialize after the meeting. When it's all over, you leave with no

The 12 Steps

1. *We admitted we were powerless over alcohol*—that our lives had become unmanageable.*
2. *Came to believe that a Power greater than ourselves could restore us to sanity.*
3. *Made a decision to turn our will and our lives over to the care of God as we understood Him.*
4. *Made a searching and fearless moral inventory of ourselves.*
5. *Admitted to God, to ourselves, and to another human being the exact nature of our wrongs.*
6. *Were entirely ready to have God remove all these defects of character.*
7. *Humbly asked Him to remove our shortcomings.*
8. *Made a list of all persons we had harmed, and became willing to make amends to them all.*
9. *Made direct amends to such people wherever possible, except when to do so would injure them or others.*
10. *Continued to take personal inventory and when we were wrong promptly admitted it.*
11. *Sought through prayer and meditation to improve our conscious contact with God as we understood Him, praying only for knowledge of His will for us and the power to carry that out.*
12. *Having had a spiritual awakening as a result of these steps, we tried to carry this message to alcoholics,* and to practice these principles in all our affairs.*

** This is adapted to the addiction relevant to each 12-step program.*

obligation to anyone and you probably feel better than you did when you walked in.

In a homophobic and male-dominated culture, gay men, lesbians, and feminists are always searching for places in which their sexual and gender identities can be simply facts rather than lightning rods for hostility and violence. At their best, the 12-step programs have been such places. But homophobia and sexism also exist within the programs. As far as I know, only one program—SLAA—explicitly states in its literature that sexual preference is a non-issue.

Alcoholics Together (AT) was a 12-step program founded in Los Angeles by and for gay alcoholics before the AA Central Service Committee would officially permit gay meetings to take place. Although AA has since abolished its formal policy of homophobic exclusion, AT continues to meet regularly in many places (10 times each week at Boston's Gay and Lesbian Counseling Services)—an indication that homophobia within AA may be unofficial now, but it's still there. The subtle and crude versions of sexism are also alive and well. Program literature routinely uses sexist language, although this seems to be changing slowly. A few women's meetings I attended simply replaced every instance of "God" with "Goddess." Women, however, also described feeling "unsafe" in mixed meetings with men, and lesbians and gay men talked about being "invisible" when surrounded by straight people in 12-step gatherings.

Twelve-step programs provide at least one thing that all people–but especially socially stigmatized people –are desperate to find: a predictably safe place in which to feel understood and accepted.

While homophobia and sexism may be alive and well in 12-step programs, one clear reason why feminists, gay men, and lesbians may have found 12-step programs so welcoming ultimately is their structure, which can best be described as decentralized democracy. The 12 traditions that govern the structure of 12-step programs feel familiar to people with experience in grassroots political movements. They guarantee open membership, group autonomy, financial self-sufficiency, and a non-professional and non-political status, among other things. These are the reasons women and gay people have been able to organize meetings of their own.

Twelve-step programs provide at least one thing that all people—but especially socially stigmatized people—are desperate to find: a predictably safe place in which to feel understood and accepted. Safety was almost tangibly present in many of the meetings I attended, and I believe the feeling of uncritical acceptance people find there may be one of the biggest reasons they flock to the meetings. The safe environment has been purchased at a rather high price, however: a community culture that does not allow room for direct reaction or interaction of any kind, criticism in particular.

Addiction is Addiction is Addiction?

They look alike, but are all the 12-step programs really the same? Does it make sense to change compulsive eating behavior with the same techniques alcoholics use to keep sober? Is sexual addiction different from food addiction, and are they both different from addiction to mind-altering substances?

Food is something we all need to live; none of us ever needs drugs or alcohol, but alcoholism and drug addiction are characterized by a physiological process of dependence completely unknown to most overeaters or "sex and love addicts." Food can be a way for people to establish and maintain relationships, express their cultural identities, or spend leisure time. At least one progressive political analysis of food and eating conflicts directly with the 12-step approach of Overeaters Anonymous: fat liberation.

In particular, feminists exposed cultural imperatives about the physical body—what it was supposed to weigh, look like, feel like, smell like, and act like—and pronounced accepted notions of clothing, diet, and appearance to be among the causes of women's self-hatred. Gay liberation as an organized movement has had less to say on this topic, but fat liberation is developing a voice within the gay community. Activists have pointed to ideal physical types that may be queer but are "fat-oppressive" nonetheless: the androgynous dyke with the curveless body of a teenage boy

THE CAUSES OF ADDICTION

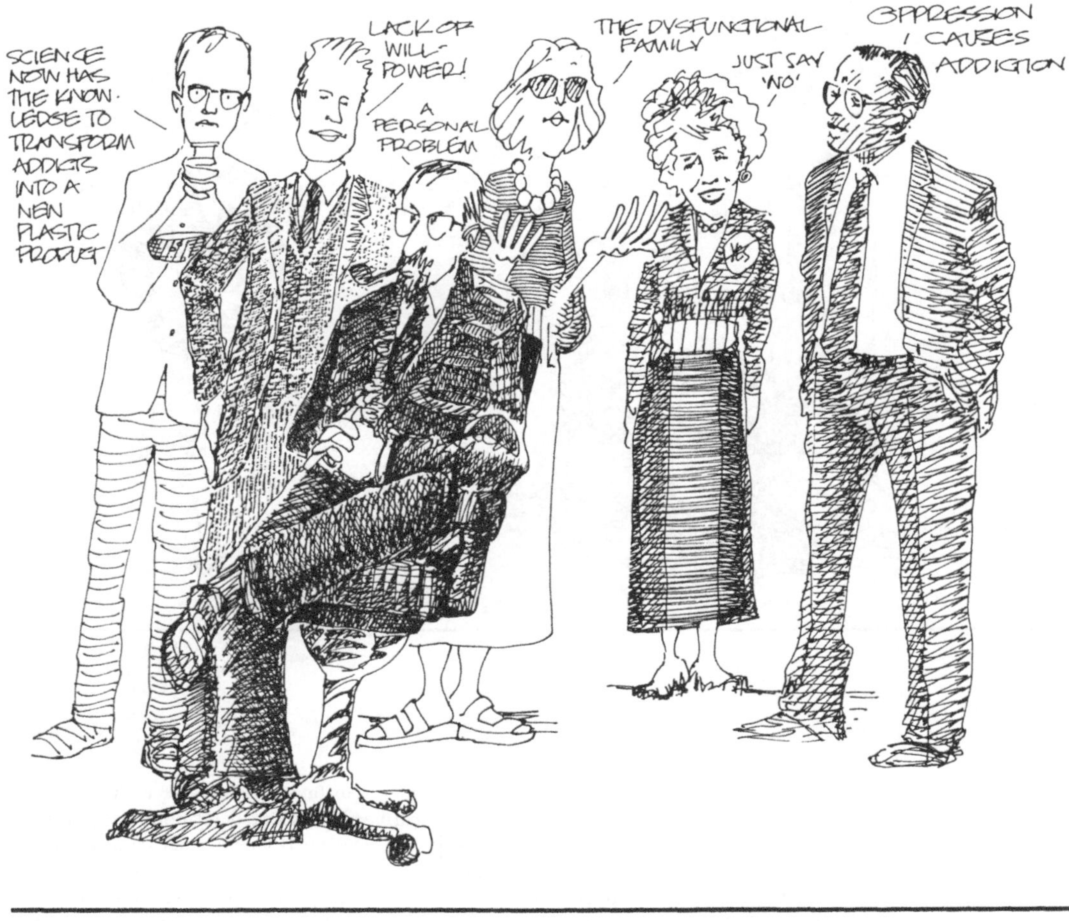

SCIENCE NOW HAS THE KNOW-LEDGE TO TRANSFORM ADDICTS INTO A NEW PLASTIC PRODUCT
LACK OF WILL-POWER!
A PERSONAL PROBLEM
THE DYSFUNCTIONAL FAMILY
JUST SAY 'NO'
OPPRESSION CAUSES ADDICTION

and the clone with a mania for Nautilus machines and the muscles to prove it. Fat liberationists have developed the very convincing argument that fat itself is far less of a health or self-esteem issue in the lives of fat people than are endless cycles of debilitating diets or stereotypes about what fat (and thin) people must be like.

Sex is no more a survival need than alcohol. Yet like the desire for food, the desire for sex often exceeds the body's need to satisfy the basic hungers of human emotion and spirit. It can be a tremendous source of pleasure, and so most people do not choose long-term celibacy. That people are "dependent" on sex because they enjoy how it makes them feel about their partners or simply look forward to the next time they have an orgasm can be considered perfectly ordinary, slightly neurotic, or completely obsessive. Whether an individual feels sexually "normal" or "abnormal" is determined by social attitudes as much as by the

THE BIOLOGICAL MODEL

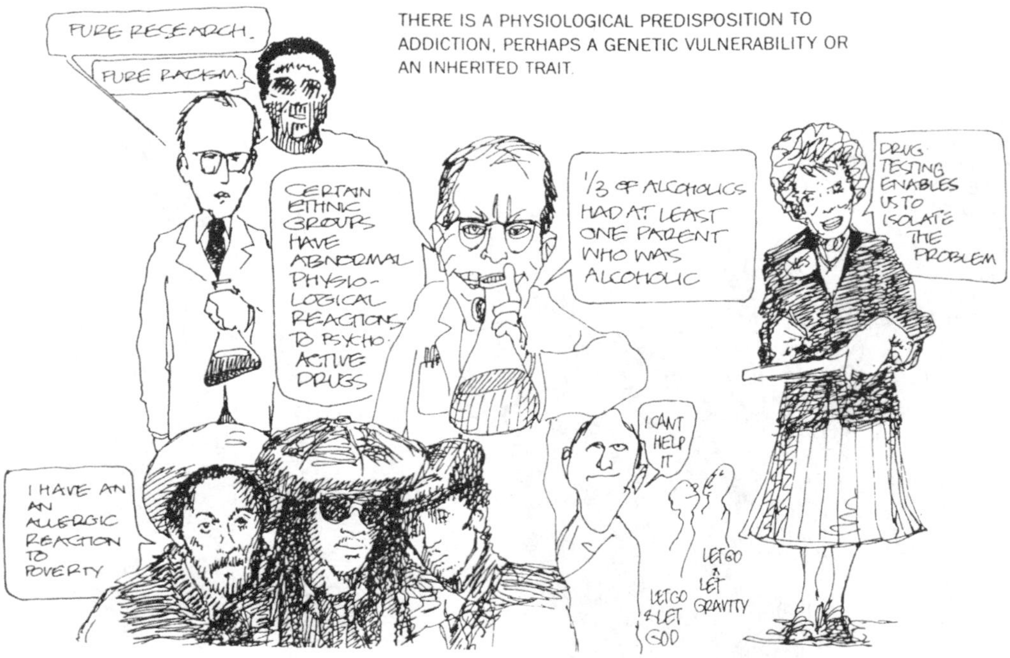

THERE IS A PHYSIOLOGICAL PREDISPOSITION TO ADDICTION, PERHAPS A GENETIC VULNERABILITY OR AN INHERITED TRAIT.
PURE RESEARCH.
PURE RACISM.
CERTAIN ETHNIC GROUPS HAVE ABNORMAL PHYSIOLOGICAL REACTIONS TO PSYCHO-ACTIVE DRUGS
1/3 OF ALCOHOLICS HAD AT LEAST ONE PARENT WHO WAS ALCOHOLIC
DRUG TESTING ENABLES US TO ISOLATE THE PROBLEM
YES
I HAVE AN AN ALLERGIC REACTION TO POVERTY
I CAN'T HELP IT
LET GO & LET GOD
LET GO & LET GRAVITY

specifics of sexual pain and pleasure in her or his own life.

SLAA (Sex and Love Addicts Anonymous) is a relatively new program; it was founded in Boston in 1976 by recovered alcoholics. The SLAA pamphlet entitled "40 Questions for Self-Diagnosis" asks: "Have you ever wished you could be less emotionally dependent?...Do you find yourself in a relationship you cannot leave?...Do you believe that sex and/or a relationship will make your life bearable?" I think many people—certainly large numbers of women—would be inclined to answer yes to questions such as these. Does that make us all "sex and love addicts"?

What exactly does recovery involve for an SLAA member? According to members, the goal is to find love and sex within a "true partnership," a kind of relationship (generally understood to be monogamous) that does not fuel the addiction. If no committed, continuing relationship is possible, then total sexual abstinence is called for as the only method of maintaining "sexual sobriety." Clearly, a traditional hierarchy of sexual values is being upheld: monogamy is the healthy ideal, and celibacy is preferable to promiscuity.

Many of the gay men with whom I spoke about SLAA said the program is a way for them and others to cope with AIDS and AIDS anxiety. At a time when sexual desire itself has started to feel lethal, and a virus that is transmitted sexually is killing incredible numbers of gay men and others, it is not surprising that people have started identifying sexual feelings as symptoms of uncontrollable disease or addiction.

Whatever one thinks about overeating or sexual "addiction," it is clear that feminists, gay men, and lesbians in OA and SLAA are dealing with food, sexuality, health, and other important issues that were and are explored politically within the women's and gay liberation movements. Likewise, the insights adult children of alcoholics have developed about the emotional consequences of growing up in "dysfunctional" families can be traced, at least partially, to a feminist analysis of the family, which understood that institution to be oppressive to women, children, and gay people.

The 12-step approach does not take up the significant differences between addictions or people. Although I assume that differences do exist, 12-step programs simply consider them to be beside the point.

The War on Excess

The programs level contradictions and differences by implying that all substances and activities are addictive when they enable the user (or doer) to "numb out," and suggest that people are trying to fill painful psychological/spiritual voids that no substance or activity can actually satisfy. Can and should all human pain be collected into one big bundle labeled addiction? What about the feelings of pleasure that people derive from food, drugs, alcohol, sex, and a host of other substances and activities? Are these merely self-delusions, the sneaky evidence of addictions-in-the-making? Or are 12-step programs just adding to the dose of guilt we are already handed by a pleasure-phobic culture?

If defining addiction is tough, the "just say no" campaign has made it even tougher by throwing every manner of "excess" into the addiction pot and suggesting that a stiff upper lip can lick everything from a monster federal deficit to urban crime. "Just say no" sounds catchy and you have probably seen it on everything from milk cartons to football stadium billboards, but what the slogan is really saying is that self-control is the entire answer, that standing up to ____________ (fill in the blank) is an act of moral significance, and that the people who do so are strong and true, whereas people who don't are unable to because they are pathetic weaklings. This trend toward championing the heroism and romanticizing the virtue of sheer will is probably a significant contributing factor to the growth and popularity of 12-step programs.

The current war on drugs, sex, and other modern "evils" is a hypocritical effort to rub out the cultural changes of the past two decades by masquerading as a caring crusade. Take, for example, the dismal state of sex education. The Reagan administration has suggested that parents instill "chastity" in their children by whatever means they see fit. Millionaire John LaCorte recently made national headlines with his modest contribution to the "just say no" campaign: an offer to pay $1000 to any girl who guarded her virginity until age 19.[5]

The current war on drugs, sex, and other modern "evils" is a hypocritical effort to rub out the cultural changes of the past two decades by masquerading as a caring crusade.

AIDS educators know that they too must play by rules that put them in an impossible bind. They can squeak by only as long as they say "no" to frank discussions about sexual pleasure, as a recent case in Massachusetts clearly illustrates. In November 1987, when it looked like a long-fought-for state gay rights law might finally pass, opponents of the bill created extensive publicity about sexually explicit AIDS education materials and succeeded in killing the bill for yet another year. Even "friendly" legislators and liberal governor Michael Dukakis self-righteously demanded an explanation from the AIDS Action Committee for a pamphlet distributed to gay men in the bars called "Safer Sex Can Be Sensuous." Dukakis and the legislators said they were offended.

As for alcohol and drugs, if our government were really interested in eradicating substance abuse, it would be spending time and money on rehabilitation, but it is not. In January 1987, while Nancy Reagan was having her picture taken with born-again drug addicts, her husband cut nearly $1 billion from the national anti-drug budget and actually

The programs' core concept–accountability for one's actions –is decidedly apolitical: the responsbility for both addiction and recovery rests squarely within the individual.

recommended that not a single federal dollar be spent on treatment programs.[6] Meanwhile, 30 million Americans undergo drug screening today—in prisons, workplaces, sports, the military, and on campuses—and some estimates hold that 50 percent of the working population will be tested regularly for drugs by 1992.[7]

Douglas Ginsburg is the most ironic casualty in the war on drugs to date. Nominated to the Supreme Court in the aftermath of the Bork defeat, revelations that he smoked marijuana while teaching at Harvard Law School not only forced him to exit the confirmation process before it began (his swan song was a half-hearted call for young people to "just say no" in spite of Ginsburg's own errors), but brought forth a chorus of unsolicited confessions from politicians across the political spectrum that might have been comical if it hadn't seemed so mandatory. Dope-smoking has clearly become a litmus test that all public figures must pass. "Do you now or have you ever...?" may have conveniently eliminated the prospect of a Supreme Court justice with libertarian to right-wing views, but the point of the question was as much to stamp out the radical political legacy of the 1960s as it was to stigmatize anyone caught red-handed with drugs.

It was a coded warning to anyone who remains attached to values associated with the counterculture: personal freedom, experimentation, and pleasure, to name just a few. Politically, that means us—feminists, lesbians, and gay men. We have little to gain from jumping onto a "just say no" bandwagon that equates pleasure and experimentation with addiction. We and all that we represent will be among the first things sacrificed.

No matter where the political winds are blowing, however, the 12-step programs are determined to ignore them. In fact, avoiding public controversy at all costs is one of the programs' most consistent structural features. The tenth tradition specifies: "Our fellowship has no opinions on outside issues, hence our name ought never be drawn into public controversy." This tradition implicitly recognizes that diverse individuals with conflicting viewpoints participate in 12-step programs, and it concludes that a formal, non-political identity is the only logical way to preserve internal unity and prevent groups from being diverted from their purpose by secondary issues. Some important questions do remain, however, about the political implications of 12-step philosophy and structure.

The programs' core concept—accountability for one's actions—is decidedly apolitical: the responsibility for both addiction and recovery rests squarely within the individual. In particular, the programs' philosophy that addiction is a "disease" emphasizes the person and problem in isolation from any outside social forces. This may ease some of the guilt that people feel for pain that they and others have experienced. One Al-Anon member, in great relief, told me: "I make no decisions. The disease does. I am sick." This kind of language and the steps themselves constantly refer people back to themselves with the message that their old negative ways of thinking and behaving are the sources of their pain. Consequently, only new, positive approaches, nurtured by the programs themselves, will produce serenity.

I rarely heard any speakers in meetings—whether recounting stories of assault, workplace hassles, or matters of the heart—mention directly the realities of physical power, economic inequality, racial bigotry, or sexual coercion, even in instances where these were clearly being described. This is true even in Women for Sobriety (WFS), a "new life" program for women alcoholics that differs from 12-step programs in that it tries to identify the unique recovery needs of women. For example, one WFS member was talking happily about her new job as a clerical worker in a big law firm but started sounding anxious when she described her new boss as "a man with a bad reputation for kicking his secretaries around like dogs." She concluded that this worrisome situation was really a test of her sobriety and she resolved to "meet the challenge to be a pleasant person, no matter what." Because meeting rules do not permit direct responses from others present, and also be-

THE SOCIOCULTURAL MODEL

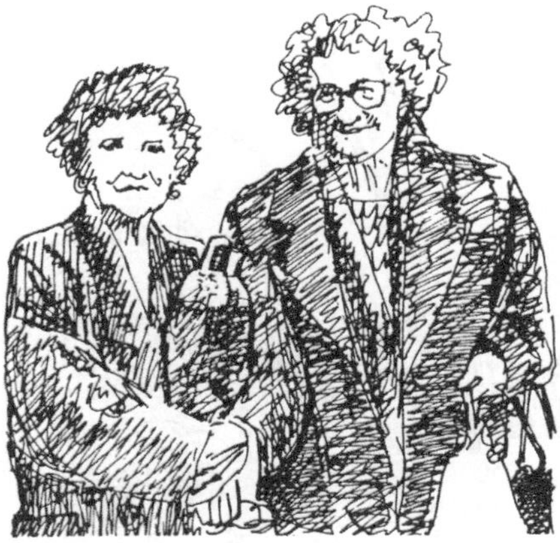

IF THE CULTURE PUTS A HIGH DEGREE OF VALUE IN ALCOHOL, THE INCIDENCE OF ALCOHOLISM WILL BE HIGH. IF CERTAIN GROUPS AREN'T VALUED, THEY ARE MORE LIKELY TO BECOME ADDICTS.

MANY WOMEN BEGIN THEIR IMMODERATE DRINKING WHEN LIFE-SITUATION CHANGES ARE COMMON: DIVORCE, MENOPAUSE, EMPTY-NEST SYNDROME.

cause no larger social context is officially recognized, no one in the room suggested to this young woman that she did not deserve to be treated like an animal or that she was the potential object of sex discrimination. As far as the program went, the answer was for her to "think positive."

"Powerlessness is My Goal"

The conflict between seeing responsibility in purely individual or purely political terms comes up right away, in the first of the 12 steps: "We admitted we were powerless over __________[8] —that our lives had become unmanageable." For many feminists, lesbians, and gay men in these programs, this step is problematic because it turns a progressive political practice of empowerment on its head. Unlike the women's or gay movement, 12-step programs are anything but laboratories in which to experiment self-consciously with forms of personal and political power. But because people generally do not like living with intense contradictions, politically aware and active 12-step members creatively manage the conflicts between their politics and their 12-step experiences. Here is how one politically sophisticated lesbian explained the importance of taking the first step, admitting powerlessness, and another sticky concept, the Higher Power.

> When I was first getting sober, AA was completely in opposition to my experience as a politico because one of the big words was powerlessness. Every activist's hair stands on end at the idea of embracing powerlessness, which you're supposed to be wild about in AA....I found a way to rework the philosophy. It was clear to me that the minute you "give up," you begin a process of empowerment....The big stumbling block for me was the whole God thing....To me, this was completely patriarchal and repugnant. So someone suggested a concept of God that wouldn't offend me—historical materialism [the orthodox Marxist theory of history].

Members who aren't quite as good at fine-tuning the 12-step approach to their own personal philosophies are simply reminded to "take what you need and leave the rest," a handy slogan designed to minimize conflict and help people feel comfortable.

Ironically, the programs seem to be places where women in particular can safely express the feelings that the women's movement first identified as the result of sexism and then criticized in individuals: passivity, confusion,

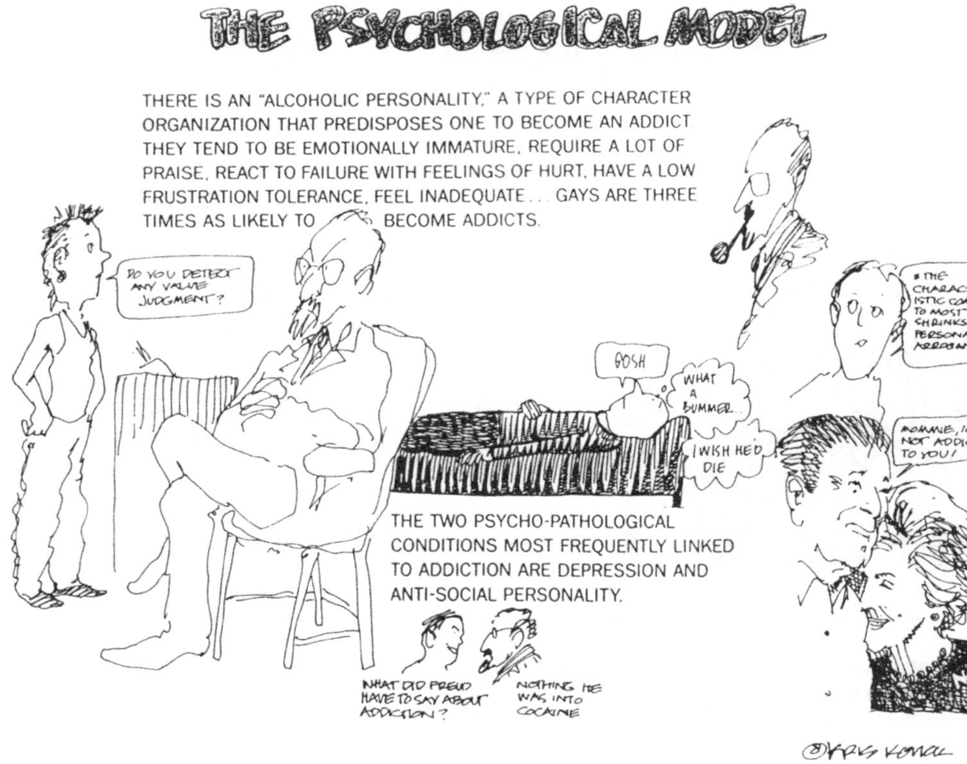
THE PSYCHOLOGICAL MODEL
THERE IS AN "ALCOHOLIC PERSONALITY," A TYPE OF CHARACTER ORGANIZATION THAT PREDISPOSES ONE TO BECOME AN ADDICT. THEY TEND TO BE EMOTIONALLY IMMATURE, REQUIRE A LOT OF PRAISE, REACT TO FAILURE WITH FEELINGS OF HURT, HAVE A LOW FRUSTRATION TOLERANCE, FEEL INADEQUATE . . . GAYS ARE THREE TIMES AS LIKELY TO BECOME ADDICTS.
DO YOU DETECT ANY VALUE JUDGMENT?
GOSH
WHAT A BUMMER
I WISH HE'D DIE
* THE CHARACTERISTIC COMMON TO MOST SHRINKS IS PERSONAL ARROGANCE
MOMMIE, I'M NOT ADDICTED TO YOU!
THE TWO PSYCHO-PATHOLOGICAL CONDITIONS MOST FREQUENTLY LINKED TO ADDICTION ARE DEPRESSION AND ANTI-SOCIAL PERSONALITY.
WHAT DID FREUD HAVE TO SAY ABOUT ADDICTION?
NOTHING. HE WAS INTO COCAINE
NO
©KRIS KOVICK

Kris Kovick is a cartoonist from San Francisco. Her work reflects her experience as an Adult Child of Parents.

powerlessness. As one woman explained:

> I have finally learned to accept fear. I have finally learned to accept confusion. I have finally learned to accept passivity. I think that powerlessness is the whole point of the program, overcoming the will, giving in, giving up. Powerlessness is the same as serenity. It is my goal.

The consciousness-raising groups of the early women's movement were also extremely supportive spaces where personal sharing contributed to a sense of common female experience, which in turn generated commitment and community among individuals who had previously felt alone. Personal transformation, when it occurred, was simply considered to be one logical consequence of developing an analysis of gendered power and making social changes on behalf of women. Powerlessness in all its forms was challenged. Living a serene life was not the point; personal and political liberation were.

The custom fit of the 12-step experience is undoubtedly part of its appeal, but in the context of a "just say no" culture, it risks distorting personal pain to the point where people who really do not have addiction problems are encouraged to think they do. The most striking evidence of this is that many people who do not fall into any of the programs' target groups (such as alcoholics, overeaters, drug addicts) are regularly attending meetings and adopting the 12-step philosophy as their own. The presence of "non-addicts" is controversial in some, but not all meetings, where addicts consider them to be "diluting" the program and distracting members from their main goal of recovery.

> There are some people—I won't say they're addicted to the programs because that's not an appropriate use of the word—who do use the programs as a crutch. The meetings aren't about making friends. They're about changing your life.

But for many, the programs *are* about making friends, and it is not at all unusual for members' friendship networks to change radically, even completely, after entering the program. For some, this is a necessary part of learning that friendships that do not revolve around alcohol or drugs are possible. For others, the programs are just new ways of feeding never-to-be-satisfied hungers for visibility and recognition and a place to experience unrealistic interactions dressed up as recovery. The latter experience is nothing but a new form of dependency.

Getting to Serenity

Substance and other abuses clearly exist, taking horrible tolls on individual lives, and total abstinence must be supported for those who feel it is their only non-abusive option. But just because many things can be dangerous does not mean that they always are. Positive and negative potentials exist side by side. Drugs, sex, food, and other things can be quite wonderful. We should be as determined to defend our right to pleasure as we are to eradicate the reality of our pain. To some degree, our dignity as a society will be measured by our success or failure.

Progressive political movements should be taking notes on what is so appealing about the recovery movement. Political leaders and artists inspire us with visions of peace and social justice; activists discuss and strategize; foot soldiers do the work of getting us from here to there. Meanwhile, we all have to get through the day. Getting through the day might mean staying away from a bar, finding a friend to cry with in a moment of sadness, or having wonderful sex all afternoon. It might just be another day at work. Whatever it means, it is what the women's movement and the gay movement should be about. Changing the structure of political power is not as possible, certainly not as meaningful, when changing ourselves is absent from the agenda.

There is no doubt that 12-step programs have helped people get through a lot of days. But they do nothing to decipher or change the larger context in which time passes, especially in a "just say no" culture that would like to wipe out progressive gains for good.

Political movements can address the larger context, and they have something unique to contribute to the recovery process: an understanding that prevailing cultural messages affect how people feel about themselves just as much as "think positive" slogans do. Self-hatred and self-love are not matters of luck or fate; they do not come and go only on uncontrollable tides of will power. People struggle for and against them, and they will be won or lost just as all contests of power are won or lost. We must keep our eyes on the prize of pleasure even when we are in pain, not allowing suffering to become a symbol of sin or sainthood, not endorsing sickness as a test of moral character, and not making addiction a pre-requisite for support and community. If we succeed, we may all get to serenity. ▼

We should be as determined to defend our right to pleasure as we are to eradicate the reality of our pain.

---

[1] This list is not intended to be comprehensive. Because of the autonomous structure and self-help philosophy of 12-step programs, new ones seem to spring up with great regularity.

[2] *The Twelve Steps for Everyone...who really wants them* by Grateful Members (Minneapolis, MN: CompCare Publishers, 1975), p. 13.

[3] Susan Greenwood, Gay and Lesbian Counseling Services in Boston, personal communication.

[4] The Cambridge Women's Center, for example, currently provides space for weekly meetings of Women for Sobriety, NA, and lesbian Al-Anon.

[5] "Just Say No—Till You're 19," *Newsweek*, December 7, 1987, p. 75.

[6] *Steal This Urine Test: Drug Hysteria in America* by Abbie Hoffman with Jonathan Silvers (New York: Penguin Books, 1987).

[7] *Ibid.*, p. 4, and press release.

[8] Each program uses different words. AA uses "alcoholism"; OA uses "food," and so on.

The International Journal of the Addictions, 18(8), 1085–1107, 1983

Homosexuality as a Cause of Alcoholism: A Historical Review*

S. Israelstam,† MA

S. Lambert,† BA

Addiction Research Foundation
Toronto, Ontario, Canada M5S 2S1

The definitions of homosexuality and of alcoholism have exercised therapists since they first found themselves dealing with the respective behaviors. In both cases, the definition has changed with the change in attitude toward the behavior. Both behaviors have been subject to sanctions of the law. Both have been subdivided into numerous types. Both have social implications that have kept the behaviors "hidden" or "closet." The definitions of both are still not fixed, the underlying causes not fully understood, with consequent confusion as to what homosexuality and alcoholism are and confusion therefore in how we view and deal with them.

The reason we are looking at these two subjects conjointly is because the psychoanalysts developed a theory that linked alcoholism causally with homosexuality. In this paper we attempt to delineate the various aspects of the theory and review work of psychiatrists and social scientists whose work supported or refuted the idea of a causal relationship.

PSYCHOANALYTIC THEORY

Psychoanalysis (see Note 1) opened up the study of human sexuality. With a fervor matched only by the astigmatism of the convert to a new dogma, psy-

*The views expressed in this article are those of the authors and do not necessarily reflect those of the Addiction Research Foundation.

†Requests for reprints may be directed to S. Israelstam, Research Associate, or Sylvia Lambert, Epidemiology Section, Social Policy Research Department, Addiction Research Foundation, 33 Russell Street, Toronto, Ontario, Canada, M5S 2S1.

 0020-773X/83/1808-1085$3.50/0

choanalysis related all behavior and all personality characteristics to sex, and built theories on the basis of a small (usually one or a few case studies) sample from middle-class Western cultures. Deviation from the norm of this relatively small group was explained not in terms of cultural or social or biological differences but in relation to the psychoanalytic concepts of stages of sexual development. Homosexuality was first linked with alcoholism at the beginning of the 20th century by Karl Abraham, the first German psychoanalyst. In 1908 he published the paper (English translation, 1926) "The Psychological Relationship between Sexuality and Alcoholism," which was "the first psychoanalytical view of alcoholism, offering the theory of homosexuality on the Freudian [Note 2] basis as the underlying cause. With the passage of time, that paper remains the classical exposition of the subject" (Smalldon, 1933, p. 650). Two statements of Abraham (1926) became basic to much of the psychoanalytic thought which followed: "Alcoholic drinks have an effect on the sexual instinct, for they dispel the resistances present and increase sexual activity" (p. 3). And "To a healthy minded man any kind of tender contact with other men is repugnant.... These feelings are dispelled by alcohol" (p. 4).

As we have indicated, homosexuality is as hard to define as alcoholism. This is partly because of the variations and shades of meaning given the term by analysts and others. For instance, it appeared to be viewed both as something abnormal and perverted, and as a normal type of behavior involving affection between members of the same sex. Thus the psychoanalyst Wholey (1918) wrote: "The suggestion that every social gathering of men is interpreted by us as evidence of homosexuality *in a degenerate sense* [italics added], is a misinterpretation of our [psychoanalysts'] position" (p. 447).

However they defined or subdivided the term, psychoanalysts of the strict neo-Freudian school appeared to believe that homosexuality caused or was linked to alcoholism. They argued that alcohol caused regression (Note 3) to various levels of psychosexual development—to a level of lewdness, to one where sadistic and masochistic tendencies are released, to a stage where latent (unconscious) homosexuality is released. "According to the amount of alcohol taken, different degrees of regression may occur, and at the level reached different conflicts may be unearthed" (Read, 1920, p. 236).

According to Read (1920), who was a British physician, alcohol is originally taken "to promote the social instincts and alleviate and narcotize the many mental conflicts to which we must all to some extent be victims" (p. 242). However, as we take it to excess "its effect tends to destroy sublimation and aid mental regression . . . and thus bring into active conflict with the personality different impulses and desires previously more or less successfully repressed. Of these the homosexual impulse is found by analysis to be most frequent" (p. 243).

It seems to have been only the psychoanalysts and, following their lead, psychiatrists who related alcoholism to homosexuality in the first part of this century. For example, Smalldon (1933), a British physician, gave physical, environmental, psychogenic, and hereditary points of view in his review of the etiology of alcoholism but did favor the psychoanalytic. The analysts played around considerably with the more dramatic aspects of alcoholism: alcoholic hallucinosis, alcoholic paranoia, alcoholic psychosis, and dipsomania–very much as Bynum (1968) described the "German romantic psychiatrists" of the 19th century who, he said, "although they recognized chronic alcoholism as a cause of disease, were much more interested in the mental states which acute intoxication produced" (p. 163–164). Many early psychoanalysts and psychiatrists (e.g., Kraepelin and Gaupp–see Read, 1920; Riggall, 1923) believed dipsomania (i.e., recurrent and uncontrollable desire for drink) to be closely allied to epilepsy. Several (e.g., L.P. Clark, 1919; Lewis, 1941) built elaborate theories around the etiology of paranoia. Clark (1919), an American physician, for example, stated that alcoholic hallucinations, both acute and chronic, "can be found to be a form of persecution mania arising from unconscious and denied homosexuality" (p. 931). Delirium tremens added grist to their mill. It is accompanied, according to Riggall (1923), a British neurologist and psychoanalyst, "by fear of men and of attacks from men. This fear, of course, is projection of the desire for male companionship" (p. 166). (Whether this applied to women he does not specify.) Clark (1919) said that delirium is accompanied by fear hallucinations not only of men "but animals–well known sex symbols" (p. 931).

Sexual Development and Alcohol

"Homosexuality is a normal instinct and plays an important role in the development of the individual's heterosexuality" (Wholey, 1918, p. 447). This view seems to follow Freud's theory of bisexuality (1898) and that of Juliusburger (Jelliffe, 1917) with its subsequent sublimation or repression (Notes 4 and 5) of the sexual attraction to one's own sex.

How the homosexual becomes involved with alcohol, following upon this viewpoint, is described by Emanuel Miller (1931), who was not only a surgeon and clinical psychologist but also a psychoanalyst (and something of a litterateur).

> Every individual, according to the Freudian psychology, passes through a phase of homosexuality in his attempts to deliver himself from the thraldom of his own oedipus complex. In most of us it survives as an aroma of friendships with members of our own sex, and blossoms furtively and momentarily in the exuberances of the taphouse and the bar. But in some who become social pariahs it continues to dominate not only the sexual life, but the whole of the character. Such persons may be happy in their inversion, and continue without overt disturbances of

> behaviour. In others, however, the solution is only partly completed, and the struggle between homosexuality and other urges in the sexual life and in the life of self becomes the source of the deepest unhappiness, if not the incentive to neurosis and even such psychoses as paranoia.
>
> In such apparently blessed anodyne as alcohol the patient, quite unaware of the inner battle between homosexuality and normal sex or the higher manifestations of the self, seeks escape. In this escape the homosexuality may assert itself either in actual invert behaviour or in pseudomasculine truculence with one's own sex. On the other hand, the normal sexuality with which the patient is endowed wins through and the victim may have sexual successes of transitory character. And, again, the ideal of the self may conquer over both forms of sexuality and emerge in grandiloquence of sublime detachment from all calls of the flesh. Such escapes in alcoholism occur only to the poet and the painter. They are rare amongst ordinary men. (pp. 110–111)

Others (Bigelow et al., 1939; Lewis, 1941; Tabori, 1933; Weijl, 1944) reiterated these viewpoints with variations. Tabori, for example, claimed that the psychic reason for alcohol addiction was the incompletely repressed homosexuality which the id (Note 6) is unable to sublimate.

The American neurologist and psychiatrist Hart (1930), however, was an early dissenting voice. He used a sample of 30 alcoholic patients of whom five were female. In the course of examining them for personality factors he looked at the available facts that might support the psychoanalytic doctrine that homosexuality is an important factor in alcoholism. Only one patient was an "outspoken example of homosexuality," and he drank less and over a shorter period than the others. However, on the basis of defining homosexuality as "a strong tendency to associate with one's own sex in preference to the opposite sex," then 11 persons (two of them women) showed such tendencies. The nine men drank almost exclusively with men or else alone. Three said their desire for women diminished under the influence of alcohol.

Hart did not draw the conclusion that such persons had homosexual tendencies: "On considering the group as a whole, there seemed little evidence of any important [*sic.* Might he have meant latent?] or overt homosexual tendency" (p. 127).

Oral Eroticism

The most obvious and popular connection between alcoholism and homosexuality made by the psychoanalysts was oral eroticism (Note 7). Thus, according to Riggall (1923):

> The craving for sweets, alcohol or tobacco is often due to the desire to satisfy the erotogenetic zone of the mouth, and it is my experience that such craving very frequently accompanies fellatio, the desire for which has obvious unconscious reference to the mother's nipple, and is only another proof of the large part a mother-fixation can play both in homosexuality and alcoholism. (p. 166)

There was no acknowledgment of the addictive quality of the substance alcohol, nor any explanation why alcohol rather than milk became the homosexual's preferred drink (Note 8).

Bergler, an American psychoanalyst, said in his book *The Basic Neurosis* (1944):

> The perversion homosexuality is genetically an oral disease. The homosexual pervert is a person who has failed in overcoming the trauma of weaning. He identifies unconsciously the breast via identification with the penis and escape to man from woman as the source of original disappointment. Thus the homosexual is an oral neurotic. As alcohol addiction has an oral basis too . . . the coincidence of drinking and homosexuality is possible. (p. 466)

However, Bergler (1944) did not see homosexuality as a cause of alcoholism. He considered it a complicated defense mechanism (Note 9):

> A person under the influence of alcohol . . . can . . . use that defense mechanism in his alibi in the battle with his inner conscience. Since every orally regressed person fights his losing battle with the image of the preoedipal mother, one of his techniques in denying that conflict can be the formula: "How can I be accused of *masochistic* submission to the mother, if I'm really interested in the man?" (p. 243)

Bergler (1944) said he would not be understood in his own time. The book was published again in 1977 with an introduction by Toronto psychiatrist Melvyn Iscove.

Another who discussed oral neurotics and drinking was Esser (1952), a Dutch alcoholism consultant:

> Sucking is the most primitive and forceful of all inborn reactions. Oral reflexes can be early conditioned sexually and can not only bring about the drinking habit but can also release sexual infantilisms like sexual oralism, the need of applicating the mouth to the sexual organs, the need for sadomasochistic activities etc. (p. 167)

Esser did not single out homosexuals here. The passage was equally applicable to heterosexuals.

Anal Eroticism

Alcoholism and homosexuality have also been related to anal eroticism (Note 10), albeit more vaguely (Weijl, 1944; Wholey, 1918). For example, Wholey (1918) commented on his case study: "The patient's overwhelming money complex revealing itself so dramatically in his psychosis, together with the marked obstinacy, orderliness, and punctiliousness characterizing the individual, present evidence of the relationship of chronic alcoholism with homosexuality and anal eroticism" (p. 442).

Maleness and Femaleness

Rigall (1923) theorized on the basic historical relationship between masculinity, the power of creation, and alcohol.

> Now, alcohol stimulates masculinity, and emphasizes the male ideas of greatness and power. Abraham deals with this characteristic in his work on creation myths. These myths, he finds, deify the male power of creation. And it is not difficult to understand how alcohol has come to be unconsciously identified with semen. So we get the "intoxication of love" idea, and a symbolic interpretation of the mythological nectar. The old-time libations to the gods probably embodied a similar unconscious idea, and to-day the common custom of drinking healths has a significant meaning. (p. 163)

L.P. Clark (1919) also discussed the drinking of alcohol in terms of manliness. "Man relies on alcohol because it gives him a feeling of manliness and flatters his manliness complex" (p. 932). On the other hand, he says, "Men drink, fall on one another's necks, feel themselves united by an inner bond and weep. In a word, their behaviour is womanish" (p. 932).

Button (1956), a psychologist, studying 87 male alcoholics of whom only two had histories of long-lasting homosexual behavior, agreed with Clark (1919) about the "manliness complex" but related it to the basic idea of *latent* homosexuality.

> Many discussions of alcoholism paint latent homosexuality as a potent force in the genesis of the condition. The position is taken here that only if by latent homosexuality is meant a pattern of incomplete and distorted masculine identifications are these discussions appropriate.

> The desire of these alcoholics is not to be a woman but rather to be a complete man. (p. 52)

When dealing with women, to further confound confusion, Riggall (1923) said that "Such women as drink will frequently show strong homosexual tendencies. Whereas men, however, drink to overcome the repression of natural homosexuality, women are more likely to drink in order to bring out the male side of their bisexuality" (p. 163).

Clark (1919) agreed that "Women who have a strong desire for liquor are likely to prove homosexual" (p. 932). Clark maintained that women's social teas were sublimated expressions of feminine homosexuality, but that alcohol, formerly reserved for men, was more satisfactory. "The virile component of women is stirred today, and this helps explain the women's increased turning to alcohol" (p. 931). (See Note 11.)

Abraham (1926) saw alcoholism as mainly a male problem; the psychosexual constitution of women, he claimed, incited them far less to take alcohol. Psychoanalysts and psychiatrists certainly appear to have centered their work on the male (see Comfort, 1967; Homiller, 1980; Leeson and Gray, 1978). Women, and lesbians in particular, even when they were included in the samples, were not usually taken into account in the conclusions regarding alcoholism and homosexuality (see, e.g., Levine, 1955). To be sure, the number of women alcoholic patients was a fraction of the number of male alcoholics. Whether it was their small number, or whether it had to do with a predominant attitude in society that women didn't "count," or whether it was too bothersome to come up with separate conclusions drawn from women's case histories, we do not know.

One American psychoanalyst, Knight (1937), however, found that there were few women alcoholics (presumably because few passed through the gates of the Menninger Clinic where he found his sample of male alcoholics). He accounted for this paucity of female alcoholics by suggesting that women, "although they may have in infancy experienced the same oral pacification and thwarting, have many more socially acceptable ways of indulging their passivity than men do and hence are not driven to drinking as the only solution" (p. 244). However, he adds that "if there is a strong active homosexual component . . . they may drink to emulate masculinity."

Female alcoholics were seldom looked at as a separate group. The year 1937, however, saw the appearance of two articles on alcoholic women, both by psychiatrists attached to a mental hospital. Although psychoanalysts might see few alcoholic women patients (Landis, 1945), the Psychiatric Division of Bellevue Hospital in New York saw them in considerable numbers. For example, over the year 1935, 1,633 women were admitted because of alcoholism (as compared to 7,506 men) (Curran, 1937). Curran's study consisted of 50 women aged 17 to 63 of low socioeconomic status, with "very severe alcoholism." Most (30) of them felt that drinking made them more socially acceptable. Two of the 50 admitted to having had homosexual experiences, one when she was 12, the other when she was 8. Only one "wanted to be a boy." Twenty felt they had satisfactory heterosexual relations, and in only 10 cases was the sexual desire or pleasure increased by drinking. In hallucinosis, homosexual remarks and threats were much less outspoken than in male alcoholics. The author summed up his findings by saying, "The evaluation of homosexuality and promiscuity in men and women differs greatly in our present society" (p. 653).

Wall, an American psychiatrist (1937), studied 50 women patients, the total consecutive admissions over the years 1920 to 1933 of women to the Bloomingdale Hospital, "in which the immediate cause of hospitalization was alcoholic indulgence" (p. 943). This followed a study of 100 men selected over the same period. Findings considered important by the author were that many of the women (32) had frequent temper tantrums in childhood and showed no strong attachment to any family members. Five cases had a history of overt homosexuality, but most said "I like men but I despise women."

Wall (1936, 1937) found distinct differences between the male and female groups in the field of psychosexual development. The males showed considerable mother attachment and preferred the company of their own sex. The women preferred male society. Wall said:

> Concerning the psychosexual development of the alcoholic patient, much emphasis has been placed on homosexuality, particularly in the psychic sense. No one with psychiatric experience doubts its significance, and its manifestations in this group of men throw some light on the problem. (1936, p. 1390)

Beyond the fact that there were 11 cases of overt homosexuality, that most of the patients indicated a preference for male drinking companions, and that those who developed alcoholic psychoses "revealed the homosexual conflict," it is difficult to ascertain just what light was thrown on the problem. The most significant and interesting finding was the differences between male and female alcoholics: For he found that the women had highly individual problems and that their alcoholism or excessive drinking was more intimately associated with some definite life situation than males (a finding similar to Lisansky's in 1957; and others: see Homiller, 1980).

Wall's paper on women alcoholics was read at the 92nd Annual Meeting of the American Psychiatric Association (1936). The discussants appeared eager for information on differences or similarities in behavior and personality characteristics, whereas Wall had made a much more profound observation: that motivation for or cause of alcoholism may be quite different for the two sexes. Dr. Karpman asked what had been learned about jealousy in women, for "As one knows, alcoholics as a group are very jealous" (Wall, 1937, p. 953). He found a homosexual factor in a man's jealousy because, although the jealousy is apparently directed at a woman, "it enables him to preoccupy his mind physically with the man" (p. 953) [a rather difficult feat?].

Another discussant, Dr. Schilder, attempted to indicate a homosexual aspect to women's alcoholism by saying that "One may speak about a homosexual relation between mother and daughter," but he did not develop this theme.

Weijl, an American psychiatrist, some 7 years later (1944), basing his statement on his own perceptions rather than quantitative data, had this to say on the subject:

> With the increasing masculinity of women, apparent in the choice of professions, in clothes, and in women's attitudes toward life, we find an increased inclination toward alcohol and drunkenness. (p. 203)

Support and Refutation in the 1950s

In 1944 Weijl summarized what psychoanalysts who came before him had to say about homosexuality and alcoholism. He concluded, like so many others, that the latent homosexual drives are directly connected with the causes of compulsive drinking. In the 1950s analysts such as Tähkä (1954) and Parland (1957) were still in agreement with this stand. Parland (1957) did say, however, that overt homosexuality could emerge in some cases. Levine (1955), a psychiatrist, also supported the theory. He studied the records of 63 male and 16 female (two overt homosexual and one lesbian interest) alcoholics. He found that a decided majority of these patients showed diminished interest in heterosexual relationships. Rather than attempting to determine if this were simply a general loss of sexual appetite, he looked for a change to homosexual interest. This he found, by inference only: 75% exhibited the "strong mother/weak father" syndrome. "With such strong feminine identification the development of a passive homosexual male is understandable" (p. 680). He continued, "This is consistent with the scientific hypothesis [Abraham's] that the alcoholic has a basic homosexual problem" (p. 680). He did not mention whether the females in his sample fitted into this explanation, and he appears to have ignored any findings on them in his conclusions.

Esser (1952) was not so sure of the direct relationship between alcoholism and homosexuality. He wrote:

> According to many writers there seems to be a deeper relationship between alcohol and behavior patterns of homosexual character. But it is difficult to know what this relationship is, since there are many theories and probably no single one is fully explanatory. (p. 168)

He went on to say that the homosexual used alcohol either to release his inhibitions to "help him to make contact which he would not dare to make when sober" (p. 168) or simply to dampen the misery and unhappiness to which the homosexual, he says, is usually subject. There were those in the 1950s who refuted the homosexuality-alcoholism connection. Gerard (1955) maintained that latent homosexuality had nothing to do with alcoholism. He noted that many overt homosexuals were alcoholics. He believed that alcohol (and opiate) addicts had failed in varying degrees to develop a definite sex role or identification. When Scott (1958) studied the personalities and backgrounds of 300 alcoholics (33 females) by looking at case records, he concluded somewhat similarly to Gerard that the fundamental characteristic of the alcoholic is not homosexuality but immaturity—an inability to face a responsible relationship with a person of the opposite sex. Another American psychiatrist who refuted the connection was Levy (1958). He found that the same range of latent homosexual factors are found in alcoholic patients as in any mixed group of psychiatric patients.

> Transient overt homosexual contacts while drinking, on the other hand, are not uncommon among our patients. In most cases this represents the lack of concern with, and clear perception of the nature and needs of the sexual object. In most cases a woman or a sheep might have done as well. (p. 656)

TOWARD A BROADER PERSPECTIVE

The emphasis of the psychoanalysts was on personality factors in alcoholism (Jelliffe, 1917), which, as we have attempted to point out, were explained or interpreted in psychoanalytic terms using psychoanalytic language. The language of psychoanalysis was literary, full of poetic allusions, and the concepts themselves were derived from mythology. Needless to say, both the layman and the mainstream scientists found the concepts (as well as the language) obscure, enigmatic, imprecise, and a barrier to understanding. This was evident already in 1918 (Wholey) at the 73rd Annual American Medico-Psychological Association Conference when alcoholism and homosexuality were discussed. A Dr. White said:

> The alcoholic hallucinosis is almost invariably an outgrowth of the homosexual life. The tendency of hallucinations invariably points to the homosexual level.

In reply, a Dr. McDonald said:

> It seems to me that using terms such as the homosexual level and the like, that such speech is meaningless.... It is symbolic talk and idle interpretation.

Dr. White defended his position by saying:

> If we are going to bother about the literal meaning of words, meanings which hark back to infantile ways of thinking, we will not understand.

As far as their expertise in the field of alcoholism is concerned, Landis (1945), a psychologist, pointed out that although "Psychoanalysts attempted to provide a deeper understanding of the true nature of the personality of the alcoholic" (p. 134), they were somewhat hampered by the fact that they seldom saw a true alcoholic. Landis reported that over a period of 10 years (Note 12) the Institute of Psychoanalysis in Chicago saw only 36 persons diagnosed as alcoholism or drug addiction—and of these only four were analyzed. In general the early psychoanalysts mentioned above used very small samples or just one or a few case studies (e.g., Clark, 1919; Reed, 1920; Wholey, 1918). Social scientists such as Landis called for the use of larger samples of alcoholics, objective language, and quantitative methods.

Thus by the 1940s two important things were happening that influenced the homosexuality-alcoholism concept. One was that alcohol addiction was becoming a field of study in itself. The emphasis was on alcoholism as a disease rather than a symptom or a personality defect. It was suggested that there was more than one type of alcoholism, and many branches of science were brought to bear on this study (Browman and Jellinek, 1941). The other was that psychology, as part of a broader trend among the social sciences to objectify and quantify their methods for purposes of prediction, was inspired to find more objective approaches to the study of the individual than psychoanalysis appeared capable of. The immediate result was a spate of psychometric tests for measuring personality, attitudes, and various aspects of individual human behavior.

Psychometric Tests

Although intended to be objective, in fact psychometric tests were often subjective and lacking in reliability and validity. However, the first faulty tests encouraged the formulation of better ones and, more important, encouraged theorists to use more than a few case studies to formulate theories that were meant to apply to a whole group or subculture.

One such test was the Minnesota Multiphasic Personality Inventory (MMPI) masculinity-feminity test (Hathaway and McKinley, 1943), which was considered to be objective as it used quantitative methods to determine what was masculine and what was feminine. Since feminine interest was believed to show homosexuality in the male, the psychologist Hewitt (1943) gave this test to members of Alcoholics Anonymous to test the alcohol-homosexual theory. He concluded that neither latent nor overt homosexuality was typical of the alcoholic. (He pointed out, however, that AA, aware that homosexuals might be attracted to their groups, discouraged those whose appearance was suggestive of abnormality from becoming members.)

More and more psychologists, mainly in the United States, began to disagree with the psychoanalytic view of alcoholism and homosexuality. Quarantana (1947), using two different personality tests, found no correlation between alcoholism and homosexuality. Botwinick and Machover (1951) also used a masculine-feminine interest test to examine the hypothesis that alcoholism involved a homosexual component. They found no differences in the masculine-feminine scale for alcoholics and controls, and concluded that "Homosexuality, latent or otherwise . . . cannot be an essential factor in alcoholism, although it may play a dynamic role in individual cases" (p. 272). They did, however, point out the obvious fallacy that "feminine interest" may not measure homosexuality.

In 1953 a Canadian psychologist, Robert Gibbins, reviewed the major areas of theoretical work on the etiology of alcohol addiction. Although not all psychoanalytical theories involved homosexuality, he found that "the majority of analysts assign the homosexual theory a prominent position in the etiology picture" (p. 8). Psychologists, on the other hand, were more likely to see a person's drinking as an attempt to overcome inhibition or inadequacies, or as an escape mechanism, although in general Gibbins found that they were content to enumerate personality traits of the alcoholic and describe his behavior rather than attempt to discover his motivation for pathological drinking.

One psychoanalyst who did not fit Gibbins's description was Sherfey (1955). She maintained that psychoanalytic literature is full of unproven theories about alcoholism, including the theory that homosexuality is the sole cause of it. Sherfey applied more rigorous standards to her study (1955) and used almost as many female as male alcoholics in her sample. In 89 male and 73 female case studies of alcoholics she found 11 diagnostic groups, among which was a variety of types of sexual adjustment. She concluded that alcoholism is a symptom which may be associated with several illnesses or syndromes.

The British psychologist Grygier (1957), in a paper entitled "Psychometric Aspects of Homosexuality," described and assessed the most popular psychometric tests such as the various personality inventories (MMPI, Terman-Miles, etc.), semantic, perceptual projective (e.g., the Rorschach), and interpersonal relationships (e.g., Thematic Apperception Test [TAT]). He concluded that the claims of these tests "to detect the dynamic aspect of homosexuality and therefore to help in the understanding of the origin of sexual inversion" were difficult to validate, given the state of knowledge of the time. Such tests, however, continued to be used by psychologists in their ongoing search to find homosexual trends among alcoholics.

Using three different tests and a sample of "remitted" and "unremitted" alcoholics, Machover et al. (1959) found that homosexual trends *were not* more prevalent among the alcoholics than among nonalcoholic, nonhomosexual controls, but they *were* more evident among the alcoholics who had stopped drinking. In attempting to explain, the authors conjectured that the alcoholics who had stopped drinking were less defensive, and so had incorporated their homosexuality into their personality, whereas the alcoholics who were still drinking were able to conceal their homosexuality through their defensive organization to a greater extent. This certainly vindicates Grygier's (1957) scepticism regarding the tests—since the whole point of them is to show up what is hidden.

A paper published the same year in the *American Sociological Review* (Parker, 1959) made even less sense logically. The author used the M-F Test of Terman and Miles [who gave a most emphatic warning against the assumption "that an extremely feminine score for males or an extremely masculine score for females can serve as an adequate basis for the diagnosis of homosexuality, either overt or latent" (Grygier, 1957, p. 524)] to show that his sample of 50 alcoholics scored more "femininely" than the 50 moderate drinkers. He then carried this information forward to the equivocal conclusion that "the dynamics leading to compulsive drinking can be formulated in such a way that homosexuality and femininity of temperament become functionally equivalent, playing the same role in the addictive processes" (p. 371).

Gibbins and Walters (1960) conducted three experiments to test the following psychoanalytic hypothesis: "The early ontogenetic development of each individual is believed to contain a homosexual component which is, under favourable circumstances, sublimated. In persons who become addicted to alcohol this sublimation has failed to occur and latent homosexual trends remain in the personality" (p. 620). The samples were composed of arrested homosexuals, psychiatric patient alcoholics, and controls from the YMCA. The authors used three tests, a visual recognition test, speed of recognition test, and a test of responses to pictures of symbols of male and female genitalia. In spite of the fact that "the experiment as a whole does not provide strong evidence for the psychoanalytic theory," that the sample was a very biased one (no nonarrested homosexuals and no nonhomosexual psychiatric patients as controls), and that the tests were not known to be reliable or valid, the authors felt that "this theory should not be lightly discarded" (p. 640).

Methodological problems of using psychometric tests for studies of homosexuality and alcoholism were pointed out in a paper by the Canadian psychologist Smart (1959), who also mentioned that many psychoanalytic studies appeared to have been based on single case histories (e.g., Reed, 1920; Rigall, 1923; Robbins, 1935). Smart himself used projective techniques on 12 homosexual prisoners, 12 heterosexual psychology students, and 12 alcoholics. He concluded that "alcoholics and homosexuals do not differ in the frequency of 'homosexual' signs" but added that this result may be due to sampling.

Two sociologists, McCord and McCord (1960), were in favor of discarding the psychoanalytic theory altogether, quoting case studies (e.g., Landis.

1945) and psychometric studies (e.g., Quarantana, 1947) that go against the theories of Freud (1898) and Abraham (1908/1926). Their own study of six overt homosexual boys, 24 feminine boys, and 166 normal masculine boys (as defined by their culture) showed that the overt homosexuals were most likely to become alcoholics. In spite of the obvious sampling problem, they felt their results did not support the belief that alcoholics have latent homosexual personalities.

The Theory in the 1960s

Testing and criticism of the work of the psychoanalysts did not prevent elaboration of the old theme (Bergler, 1959; Cappon, 1965). Cappon, a Canadian psychiatrist, for example stated: "The natural history of the homosexual patient seems to be one of frigidity, impotence, broken personal relationships, psychosomatic disorders, alcoholism, paranoid psychosis (i.e., the mental illness of suspicion and persecution) and suicide" (p. 126).

Although this may well be true for the homosexual who seeks psychoanalytic help, the danger is that this "natural history" may be extrapolated to all homosexuals. When Cappon (1965) added that "Alcohol is used as an escape from conflict; to brave the world of normalcy, to gain Dutch courage and compete, to anesthetize feelings of fear and inadequacy and, most of all, to numb one's perception and so escape from ones self, until the next morning" (p. 126), one can only believe such insight was deduced from a variety of alcoholic or drinking neurotic patients, not just homosexual ones.

Eva Blum (1966), in an article which gives a clear account of how the basic concepts of psychoanalysis were applied to the development of the theory of alcoholism, spells out what is implicit in the works cited thus far:

> In psychoanalytic writing the term addiction is not used in the strict sense of dependence upon a pharmacologically active substance. . . . Rather, in speaking of addiction, psychoanalysts refer to dependence on a substance, an activity or a person, believed to provide pleasure on the one hand and relief from psychic pain (anxiety, etc.) on the other hand. Such dependence is conceived of as resulting from developmental failure. (p. 263)

Addiction supposedly protects the individual from the "graver consequences of this failure: suicide, psychosis, asocial or criminal behaviour" (Blum, 1966, p. 263). However, according to Cappon (1965) (see above), addiction does not protect the individual, or at any rate the homosexual, from any of these behaviors except perhaps the criminal one.

Blum (1966), having shown how the analytic theory of alcoholism developed, then said it would be an error to attribute a unitary theory of alcoholism to the psychoanalysts, that the framework of psychoanalysis is too complex for a single-factor explanation. It is this complexity that makes the experiments (she mentions those of Smart, 1959, and Gibbins and Walters, 1960) disproving psychoanalytic theory "regrettable" because they have isolated a single factor out of this great complex structure. In her reading of the literature–although she pointed to many writers who believed that the alcoholic is arrested at or regressed to the oral stage of growth–analysts related homosexuality only to the alcoholics fixated at the anal stage.

A third stage discovered through case studies of alcoholics, says Blum (1966), is the phallic-oedipal stage:

> These patients have progressed beyond a homosexual love choice to a heterosexual one and have come to grief over the conflicts arising from their very progress. They have not been able to come to terms with the emerging sexual feelings toward their mother. (p. 267)

Blum (1966) summed up by saying "psychoanalytic theory may be seen to have made a very considerable contribution to the developmental theory of alcoholism and to the differential classification of alcoholics" (p. 288), and she predicted a great future for psychoanalysis in cross-disciplinary research and treatment.

Changing Attitudes Toward Homosexuality and Alcoholism

Several interrelated movements incorporating modern psychological models or schools of thought were occurring in society and in the literature of the '60s and '70s which tended to undermine the position of psychoanalysis and the medical model which viewed alcoholism and homosexuality as diseases to be cured. Of major influence was the humanistic model–for example, as expressed in the work of Carl Rogers (1951, 1961), which concentrates on the human potential and the positive side of the human condition, rather than the pathological. Another influence was the existential model, which stresses the uniqueness of the individual and freedom of self-fulfillment. Its most modern proponent is British psychiatrist R.D. Laing (Laing, 1967; Laing and Esterson, 1964).

The emergence of labeling theory in the literature on the sociology of deviance had a great effect as well: Behavior was criminal or sick only insofar as it was labeled such by society (Becker, 1963; Goffman, 1965; Kitsuse, 1962; Schur, 1971; Szasz, 1965).

Another undermining influence was the work of several social scientists and clinicians, many homosexuals themselves, who complained in their writings of the pernicious effects of psychoanalysis on patient and public alike (e.g., Altman, 1971; Churchill, 1967; Lee, 1978; Weinberg, 1972; Ziebold, 1979). The voice of gay liberation was heard in the '50s (Cory, 1951) but became more vociferous in the '60s (Hoffman, 1969) and '70s (*The Body Politic*, 1972-). One result of these various forces was that homosexuality began to lose its sickness label. In 1973 the "official" classification of homosexuality by the American Psychiatric Association was changed from "psychiatric disorder" to "sexual orientation disturbance," and Socarides (1978) lamented the fact that homosexuality was not even considered a disturbance in the 1974 printing of the American Psychiatric Association's diagnostic manual.

Alcoholism, considered as a symptom of a disease by the psychoanalysts and as a disease (psychiatric or physiological or both) by most alcohologists, is thus still generally handled on the medical model–not unreasonably in view of the heavy investment in treatment. However, because of the seeming ineffectiveness of treatment (Davies, 1979) and lack of understanding of the genesis of alcoholism (Gordis and Sereny, 1981), and perhaps because the medical model is irrelevant in terms of social policy regarding availability, alcoholism may gradually be losing the sickness label. It is also possible to give treatment to alcoholics without considering them sick by following the learning theory principles of the behaviorists (Bandura, 1969): Drinking is seen as learned behavior, and excessive drinking can be "unlearned" or deconditioned by desensitization and aversion techniques (Rimm and Masters, 1974).

In general, the study of the effects of alcohol on large samples and even whole populations was well underway by the '70s, showing the diversity both of causes of alcohol problems and also of the types of individuals involved. Thus speculation on and research into the causal relationship between alcoholism and homosexuality has all but disappeared over the past 10 years from the pages of psychiatric, psychoanalytic, and addiction journals.

If the *American Journal of Psychoanalysis* is taken as an indication of trends of psychoanalysis, then it would seem that several changes in attitudes or emphasis have taken place regarding both homosexuality and alcoholism in the last decade. In 1972 an article appeared (Miller) which put an entirely different, and somewhat more rational, interpretation on male conviviality. Miller wrote:

> Men's tendency to pursue ties to other men need not rest on a basic homosexual drive, as such. It seems much more likely that it rests on a societal definition of women as a different and less significant order of being. (p. 156)

Homosexuality was no longer necessarily considered a pathology (T.R. Clark, 1975), and the emphasis shifted from changing the homosexual patient to fit into society to making him comfortable with himself (Gilberg, 1978). Articles on alcoholism appear to have ceased in this journal.

On the other hand, the *American Journal of Psychotherapy* seems to follow the more traditional view that sees both homosexuality (e.g., Lesse, 1973, 1974; Socarides, 1978) and alcoholism (Khantzian, 1980) as psychiatric disorders.

The importance of the psychoanalysts, especially the earlier ones, regarding this theory rests in how they affected the theorizing and choice of research topics of their peers and those who came after them. It can be seen that a great deal of effort was put into studying the homosexuality-alcoholism connection. Also of importance was how the theory and the research it fostered affected patients in particular and laymen in general. Very little was found on public attitudes or feelings about the theory (e.g., if those who drank worried that they were homosexual). Cory (1951), however, an early advocate of gay liberation in the United States, was of the opinion that the American public associated homosexuality with drunkards. An example of how the homosexuality-alcoholism theory filtered down to the layman is the novel *Lost Weekend* by Charles Jackson (1944) (Note 13). In this book the traditional psychoanalytic association is made between homosexuality and alcoholism. As far as homosexual and alcoholic patients are concerned, whether a therapist would see them as having a personality disorder or not would depend to a large extent on how much the therapist followed the views of the psychoanalysts.

NEEDED FUTURE RESEARCH

Although research into homosexuality has expanded since the beginning of the 1970s, there is relatively little on the alcohol problems of the homosexual. Beaton and Guild (1976), Weathers (1976), and Small and Leach (1977) have done some research into therapy; and some research into the nature and extent of the problem has been undertaken by Fifield (1975) and Lohrenz et al. (1978). However, there are no full-scale demographic or epidemiological studies.

Changing attitudes among psychoanalysts and psychiatrists toward homosexuality (Bayer, 1981) and input from psychology, sociology, and related disciplines, together with the accumulation of research material on alcoholism in general, have tended to make obsolete the belief that homosexuality and alcoholism are causally connected through regression to an earlier developmental stage. The only reference we found from the '70s alluding to the connection was in *A Concise Encyclopedia of Psychiatry* (Leigh et al., 1977), which stated that "Some latent homosexuals seek solace in alcohol" (p. 184).

Some researchers in the 1980s (Hudson and Ricketts, 1980; Woodman and Lenna, 1980) are viewing problems of homosexuals within the framework of "homophobia"–fear of homosexuality. Homophobia is a problem found throughout society–in patients, therapists, homosexuals, and heterosexuals alike (Woodman and Lenna, 1980)–and relates to the previously mentioned statement of Leigh et al. (1977). Research exploring the relationship between drinking and homophobia could be conducted using the homophobia scale developed by Hudson and Ricketts (1980).

There has been even less research on the drinking habits and problems of lesbians than on male homosexuals (Diamond and Wilsnak, 1978; Weathers,

1976). Drinking patterns among lesbians as compared to those of male homosexuals, or heterosexual female alcoholics, is another fertile field of research investigation.

The most-quoted statistics on homosexuality and alcohol problems are: 10% of the population are homosexual (Kinsey et al., 1948, 1953), 30% of the openly homosexual population have drinking problems (Fifield et al., 1975; Lohrenz et al., 1978), and 10% of the general population are problem drinkers (NIAAA, 1978). These figures mean that 30% of persons with drinking problems are homosexuals; yet only one study was found that relates, however vaguely, to such a percentage: Small and Leach (1977) reported that in their clinical experience "almost one third of men seeking counselling or treatment for alcoholism are concerned about homosexuality" (p. 2077). Even allowing for discrepancies in terminology as well as imprecise definitions, it still seems that a disproportionately high percentage of homosexuals are alcoholics or at least have drinking problems. Research is needed to give more precision and delineation to the numbers quoted in the field of alcohol problems and homosexuality for practical purposes of education, prevention, and therapy.

Drinking in bars plays a central part in the life-style of the contemporary homosexual (Israelstam and Lambert, 1982). This and various other aspects of the homosexual experience might be looked at with a view to understanding the high rate of alcohol problems. Colon et al. (1981) pointed out that anomie is a factor that should be looked at when studying the drinking habits of socially isolated groups. Many homosexuals are cut off from their families and may lack the usual support systems such as family, church, and work peers. Do these environmental factors play a role in the drinking problems of the homosexual?

Fifield et al. (1975) showed that alcohol treatment agencies at that time in Los Angeles were either ignorant of the gay drinking problem or were likely to ignore it. Other literature (Beaton and Guild, 1976; Wellisch et al., 1981) suggests that therapists attempt to treat a homosexual's gayness rather than the alcohol problem; these authors feel that this bias disuades homosexuals from seeking treatment. Research is needed to see whether such a bias still exists, how to get treatment to those who need it, and whether homosexuals need different treatment approaches than other groups.

NOTES

1. Psychoanalysis: A theory of the psychology of human development and behavior, a method of research, and a branch of psychotherapy originally developed by Sigmund Freud. The unconscious is looked at through analysis of free associations and the interpretation of dreams.
2. Freudian theory of homosexuality: Homosexuals suffer from castration anxiety and identify with the opposite-sex parent. The homosexual refuses to admit that there are beings without penises and therefore devotes attention to males (from P. Kline, *Fact and Fantasy in Freudian Theory.* London: Methuen, 1972).

3. Regression: The partial return to more infantile patterns of reacting.
4. Sublimation: A defense mechanism operating unconsciously by which instinctual drives, consciously unacceptable, are diverted into personally and socially acceptable channels.
5. Repression: The unconscious defense mechanism that banishes unacceptable ideas or impulses from consciousness.
6. Id: That part of the personality which holds the instinctual desires and strivings of the individual.
7. Oral eroticism: Part of the oral phase of infantile psychosexual development lasting from birth to 12 months or longer. It relates to the pleasurable experience of sucking.
8. The psychoanalyst Simon Weijl (1944) addressed himself to this question. He claimed that alcohol was a substitute for milk, which in its turn symbolized the mother. "Because the taste of alcohol is so different from milk [but so, surely, is apple juice or coffee] it camouflages the unconsciously desired milk." Weijl carries his argument on by saying that a diminution of inebrriety goest hand in hand with an acceptance of milk drinking by males. He then points out that in the United States there is much more milk drinking by men than in Europe. With the sublime disregard for facts that seems to be typical of psychoanalysts of the time, he brings no statistics to bear on his case. In fact, inebriety cannot be said to have been diminishing in the United States in 1944 since the number of gallons of absolute alcohol consumed per person aged 15 years and over in the period 1942 to 1946 increased to 2.06 from the period 1936 to 1941 when it was 1.54.
9. Defense mechanism: Unconscious intrapsychic process serving to provide relief from emotional conflict and anxiety.
10. Anal eroticism: The pleasurable part of the anal phase of development—from 1 to 3 years of age. The child has particular interest and concern with the process of defecation and sensations connected with the anus.
11. It is of interest to note that Clark wrote this in 1919, the beginning of an era not dissimilar from the late 1970s in terms of women's rights, women's suffrage (gained in 1920 in the U.S.), and the general emancipation of women, as many began to enter the business and professional worlds.
12. Landis does not say what years the decade spans, but it would have been prior to 1945.
13. The public was not as wide as it might have been, however, as the homosexuality was removed from the movie version of *Lost Weekend* because of rules of censorship.

REFERENCES

ABRAHAM, K. The psychological relationships between sexuality and alcoholism. *Int. J. Psycho-Anal.* 7: 1–10, 1926.

ALCOHOLICS ANONYMOUS WORLD SERVICES, INC. *Do You Think You're Different?* New York: A.A. Grapevine, 1976.

ALTMAN, D. *Homosexual Oppression and Liberation.* New York: Outerbridge and Dienfrey, 1971.

BANDURA, A. *Principles of Behavior Modification.* New York: Holt Rinehart and Winston, 1969.

BAYER, R. *Homosexuality and American Psychiatry.* New York: Basic Books, 1981.

BEATON, S., and GUILD, N. Treatment for gay problem drinkers. *Soc. Case Work* 57: 302–308, 1976.

BECKER, H.S. *The Outsiders: Studies in the Sociology of Deviance.* New York: Free Press, 1963.

BELL, A.P., and WEINBERG, M.S. *Homosexualities: A Study of Diversity among Men and Women.* New York: Simon and Schuster, 1978.

BERGLER, E. *The Basic Neurosis: Oral Regression and Psychic Masochism*, 1977 ed. New York: Grune and Stratton, 1944.

BERGLER, E. *One Thousand Homosexuals: Conspiracy of Silence or Curing and Deglamorizing Homosexuals?* Paterson, N.J.: Pageant Books, 1959.

BIGELOW, N.J.T., LEHRMANN, S.R., and PALMER, J.N. Personality in alcoholic disorders: Acute hallucinosis and delirium tremens. *Psychiatr. Q.* 13: 732–740, 1939.

BLUM, E.M. Psychoanalytic views of alcoholism. *Q. J. Stud. Alcohol* 27: 259–299, 1966.

BODY POLITICS COLLECTIVE. *Body Politic.* Toronto: Pink Triangle Press, 1972+.

BOTWINICK, J., and MACHOVER, S. A psychometric examination of latent homosexuality in alcoholism. *Q. J. Stud. Alcohol* 12: 268–272, 1951.

BROWMAN, K.M., and JELLINEK, E.M. Alcoholic mental disorders. *Q. J. Stud. Alcohol* 2: 312–390, 1941.

BUTTON, A.D. The psychodynamics of alcoholism. A survey of 87 cases. *Q. J. Stud. Alcohol* 17: 443–460, 1956.

BYNUM, W.F. Chronic alcoholism in the first half of the 19th century. *Bull. Hist. Med.* 42: 160–184, 1968.

CAPPON, D. *Towards an Understanding of Homosexuality.* Englewood Cliffs, N.J.: Prentice-Hall, 1965.

CHURCHILL, W. *Homosexual Behaviour among Males.* New York: Prentice-Hall, 1967.

CLARK, L.P. Some psychological aspects of alcoholism. *N. Y. Med. J.* 109: 930–933, 1919.

CLARK, T.R. Homosexuality and psychopathology in nonpatient males. *Am. J. Psychoanal.* 35: 163–168, 1975.

COLON, I., CUTTER, H.S.G., and JONES, W.C. Alcohol control policies, alcohol consumption, and alcoholism. *Am. J. Drug Alcohol Use* 8: 347–362, 1981.

COMFORT, A. *The Anxiety Makers.* London: Nelson, 1967.

CORY, D.W. *The Homosexual in America: A Subjective Approach.* New York: Greenberg, 1951.

CURRAN, F.J. Personality studies in alcoholic women. *J. Nerv. Ment. Dis.* 86: 645–667, 1937.

DAVIES, D.L. Defining alcoholism. In M. Grant and P. Gwinner (eds.), *Alcoholism in Perspective.* Baltimore, Md.: University Park Press, 1979.

DIAMOND, D.L., and WILSNAK, S.C. Alcohol abuse among lesbians: A descriptive study. *J. Homosexuality* 4: 123–142, 1978.

ESSER, P.H. Drinker types. *Folia Psychiatr. Neurol. Neurochir. Neerlandica* 55: 161-179, 1952.

FIFIELD, L., DE CRESCENZO, T.A., and LATHAM, J.D. *Alcoholism and the gay community.* Summary of "On My Way to Nowhere: Alienated, Isolated Drunk; An analysis of gay alcohol abuse and an evaluation of alcoholism rehabilitation services for the Los Angeles County." Los Angeles: Gay Community Services Center, 1975

FREUD, S. Sexuality and the aetiology of neurosis. In E. Jones (ed.), *Collected Papers.* London: Hogarth, 1953 (originally published, 1898).

GERARD, D.L. Intoxication and addiction: Psychiatric observations on alcoholism and opiate drug addiction. *Q. J. Stud. Alcohol.* 16: 681-699, 1955.

GIBBINS, R. *Chronic Alcoholism and Alcohol Addiction* (Brookside Monograph No. 1). Toronto: University of Toronto Press, 1953.

GIBBINS, R.J., and WALTERS, R.H. Three preliminary studies of a psychoanalytic theory of alcoholic addiction. *Q. J. Stud. Alcohol* 21: 618–641, 1960.

GILBERG, A.L. Psychosocial considerations in treating adolescents. *Am. J. Psychoanal.* 38: 355–358, 1978.

GOFFMAN, E. *Stigma.* Englewood Cliffs, N.J.: Prentice-Hall, 1965.

GORDIS. E., and SERENY. G. Controversy in approaches to alcoholism. In V.M. Rosender and M. Rothchild (eds.), *Controversies in Clinical Care.* Jamaica, N.Y.: SP Medical and Scientific Books, 1981.

GRYGIER, T. Psychometric aspects of homosexuality. *J. Ment. Sci.* 103: 514–526, 1957.

HART, H.H. Personality factors in alcoholism. *Arch. Neurol. Psychiatry.* 24: 116–134, 1930.

HATHAWAY, S.R., and MC KINLEY, J.C. *The Minnesota Multiphasic Personality Inventory.* Minneapolis: University of Minnesota Press, 1943.

HEWITT, C.C. A personality study of alcohol addiction. *Q. J. Stud. Alcohol* 4: 368–386, 1943.

HOFFMAN, M. *The Gay World.* New York: Bantam Books, 1969.

HOMILLER, J.D. Alcoholism among women. *Chem. Depend.* 4: 1–31, 1980.

HUDSON, W.W., and RICKETTS, W.A. A strategy for the measurement of homophobia. *J. Homosexuality* 5: 357–372, 1980.

ISRAELSTAM, S., and LAMBERT, S. *Gay Bars.* Toronto: Addiction Research Foundation, Substudy, 1982.

JACKSON, C. *Lost Weekend.* Garden City, N.Y.: Farrar, 1944.

JELLIFFE, S.E. The mentality of the alcoholic. *N.Y. Med. J.* 105: 629–635, 1917.

KHANTZIAN, E.J. The alcoholic patient: An overview and perspective. *Am. J. Psychother.* 34: 4–19, 1980.

KINSEY, A.C., POMEROY, W.B., and MARTIN, C.E. *Sexual Behaviour in the Human Male.* Philadelphia: Saunders, 1948.

KINSEY, A.C., POMEROY, W.B., MARTIN, C.E., and GEBHARD, H. *Sexual Behaviour in the Human Female.* Philadelphia: Saunders, 1953.

KITSUSE, J. Societal reaction to deviant behaviour. *Soc. Probl.* 9: 247–256, 1962.

KNIGHT, R.P. The dynamics and treatment of chronic alcohol addiction. *Bull. Menninger Clin.* 1: 233–250, 1937.

LAING, R.D. *The Politics of Experience.* New York: Pantheon, 1967.

LAING, R.D., and ESTERSON, A. *Sanity and Madness in the Family.* London: Tavistock, 1964.

LANDIS, C. Theories of the alcoholic personality. In *Alcohol, Science, and Society.* New Haven, Conn.: Q.J. Stud. Alcohol, 1945.

LEE, J.A. *Getting Sex.* Don Mills, Ont.: Musson, 1978.

LEESON, J., and GRAY, J. *Women and Medicine.* London: Tavistock, 1978.

LEIGH, D., PARC, C.M.B., and MARKS, J. *A Concise Encyclopedia of Psychiatry.* Baltimore: University Park Press, 1977.

LESSE, S. Editorial. *Am. J. Psychother.* 27: 151–154, 1973.

LESSE, S. Editorial. *Am. J. Psychother.* 28: 1–3, 1974.

LEVINE, J. The sexual adjustment of alcoholics. *Q. J. Stud. Alcohol* 16: 675–680, 1955.

LEVY, R.I. Psychodynamic functions of alcohol. *Q. J. Stud. Alcohol* 19: 649–659, 1958.

LEWIS, N.D.C. Personality factors in alcohol addiction. *Q. J. Stud. Alcohol.* 1: 21–44, 1940.

LEWIS, N.D.C. Psychiatric resultants of alcoholism, alcoholism and mental disease. *Q. J. Stud. Alcohol* 2: 293–311, 1941.

LISANSKY, E. Alcoholism in women. *Q. J. Stud. Alcohol* 18: 588–623, 1957.

LOHRENZ, L.J., CONNELLY, J.C., COYNE, L., and SPARE, K.E. Alcohol problems in several midwestern communities. *J. Stud. Alcohol* 39: 1959–1963, 1978.

MACHOVER, S., PUZZ, F.S., MACHOVER, K., and PULUMEAU, F. Clinical and objective studies of personality variables in alcoholism: III. An objective study of homosexuality in alcoholism. *Q. J. Stud. Alcohol* 20: 528–542, 1959.

MC CORD, W., and MC CORD, J. *Origins of Alcoholism.* Stanford, Conn.: Stanford Univ. Press, 1960.

MILLER, E. The psycho-pathological aspects of alcoholism. *Br. J. Inebr.* 28: 109–111, 1931.

MILLER, J.B. Sexual inequality: Men's dilemma (a note on the oedipus complex) paranoia –other psychological concepts. *Am. J. Psychoanal.* 32: 147–155, 1972.

NIAAA (National Institute on Alcohol Abuse and Alcoholism). *Third Special Report to the U.S. Congress on Alcohol and Health.* Rockville, Md.: U.S. Department of Health, Education, and Welfare, 1978.

PARKER, F.B. A comparison of the sex temperament of alcoholics and moderate drinkers. *Am. Sociol. Rev.* 24: 366–376, 1959.

PARLAND, O. Alcoholism and homosexuality. *Alkoholpolitik* Hels. No. 3: 75–80, 101–102, 1957.

QUARANTANA, J.V. *Alcoholism: A study of emotional maturity and homosexuality as related to factors in compulsive drinking.* Thesis, Fordham University, 1947 (quoted in W. McCord and J. McCord *Origins of Alcoholism.* London: Tavistock, 1960).

READ, C.S. Psychopathology of alcoholism and some so-called alcoholic psychoses. *J. Ment. Sci.* July 1920, pp. 233–244.

RIGGALL, R. Homosexuality and alcoholism. *Psychoanal. Rev.* 10: 157–169, 1923.

RIMM, D.C., and MASTERS, J.C. *Behavior Therapy: Techniques and Empirical Findings.* New York: Academic Press, 1974.

ROBBINS, B. S. A note on the significance of infantile nutritional disturbances in the development of alcoholism. *Psychoanal. Rev.* 22: 53–57, 1935.

ROGERS, C.R. *Client Centered Therapy.* Boston: Houghton Mifflin, 1951.

ROGERS, C.R. *On Becoming a Person.* Boston: Houghton Mifflin, 1961.

SCHUR, E.M. *Labelling Deviant Behaviour: Its Sociological Implications.* New York: Harper and Row, 1971.

SCOTT, E.M. Psychosexuality of the alcoholic. *Psychol. Rep.* 4: 599–622, 1958.

SHERFEY, M.J. Psychopathology and character structure in chronic alcoholism. In O. Diethelm (ed.), *Etiology of Chronic Alcoholism.* Springfield, Ill.: C. C. Thomas, 1955.

SMALL, E.J., and LEACH, B. Counselling homosexual alcoholics: Ten case histories. *J. Stud. Alcohol* 38: 2077–2086, 1977.

SMALLDON, J.L. The etiology of chronic alcoholism. *Psychiatr. Q.* 7: 640–641, 1933.

SMART, R.G. *An exploratory study of the psychoanalytic theory of alcohol addiction.* Master's thesis, University of Toronto, 1959.

SOCARIDES, C.W. The sexual deviations and the *Diagnostic Manual. Am. J. Psychother.* 32: 414–425, 1978.

SZASZ, T. Legal and moral aspects of homosexuality. In J. Marmor (ed.), *Sexual Inversion.* New York: Basic Books, 1965.

TABORI, J. Homosexuality as psychic background of alcoholism, psychoanalysis of cases. *Psychiatr. Praxia Psycho-anal.* 3: 10–19, 1933.

TÄHKÄ, V. On the psychodynamic etiology of drunkenness. *Alkoholpolitik* No. 4: 103–110, 1954.

WALL, J.H. A study of alcoholism in men. *Am. J. Psychiatry* 92: 1389–1401, 1936.

WALL, J.H. A study of alcoholism in women. *Am. J. Psychiatry* 93: 944–955, 1937.

WEATHERS, B. *Alcoholism and the Lesbian Community.* Los Angeles, Calif.: Alcohol Center for Women, 1976.

WEIJL, S. Theoretical and practical aspects of psychoanalytic therapy of problem drinkers. *Q. J. Stud. Alcohol* 5: 200–211, 1944.

WEINBERG, W. *Society and the Healthy Homosexual.* New York: St. Martin's Press, 1972.

WELLISCH, D.K., DE ANGELIS, G.G., and PATERNITE, C. A study of therapy of homosexual adolescent drug abusers in a residential treatment setting. *Adolescence* 16: 680–700, 1981.

WHOLEY, C.C. Revelations of the unconscious in a toxic (alcoholic) psychosis. *Am. J. Insan.* 74: 437–447, 1918.

WOODMAN, N.J., and LENNA, H.R. *Counselling with Gay Men and Women.* San Francisco: Jossey-Bass, 1980.

ZIEBOLD, T.O. Alcoholism and recovery: Gays helping gays. *Christopher Street* 3: 36–44, 1979.

Gynecologic Care for the Lesbian

Susan R. Johnson, MD
University of Iowa College of Medicine
Iowa City, Iowa

Jefri L. Palermo, MA
University of Iowa
Iowa City, Iowa

This article has three purposes: 1) We provide information about reproductive system problems as experienced by lesbian women and make recommendations for management. Research in this area is limited; so we also point out the gaps in our knowledge.[1] 2) Alcohol abuse is the one health problem that may be more common among lesbians than among heterosexual women. Because the obstetrician-gynecologist may see patients who are concerned about alcohol dependency, we include a section outlining current thinking about alcoholism as it occurs among lesbians. 3) The physician will not know a patient is lesbian unless she chooses to reveal this information. A variety of concerns make the decision to disclose such information difficult. We will review some of these concerns and suggest ways the interested physician can provide an atmosphere that allows patients to comfortably discuss sexual preference. Because information about sexual activity is important in the assessment of many gynecologic complaints, this skill seems particularly important for the obstetrician-gynecologist.

Gynecologic Health

In this section we will review specific gynecologic problems and suggest how management may differ for lesbians. We have relied primarily on our study at the University of Iowa in which 117 lesbians were surveyed.[2] Other relevant studies are cited where appropriate.[3-7] The reader should recognize the limited generalizability of all these studies due to the (unavoidable) use of volunteer subjects.

Vaginal Infections

Vaginal infections of all types occur even in women who are exclusively homosexual. In our study half of the women had experienced a monilial infection, a figure similar to the expected rate in heterosexuals and consistent with the epidemiology of *Candida albicans*, which does not require venereal transmission. While *Trichomonas*

Correspondence: Susan R. Johnson, MD, Department of Obstetrics and Gynecology, University of Iowa Hospitals and Clinics, Iowa City, IA 52242.

vaginalis vaginitis is frequently thought of as a heterosexually transmitted disease, this is not the case. Several women in our study who were exclusively homosexual experienced *Trichomonas* vaginitis. It is not known whether a woman can transmit trichomonads to a female sexual partner; we suggest discussing this uncertainty with the individual lesbian patient, recommending examination of any partners in whom symptoms develop. The epidemiology of nonspecific vaginitis (*Gardnerella vaginalis* vaginitis) is largely unknown. While transmission by heterosexual coitus is probable, it does not appear to be necessary. Lesbians in our study had been given a diagnosis of nonspecific vaginitis, and we have seen exclusive lesbians in our own clinic who have this problem. Again, it is not known whether a lesbian can transmit this infection to her partner.

The lesbian patient will want to know whether she needs to alter her sexual practices while she is being treated for a specific vaginal infection. It seems prudent to recommend that activities which are uncomfortable should be stopped until the infection is treated. Specific advice about the risks of transmission cannot be given because scientific information is lacking. There is, for example, the theoretic possibility that a partner could contract oral pharyngeal monilial infection after oral genital contact, but this must be rare. Treatment of each of these infections in lesbians is identical to that in heterosexual women.

Sexually Transmitted Diseases

As suggested by several studies, the traditional sexually transmitted diseases, gonorrhea and syphilis, are rarely contracted by lesbians.[2,5-7] Further, *Chlamydia*, now considered an etiologic agent in pelvic inflammatory disease, was not found in routine cultures of a group of lesbians.[7] We conclude that the diagnosis of pelvic inflammatory disease in an exclusively homosexual woman is unlikely.

Genital herpes, on the other hand, while not identified as a specific problem in any reported studies, can occur in lesbians as a result of oral-genital transmission of the virus. Lesbians need to be aware of this potential problem, and if they do suffer from either oral or genital herpes, need to take the usual precautions in order not to expose sexual partners directly to virus-shedding lesions.

Acquired Immunodeficiency Syndrome

There are no reported cases of lesbians contracting acquired immunodeficiency syndrome (AIDS) on the basis of their sexual activity. The susceptibility to this illness of homosexual men seems to be based on the increased rate of drug abuse, sexually transmitted disease, and exposure to penile-anal intercourse. Because neither of the latter risk factors affect lesbians, nondrug abusing exclusively homosexual women are not likely to be at risk for contracting this disease.

Cervical Intraepithelial Neoplasia

The prevalence of cervical intraepithelial neoplasia among women who have been exclusively homosexual would be expected to be similar to the rate found in celibate women. In our study the only woman who had significant dysplasia defined herself as bisexual, and thus her risk was presumably more similar to that of a heterosexual woman.[2] One study performed screening Papanicolaou smears on 148 consecutive lesbians and found a dysplasia rate of 2.7%, suggesting that dysplasia does occur.[7] As many as 80% of women who identify themselves as lesbian have had heterosexual intercourse in the past, thus placing them at some risk. We agree with Robertson and Schachter that Pap smear screening should be offered to lesbians, the interval between screenings determined by the patient's individual history.

Menstrual Cycle Disorders

There do not appear to be differences in reproductive hormones between lesbians and heterosexual women.[5] There is thus no theoretic reason to suspect that lesbians would have any increased risk for menstrual cycle abnormalities. In our study, only 15% of women surveyed had ever seen a gynecologist for irregular menses, a rate which does not seem unusual for a reproductive age population. Kenyon's work found that lesbians reported fewer menstrual cycle irregularities, dysmenorrhea, and premenstrual symptoms than heterosexual control subjects.[4]

Endometriosis

Because endometriosis is thought to be more common in nulliparous women, nulliparous lesbians should be at increased risk. This problem has not been examined adequately, but in our study only one woman reported this disease. While the diagnosis of endometriosis in lesbians would be made in the usual way, management might differ. For many lesbians fertility is not a major concern and earlier consideration of definitive surgical therapy might be considered.

Pregnancy-Related Concerns

A substantial number of lesbians, 23-50% in reported studies, have been pregnant and are raising children.[2,5,6] While these pregnancies may have occurred during a prior heterosexual relationship, some lesbians are choosing to have children on their own or with a female partner. We found evidence that the desire to have a child is quite common, but that the number of women who are actually successful in doing so is small.[2] Several options for obtaining a child are theoretically available: 1) adoption, 2) artificial insemination, 3) intercourse with a cooperating male, or 4) intercourse with an unsuspecting male. In our study, all four options had been considered by at least some women, with adoption and artificial insemination the most commonly considered courses.

Many adopting agencies will not consider single persons, and the option of coitus is not acceptable to many lesbians. Thus, the gynecologist may be approached about arranging artificial insemination. There is no information available about how many physicians are willing to do this, but apparently many are not. In response to this perceived lack of availability, several independent women's clinics have set up artificial insemination programs.

Unless a woman is exclusively homosexual, she may still need information about birth control methods.

Sexual Function and Dysfunction

Lesbians have available the same repertoire of sexual techniques as heterosexual men and women, with the obvious exception of the absence of a penis.[3,5,6] Manual stimulation of the clitoris and cunnilingus are reported to be the two principal methods of achieving orgasm. While use of dildos seems to be relatively uncommon, vibrators are probably used to the same extent as among heterosexual women. There is no difference in the sexual response cycle when female homosexuals and heterosexuals are compared.[5]

The prevalence of sexual dysfunction among lesbians is not known, but there is some evidence to suggest that it is no higher and may even be lower than the incidence among married heterosexual individuals.[2,5,8] When these problems occur, the approach to treatment would in general be the same as with heterosexuals.[5] The physician who is trained in office sexual counseling and is comfortable with lesbian patients should feel confident that he or she can undertake the management of sexually dysfunctional lesbian women. *Physicians without this training or comfort level should refer the patient to an appropriate source.* While this latter advice seems obvious, it has not always been followed. Masters and Johnson reported that of 151 gay men and women who came to them for treatment, 81 had sought help first from another physician; of these 81, 57 had been refused treatment, and only *one* had been referred elsewhere.[5]

Some physicians may believe that caring for lesbian patients will require counseling skills beyond their training. This belief is perhaps derived from the stereotypic notion that homosexual persons are all unhappy and would like to change their sexual orientation. In fact, this problem will rarely be encountered by the practicing physician. Recent studies on samples of the general population suggest that most gay people are satisfied with their sexual preference.[6] Bell and Weinberg suggest that those who do seek help for problems related to sexual preference usually see psychiatrists, counselors, or other mental health care professionals rather than gynecologists or general practitioners. In our view it is not appropriate for the physician to suggest therapy to a patient who has not expressed dissatisfaction.

Alcohol Abuse

The incidence of alcoholism among lesbians is estimated to be from 25% to 35%, or 5-7 times that of heterosexual women.[9-12] The three most commonly cited reasons explaining this high incidence are 1) the importance of the gay bar as a social/community center,[11] 2) the alienation and isolation lesbians experience as a result of society's rejection and oppression,[11,13] and 3) the lack of responsiveness alcoholism treatment agencies have shown for the needs of lesbian alcoholics.[13]

Background

Before discussing each of these hypotheses, we will point out three assumptions researchers often make—incorrectly, we think—about characteristics of lesbian alcoholics.

First, lesbians are assumed to be the same as gay men, and the results of studies focusing on male homosexuals are generalized to lesbians. While lesbians experience many of the same effects of homophobia, as women they experience additional stresses and expectations that gay men do not—they earn significantly less, are usually the single parent when there are children from a heterosexual marriage, and they are under greater social pressure to marry.

Second, all alcoholics are often assumed to be the same regardless of sexual orientation; the real differences that exist between heterosexual and homosexual lifestyles and experience are ignored. Treatment programs that ignore or deny the special needs of homosexual clients have had very little success.[13,14]

Third, some writers have assumed that men and women alcoholics are alike. Recent studies suggest that women's drinking patterns differ from men's in several significant ways.[15] Women abuse alcohol in response to situational crises such as battering, rape, divorce, death in the family, menopause, etc. Woods found that factors contributing to lesbian alcohol abuse include many of these same stresses, and she suggests that differences between lesbian and heterosexual female alcoholics may not be so much a difference in kind as of degree.[10]

To return to the reasons for the high relative incidence of lesbian alcoholism, we begin with the importance of the gay bar as a social center. Fifield found that a significant proportion of Los Angeles homosexuals spent up to 80% of their social time in gay bars or at parties where alcohol was served (grant proposal submitted to the NIAAA, Los Angeles, 1975). This finding is probably more descriptive of the limited social options available to gays rather than an indication of deviance, and while a lack of alternatives for socializing may encourage greater attendance in bars, alcoholism is not an inevitable result. For example, Woods found that nonalcoholic lesbians went to bars as often as abusers did, but they drank less and did not stay as long.[10]

Woods discredits the second hypothesis that lesbian alcoholism is the sole result of societal oppression[10]: "The available literature is preoccupied with the view that alcohol abuse among lesbians is mainly symptomatic of the oppressed minority status of lesbians. There seems to be a definite unwillingness on the part of such writers to consider other possible factors. . . . Perhaps a reason for this unwillingness to look at other factors is the inability to separate the subject of lesbianism from that of alcohol abuse." While it is important not to ignore the effects of the minority status of lesbians, oppression does not cause lesbian alcoholism. Lesbian alcoholics are sick not because they are lesbians but because they are alcoholics.

A lack of responsiveness of treatment programs does appear to be an important factor.[14] Three major types of negative interaction have characterized the lesbian alcoholic's experience with alcoholism agencies: 1) refusal of services if the woman's lesbianism was known or suspected: 2) provision of services on a limited basis, or with attitudes not conducive to support, self disclosure, or sobriety; and 3) isolation of lesbianism as the primary problem, with little or no attention directed to the alcoholism.

While a lack of responsiveness in an agency cannot be considered causal in lesbian alcoholism, neither is it curative. Those few agencies that do attempt to address the specific needs of gays have found that they will come for treatment. Underhill suggests that in order for treatment programs to serve lesbians effectively, they must 1) provide lesbian staff counselors, 2) do outreach to lesbian alcoholics in the local community, and 3) integrate an awareness of the damaging effects of homophobia and sexism into the traditional treatment goals of maintaining sobriety (personal communication, February 1983).

In summary, it is important to understand both the unique factors contributing to alcohol abuse among lesbians as well as the factors they share in common with alcoholic heterosexual women and with alcoholics in general.

Recommendations

Physicians should keep the following recommendations in mind when interacting with lesbian patients who abuse alcohol: 1) Do not assume that alcohol abuse is causally related to sexual preference. 2) Respect the patient's reluctance to enter into a traditional treatment program. While this cannot be used as an excuse to avoid treatment, every effort should be made to make a referral based on verification of the agency's ability to work effectively with lesbians. 3) Be familiar with gay resources, including books, organizations, lesbian or gay support groups, Alcoholics Anonymous, and Al-Anon. 4) Be willing to involve the lesbian alcoholic's significant others in her treatment. They are profoundly affected by the problem and can be critical in the success of her treatment. 5) Above all, examine your own prejudices and make an honest assessment of your strengths and weaknesses in intervening with lesbian women with alcohol problems.

Patient-Physician Interaction

There is little doubt that many lesbian patients have serious concerns about physicians.[2,16] Only 18% of the women in our study had ever revealed their sexual preference to a physician providing them with gynecologic care. Forty percent thought their health care would be adversely affected if their physician were aware of their sexual preference. Finally, 35% of the women in our sample sought out nontraditional alternative clinics for their gynecologic care.

Despite these figures, the majority of the women in our study reported that under ideal circumstances they would prefer to be open with their physicians. Why? Lesbians who feel they cannot be open may unwillingly give inaccurate or incomplete information related to their medical problems. Many lesbians would like to be open so they can obtain accurate information, especially when a problem may relate to sexual activity. The desirability of openness is supported by Dardick and Grady, who found a strong positive correlation between openness with the physician and overall satisfaction with health care.[16]

What are some of the reasons for concern? Many lesbians are put off by the assumption of heterosexuality reflected in the language of questions concerning "marital status," birth control, and sexual activity. The lesbian hearing these questions may assume the doctor is not willing to listen to her answers. In addition, each time the patient is asked a question related to sexual activity, she must decide whether to be honest or whether to withhold information.

Many of the women in our survey believed gynecologists are not well informed about lesbian health care issues. This is likely to be the case, because little has been written and most residency programs do not include specific information about this topic.

Lesbians are aware of the potential repercussions a breach of confidentiality may have on their employment, family, and even treatment by the remainder of the health care team. Our survey suggests that lesbians would be more likely to discuss their sexual preference if they were assured the information would not be recorded in the medical record. The patient's need for confidentiality may be particularly acute if the community is small, if the patient is a minor, or if she has not been open about her sexual preference with other people in her life.

Homophobia is defined as an irrational fear of homosexuals, and represents a not uncommon extreme of the range of attitudes held in our culture toward homosexuals.[5] The lesbian has no way of knowing in advance what attitude a physician may hold, and she may be concerned that her care will be compromised if the attitude is a negative one. Dardick and Grady reported that 27% of a sample of 622 gay men and lesbians had dealt with at least one primary care physician whom they thought was prejudiced against homosexuals.[16]

While the women in our study indicated that, given a choice, they would prefer to see a lesbian gynecologist, many wrote that they would prefer a caring, knowledgeable, nonjudgmental physician regardless of sex or sexual preference; we conclude that any interested physician can successfully care for lesbian patients.

Recommendations

We believe there are several steps the obstetrician-gynecologist can take that will improve his or her ability to care for lesbian patients.

1. The physician should reassess his or her own attitudes and beliefs about persons with a homosexual preference. Stereotypic images are reinforced by the media, and because many people have never known an openly gay person, they have no real basis on which to test their thinking. Recent research confirms that homosexuals are no different in appearance, job choice, pattern of friendships, or family relationships than heterosexuals. There are no physical or historical characteristics that allow homosexual men and women to be easily identified. As Bell and Weinberg point out, there is "no unique gay lifestyle, and homosexual men and women are similar in every way to heterosexual persons except in the choice of their sexual partners."[6]

2. The physician should learn about health problems and concerns of lesbians. While much is unknown, particularly in the area of the transmission of vaginal infections and in the incidence of long-term health problems, information included in the first section of this chapter will provide a beginning point for this education. It should be noted that we and others have been unable to identify any medical disorders that are unique to or appear to be more common in lesbian patients.

3. The physician should recognize the importance of confidentiality and let the patient know that information about sexual preference need not be written in the medical record.

4. The physician should recognize and utilize the lesbian patient's support system, particularly if she develops either a chronic or serious illness. This system may include

either a single "significant other" or a group of friends. While there are legal constraints on the physician in certain matterns like informed consent, other areas are within the physician's control. The physician should ask the patient whom she would like to be involved in her care, and then the physician can communicate with those persons just as he would with the family or friends of a heterosexual patient. Hospital visiting regulations can be modified to allow a significant other of the same sex to spend the same time with the patient that a heterosexual's spouse would spend. This is especially important in intensive care units, where regulations are often quite restrictive.

5. Physicians need to think carefully about what they say to patients and how they say it.[18] Recognize that questions about sexual preference are *not* necessary in every situation. This information *is* pertinent if an illness may affect sexual functioning or sexual activity may have caused the problem. If the physician asks directly about sexual orientation, the reason for the question should be made clear. All questions should be open-ended and nonjudgmental and should not imply that the patient is heterosexual. They should allow the patient to respond without embarrassment or the need to hide information. For example, instead of asking, "What kind of birth control do you use?" one should ask, "Are you using or in need of a birth control method?" The lesbian patient who senses that the physician is nonjudgmental is more likely to volunteer the information about her sexual preference if she feels that it is important.

6. The physician should find indirect ways to let patients know you accept their lifestyle choices. For example, information about lesbian health issues or organizations could be included among the brochures in the waiting area. If the physician is uncertain about whether to ask a patient about her sexual activity, information relevant to both the heterosexual and homosexual situations can be provided. For example, if the patient has genital herpes, she can be told that she is at risk of transmitting the disease to a male partner via coitus or to either a male or a female partner via oral-genital sex. The patient is provided with the information she needs without needing to disclose information and also has received a positive message about the physician's attitudes.

Summary

Lesbians constitute a significant minority in the practice of many gynecologists. No special skills are needed for physicians to care for lesbian patients—he or she need only use the skills needed for the expert care of any patient: knowledge, acceptance, and empathy.

References

1. Good RS. The gynecologist and the lesbian. Clin Obstet Gynecol 1976;19:473.
2. Johnson SR, Guenther SM, Laube DW, Keettel WC. Factors influencing lesbian gynecologic care: a preliminary study. Am J Obstet Gynecol 1981;140:20.
3. Kenyon FE. Homosexuality in gynaecological practice. Clin Obstet Gynaecol 1980; 7:363.
4. Kenyon FE. Physique and physical health of female homosexuals. J Neurol Neurosurg Psych 1968;31:487.
5. Masters WH, Johnson JE. Homosexuality in perspective. Boston: Little, Brown, 1979.
6. Bell A, Weinberg M. Homosexualities: a study of diversity among men and women. New York: Simon and Schuster, 1978.
7. Robertson P, Schachter J. Failure to identify venereal disease in a lesbian population. Sex Transm Dis 1981;8:75.
8. Frank E, Anderson C, Rubinstein D. Frequency of sexual dysfunction in "normal couples." N Engl J Med 1978;229:111.
9. Saghir MT, Robins E. Homosexuality: IV. Psychiatric disorders and disability in the female homosexual. Am J Psychiatr 1970; 127:64.
10. Woods C. Alcohol abuse among lesbians: an investigation of possible contributing

factors. Dissertation, 1981, United States International University, San Diego.
11. Hawkins J. Lesbianism and Alcoholism. In: Greenblatt M, Schuckit M, eds. Alcoholism problems in women and children. New York: Grune and Stratton, 1976;137.
12. Diamond D, Wilsnack S. Alcohol abuse among lesbians: a descriptive study. J Homosex 1978;4(2):123.
13. Weathers B. Alcoholism and the Lesbian Community. June 1976, Gay Council on Drinking Behavior, Whitman-Walker Clinic, Inc., Washington, D.C.
14. Driscoll R. A gay-identified alcohol treatment program: a follow-up study. J Homosex 1982;7(4):71.
15. Sandmaier M. The invisible alcoholics: women and alcohol abuse in America. New York: McGraw Hill Book Co., 1979.
16. Dardick L, Grady KE. Openness between gay persons and health professionals. Ann Intern Med 1980;93(Part 1):115.
17. Owen WF. The clinical approach to the homosexual patient. Ann Intern Med 1980; 93(Part 1):90.

Bioethics ISSN 0269–9702
Volume 1 Number 1 1987

AIDS, GAYS, AND STATE COERCION[1]

RICHARD D. MOHR

For Robert W. Switzer

ALARUMS AND EXCURSIONS

Of those dead and dying from AIDS three-quarters are gay men. Government funding for AIDS research was at best sluggish till the disease appeared to the dominant non-gay culture as a threat. That perceived threat has spawned state-mandated discrimination against groups at risk for AIDS in employment and access to services, allegedly on medical grounds but in pointed contradiction to the judgments of the very medical institutions to which society has entrusted the determination of such grounds (the US Department of Health and Human Services, the Centers for Disease Control, and the National Institutes of Health).[2]

[1] This paper partially overlaps 'AIDS, Gay Life, State Coercion,' *Raritan: A Quarterly Review* VI:1 (Summer 1986) 38–62. It was widely circulated in draft form. I thank the following people for offering comments which prompted revisions or amplifications: the editors and referees of this journal, Jennifer Bremer (Robert Nathan Associates, D.C.), Sandra Panem (The Brookings Institution), Ronald Bayer (The Hastings Center), Doug Mitchell (The University of Chicago Press), Thomas Edwards (Rutgers), James Rachels (University of Alabama), Michael Slote and Fred Suppe (University of Maryland), Joyce Trebilcot (Washington University), Christopher Morris (Bowling Green State University), Timothy Murphy (Boston University), Larry Thomas (Oberlin), Mark Chekola (Moorhead State University), Larry Klein (San Francisco City College), Ferdinand Schoeman (University of South Carolina), Mary Mahowald (Case Western Reserve University), Donald Levy (Brooklyn College-CUNY), David Luban, Bob Fullinwider, Claudia Mills, Judy Lichtenberg, Henry Shue and Doug MacLean of The University of Maryland's Center for Philosophy and Public Policy, where the paper was written while I was the Rockefeller Foundation Fellow in the Humanities for 1985–86, and my husband, the dedicatee.

[2] See particularly the CDC's guidelines for preventing transmission in the workplace, 'Recommendations for Preventing Transmission of Infection with Human T-Lymphotrophic Virus Type III/Lymphadenopathy-Associated Virus

Government's disregard for medical opinion and for the lives of gays strongly suggests that prejudicial forces are at work. There is of course nothing new in this, but the stakes here are high. The armed forces have already established quarantines of those at risk for AIDS on some bases (*The Washington Post*, 19 October 1985, A12; *The Advocate*, #442, 18 March 1986, p. 14). With state-mandated discriminations installed and calls for civilian quarantines circulating, it is clear that the AIDS crisis is going to test the country's mettle. Not since the Supreme Court affirmed the internments of Japanese-Americans in World War II has so live a danger existed to America's traditional commitment to civil liberties. And again the danger is created by hysteria and not a reasoned necessity.

The hysteria, when not simply an expression of old anti-gay prejudices, is based on the presumption that the disease is spread indiscriminately. This presumption permitted Jeane Kirkpatrick to begin a syndicated column by using AIDS as a metaphor for international terrorism—'it can affect anyone'—in the serene belief that her audience, educated America, already thought this about AIDS and might even be ready for extreme measures (*The Washington Post*, 13 October 1985, B8).[3]

ALLEGED HARMS TO OTHERS

For public policy purposes, the most important fact about AIDS is not that it is deadly but that it, like hepatitis B, is caused by a blood-transmitted virus. For the disease to spread, bodily fluids of someone with the virus must *directly enter the bloodstream of another*: 'It appears that, in order to infect, this virus must be virtually injected into the blood stream.'[4] But not just any bodily fluid will do. Only

in the Workplace,' *Morbidity and Mortality Weekly Report* (*MMWR*), 15 November 1985, 34:45, 682–95.

[3] If a *Los Angeles Times* poll of twenty-three hundred Americans is to be believed, the country indeed is ready for extreme measures: 51 per cent favored quarantines of people with AIDS, 48 per cent the closing gay bathhouses, 42 per cent closing gay bars and 14 per cent tattooing people with AIDS. Twenty-eight per cent thought AIDS was God's punishment for homosexuals and 23 per cent thought AIDS victims were 'getting what they deserve' (19 December 1985, I:1). For discussions of civil liberties issues raised by the AIDS crisis, see for example 'AIDS and Individual Rights,' *The New York Times*, 15 December 1985, E6 and 'Quarantines Considered to Combat AIDS,' *The Washington Post*, 16 December 1985 A1, 26–7.

[4] Krim, Mathilde. 1985. 'AIDS: The Challenge to Science and Medicine'. *AIDS: The Emerging Ethical Dilemmas, A Hastings Center Report Special Supplement*, p. 4.

blood and semen have been implicated in the transmission of the virus (*MMWR* 34:45, p. 682).

That the virus is blood transmitted means first and foremost that, in countries with reasonable sanitation, groups at risk for the disease are clearly definable—more so than for virtually any other disease known—with 96 per cent of cases having clearly demarcated modes of transmission and cause.[5] And now that blood supplies are screened with a test for antibodies to the AIDS virus, the number of these groups is indeed dropping. Hemophiliacs not already exposed and blood transfusion recipients are now no longer groups at risk.

Admittedly, in countries without adequate sanitation, blood transmitted viruses like hepatitis B are rampant. If a population prone to cuts and abrasions bathes in the same water in which it bleeds and urinates, it will have blood-transmitted viruses dispersed widely through its membership. Perhaps a quarter of the Third World suffers from hepatitis B, which in the US infects the same groups that are at risk for AIDS. Though hepatitis B has always been around, it has not been a threat to the general US population and has never caused much social or government concern, even though for high risk groups—basically gays and intervenous drug users—it is occasionally fatal. At the very least it causes weeks or months of debilitating pain and exhaustion, and threatens chronic recurrence and a greatly increased risk of liver cancer. Indeed, the very close epidemiological modelling of AIDS to hepatitis B was what first led medical investigators to hypothesize that AIDS was caused by a blood-transmitted virus, long before the virus itself was discovered.[6] Those who take Zaire as their model of AIDS contagion for the U.S. conveniently fail to weigh these facts or even mention them (e.g. Krim, p. 6).[7] Fear of general, indiscriminate

[5] 'Strictly heterosexual adult men and women who cannot be classified as belonging to any high-risk group' constitute but one per cent of AIDS cases and this figure has been constant (Krim, p. 6). See also Norman, Colin. 'AIDS Trends,' *Science* 230, 29 November 1985, 1021.

[6] For a comparison of AIDS virus transmission to that of the hepatitis B virus, see *MMWR*, 34:45, 682–3. The close modelling of the two viruses continues to be the chief basis of the CDC's guidelines for AIDS prevention.

[7] The much reported finding that AIDS occurs in Zaire in equal numbers between men and women weighs no more in favor of the thesis that heterosexual transmission is the chief cause of African AIDS cases than that lack of sanitation is the chief cause.

Alternatively, the widespread practices in central Africa of female circumcision, excision and infibulation and attendent consequences for sexual behavior may account for the high incidence of AIDS in central African women (see 'AIDS in Africa,' *Science* 231, 17 January 1986, 203). If so, again the circumstances of blood-borne contagion in Africa are strongly disanalogous to those in America.

contagion by AIDS is unwarranted—though it makes for terrific press.

The July 1985 cover of *Life* informed the nation in three-inch red letters that 'NOW NO ONE IS SAFE FROM AIDS.' The magazine used as its allegedly compelling example a seemingly typical Pennsylvania family all but one of whose members has the disease. But it turns out that all those members with the disease were indeed in high risk groups. The father was a hemophiliac, his wife had sex with him, and she conveyed the virus to a child in the process of giving birth. No one got the disease either mysteriously or through casual contact. The family example in fact was evidence *against* the article's generic contagion thesis. Equally irresponsible journalists, lobbyists, and elected officials have compared AIDS to air-borne viral diseases like influenza and the common cold.[8]

The case for general contagion cannot be made. In consequence government policy which is based on that fear is unwarranted. The extraordinary measures—including the suspension of civil liberties — which government might justifiably take, as in war, to prevent wholesale slaughter simply do not apply here. In particular, quarantining the class of AIDS-exposed persons in order to protect society from indiscriminate harm is unwarranted.

HARM TO SELF

The disease's mode of contagion assures that those at risk are those whose actions contribute to their risk of infection, chiefly through intimate sexual contact and shared hypodermic needles.[9] In the transmission of AIDS, it is the general feature of self-exposure to contagion that makes direct coercive acts by government—like bathhouse closings—particularly inappropriate as efforts to abate the disease.

If independence—the ability to guide one's life by one's own

[8] For an irresponsible analogy of AIDS to air-borne disease, see Dr. Richard Restak's widely reprinted op-ed piece 'Worry about Survival of Society First; Then AIDS Victims' Rights,' *The Washington Post*, 8 September 1986, C1. For claims of casual transmission, see Johnson, Tom. 1986. 'Congressman AIDS'. *Los Angeles*. 125 ff. especially 199. For a history of irresponsible and hysteria-pandering reportage in the mass media, see Check, William. 'Public Education on AIDS: Not Only The Media's Responsibility'. *Special Supplement* (see n. 4 above), pp. 27–31. For a readable social history of the disease, see Altman, Dennis. 1986. *AIDS in the Mind of America*, Doubleday, New York.

[9] A small exception is those whose well-being and life chances are already substantially at the mercy of the person who infects them—newborns of infected mothers. For this set of cases social policy should be what ever it already is for cases of parents who pass fatal congenital disease to their children.

lights to an extent compatible with a like ability on the part of others—is, as it is, a major value, one cannot respect that value while preventing people from putting themselves at risk through voluntary associations. Voluntary associations are star cases of people acting in accordance with the principle of independence, for mutual consent guarantees that the 'compatible extent' proviso of the principle is fulfilled. But the state and even the courts have not been very sensitive to the distinction between one harming oneself and one harming another— nor has the medical establishment.[10] It appears to all of them that a harm is a harm, a disease a disease, however caused or described. The moral difference, however, is enormous. Preventing a person from harming another is required by the principle of independence, but preventing someone from harming himself is incompatible with it. While no further justification is needed for the state to protect a person from others, a rather powerful justification is needed if the state is to be warranted in protecting a person from himself.

In the absence of such a justification, the state sometimes tries to split the moral difference and argues that state coercion *may* be used when the harm to others is remote and indirect. Such an argument from indirect harms runs to the effect that state-coerced use of, say, seatbelts and motorcycle helmets is warranted, for helmetless motorcycle crashes and seatbeltless car accidents harm even those not involved in the accidents, by raising everyone's insurance costs and burdening the public purse when victims end up in county hospitals. Here state coercion comes in through the backdoor.

This line of argument has been used with increasing frequency even by self-described liberals like New York's Governor Cuomo, and it is beginning to be heard in AIDS discussions. This is not surprising, for the cost of AIDS patient care from diagnosis to death is somewhere between $35,000 and $150,000. Private funds are often quickly exhausted, and the patient ends up on the dole—harming everyone, and so allegedly warranting state coercion of the means of possible AIDS transmission.

J. S. Mill's rule-of-thumb for appraising such appeals to indirect harms is exactly on target: an indirect harm counts toward justifying state coercion only when the harm grows large enough to be considered a violation of another person's right. This understanding of harm to others is necessary so that independence is not

[10] For instance, Mervyn F. Silverman, former Director of Health for San Francisco, shows no cognizance of the distinction in his argument for his unsuccessful 1984 attempt to close that city's bathhouses: Silverman, Mervyn F. and Silverman, Deborah B. 'AIDS and the Threat to Public Health' *Special Supplement* (see n. 4 above), pp. 21–2.

rendered nugatory and, *as a right*, is only outweighed by something comparable to it. Now, while it is nice if products (like insurance) are cheap and taxes low, the considered opinion of our society is not that one's rights have been violated when taxes or the price of milk goes up. Indeed, in the case of taxes, the considered opinion is cast as a Constitutional provision. So arguments that smuggle coercion in through the backdoor of indirect harms are not successful.[11,12]

In general, heed should be given to Douglas's warning in his dissent to *Wyman* that the welfare state is gradually being allowed to buy up rights. In *Wyman* the Court ruled, among other horribles, that an indigent woman in accepting welfare for her child had simply waived her Fourth Amendment rights.[13] Actions infringing upon rights are most likely to go unnoticed or be misperceived, and so be most insidious when they are performed for an end that is good. Many addressing the AIDS crisis seem to be operating with bad motives. They generally can be easily spotted; appeals to consistency are usually enough to trip them up. But those with good motives yet anxious to do something quickly are those most likely to effect policies which destroy rights. The problem identified

[11] Whether it is legitimate for the state to condition, for instance, motorcyclists' access to county hospitals upon the wearing of helmets, cannot be determined independently of an assessment of the arguments for such free health care in the first place. The arguments advanced in 'AIDS, Gay Life, State Coercion' (see n. 1 above, pp. 50–8) for AIDS patient funding bar any such conditioning of relief upon cost-reducing conformity.

[12] A wife who contracts AIDS from a bi-sexual husband does not have a right that has been violated by the bathhouse where he may have been AIDS-exposed. Rather if she has a legitimate plaint, it is against the direct harm caused by the husband or against the institution of marriage itself if it has kept her in a position of enforced ignorance. But, it should be remembered that traditional marriage vows pledge the participants to joint risk taking and place commercial and medical risks on a par. The institution of marriage itself, then, acknowledges what is independently true: it is as little a good reason to shut down bathhouses to protect 'innocent' wives as it is to shut down stock-markets to spare them lost spousal income.

Further, it is wholly unfair to coerce one institution, because of the patent immoralities of another. The immoralities which occur within marriage (lying, cheating, promise-breaking, willful ignorance) or which are endemic to it (enforced ignorance, indenture) cannot ground the coercion of gay bathhouses. For an excellent discussion of the procedural and substantive abuses inherent in traditional marriage contracts, see Ketchum, Sara Ann. 1977. 'Liberalism and Marriage Law' in Mary Vetterling-Braggin (ed.), *Feminism and Philosophy*. Littlefield, Adams, Totowa, NJ, pp. 247–76.

[13] *Wyman* v. *James*, 400 US 309, 328 (1971) J. Douglas, dissenting: 'The central question is whether the government by force of its largesse has the power to "buy up" rights guaranteed by the Constitution. But for the assertion of her constitutional right, Barbara James in this case would have received the welfare benefit.'

by Justice Douglas is part of a wider problem detected in Justice Brandeis' vindicated dissent in *Olmstead*: 'Experience should teach us to be most on our guard to protect liberty when the Government's purposes are beneficent. Men born to freedom are naturally alert to repel invasion of their liberty by evil-minded rulers. The greatest dangers to liberty lurk in insidious encroachment by men of zeal, well-meaning but without understanding' (*Olmstead* v *US*, 277 US 438, 479).

STATE PATERNALISM CONSIDERED

The important question remains whether AIDS warrants paternalistic state coercion to prevent those not-exposed from harming themselves, through banning or highly regulating the means of possible viral transmission. Usually paternalistic arguments cannot be made sensible and consistent. For example: federal AIDS funding for FY 1986 in the House came with a paternalistic rider giving the surgeon general a power he already has—to close bathhouses, gay social institutions, if they are determined to facilitate the transmission or spread of the disease, which indeed they do. (So do parks and bedrooms.)[14] The sponsor of the rider

[14] A directive from New York's Governor Cuomo mandated in late 1985 the closing of public accommodations where oral or anal sex occur. But the distinction between a public accommodation and a private dwelling, given the nature of the disease, is medically irrelevant. So is the distinction between providing for profit a location for sex and providing one for free. Public accommodations, private clubs, parks and bedrooms—even marital ones—are medically all equally suspect. The line of thought that has led to bathhouse closings, if carried out consistently, would require shutting down relator's offices that make a profit from selling homes to gays.

Further, the directive curiously enough omits banning vaginal sex. Though there is some reason to believe that anal sex is extremely risky, there is no evidence that vaginal penetrations are any less likely a mode of transmitting the virus than oral sex. Cuomo's directive disingenuously recriminalizes sodomy in New York (*The Washington Post*, 31 October 1985, A1). New York City's corporation counsel has argued that restrictions on oral and anal sex do not discriminate against gays because they also apply to non-gays (*The New York Times*, 15 December 1985, IV 6). One could as well argue that a law against sleeping under bridges does not discriminate against the poor because it also bars the wealthy from sleeping there.

In applying the directive both the Governor and New York City's Mayor Koch claimed that their acts were not to be construed in any way as assaulting the gay community. But instead of showing good faith in this regard by doing something that would be politically unpopular (like first shutting down, say, a marriage with an AIDS-exposed hemophiliac member), they chose instead to shut down as their very first target a central part of gay male mythology—the notorious private membership sex club—The Mineshaft (*The Washington Post*, 8 November 1985, A7).

Subsequently, New York state's health commissioner reported that 'his

argued that it was 'a small step to help those who are unable or unwilling to help themselves' (*The Washington Blade*, 4 October 1985, p. 1). Cast *so* baldly, the argument simply denies independence as a value. For it is consistent with the presumption that the majority gets to determine both what the good life is and to enforce it coercively. The argument could as well be used to justify compulsory religious conversion—those who are unable or unwilling to see the light are helped to see it.

REASON ASSURED

Occasionally, to be sure, the case for paternalism can be made to work. One legitimate way to justify paternalistic coercion is to claim as warrant a lack of rationality on the part of an agent (say, a child). By 'rationality' here I mean having relevant information and certain mental capacities, including the ability to reason from ends to means, but I do not presume that making the best possible assessment of means to an end is a requirement for rationality—error is compatible with rationality.

A presumption of an agent's rationality is a necessary condition for the very respect which is owed to his making his own decisions and guiding his life by them. Thus, paternalistic interference is warranted when a person is operating at risks which he is unable to assess due to diminished mental skills or lack of information. But education, not coercion, is the solution which is tailored to, and so appropriate for, such incapacities. Coercion in such cases is warranted only temporarily, to permit a check of whether a person indeed knows the risks he is taking. Thus (to borrow an example from Mill) it is justified to forcibly detain someone about to cross a structurally-compromised bridge just long enough to inform him of its condition. Dilated to an extreme, this line of argument permits paternalistic labelling of possibly dangerous products and other means of placing a decision-maker in a reasonable position to make decisions for himself.

But far from justifying major paternalistic coercion of gay institutions, say, closing gay baths, the argument from rationality here indeed suggests that paternalistic arguments surrounding AIDS are not even being advanced in good faith. For though

investigators will enter hotel rooms if necessary to stop sexual activities linked to the spread of AIDS' (*The Washington Post*, 18 November 1985, A4). His office has assured gays that the free enterprise system will preclude discrimination against gays in hotel accommodations (*The Washington Blade*, 22 November 1985, p. 12). New York, like forty eight other states, has no legislation that would bar such discrimination against gays.

education is one of government's highest spending priorities, governments have made no serious attempt to educate people about medically-informed risk of AIDS and of safe alternatives to high-risk sexual practices. It took the federal government five years even to put out bids for studies of ways in which programs of AIDS education might be effected (see *Federal Register* 50:143, 25 July 1985, p. 30298). The government then stalled in releasing the funds and finally barred their use for sexual messages that would be explicit enough to be effective. James Mason, the director of the CDC, which administered the grants, claimed 'We don't think that citizens care to be funding material that encourages gay sex lifestyles' (*The Advocate*, #437, 7 January 1986, p. 20).

Local governments in many cases have positively hampered private attempts at such education. In Los Angeles and Philadelphia, for instance, government sponsorship of private-sector distribution of safe-sex literature was denied or withdrawn when some officials branded the literature as pornography—neo-feminists take note. Thus one is probably justified in seeing as disingenuous any governmental argument for the coercion of gay institutions on paternalistic grounds. At most the argument from rationality warrants placing warning labels on baths as they are placed on cigarettes, the use of which also threatens death.[15]

SELF-INDENTURED GAYS?

The other legitimate argument for paternalistic coercion is that one should be protected from ceding away the very conditions that enable one to be an independent agent. Thus one cannot legitimately contract to become a slave or to sign away rights to the fair administration of the enforcement of contracts or more generally the equitable administration of justice.

When dilated to the extreme, this line of justifying paternalistic coercion is used to support legislation mandating seat-belt use: it's good for you, since it preserves you as an independent agent (though usually politicians cast the argument in terms of indirect harm to others). How does putting oneself at risk for AIDS weigh

[15] Whether warning labels *should* be placed on bathhouses turns on considerations of consistency: some dangerous products are labelled, others not. What gets labelled should not depend on ideology, prejudice or politics. Getting right on this point is particularly important in the case of bathhouses since such labelling, even when carried out in good faith, will have the side-effect of saying to most people that gay sex is bad. The relevant question, one for which I do not have an answer, is whether bathhouses present the same degree of risk to the user as other products that are already so labelled.

into this conceptual scheme? Does AIDS, invariably fatal in full-blown cases, rise to a level of seriousness to warrant on these paternalistic grounds a state-imposed bar to putting oneself at risk for it?

Admittedly, minimally good health is a central personal concern and its possession a necessary condition for being viewed seriously as an independent agent. So at first blush the AIDS case may seem relevantly similar to the contracting-to-slavery case. It differs, however, in two significant, severally decisive ways.

First, slavery *by definition* is a condition of lost independence. However, as with other venereal diseases, not every sexual encounter with a virus-exposed person exposes one to the AIDS virus, and even exposure to it is nowhere near a guarantee of actually contracting AIDS, since only some portion of those exposed actually get the disease (Krim, pp. 4, 5). Because the risk is high but the results not invariably catastrophic, putting oneself at risk for AIDS becomes less like contracting into slavery and more like being a race car driver, mountain climber or astronaut. In the absence of inevitability, the assessment of risk should be left to the individual, and indeed, as the examples of space flight, mountaineering and race car driving show, this is the considered standard of society as well. Deviations from the standard in other similar cases are likely to be motivated by something other than honest paternalistic concerns.

Second, it is hard to imagine even dispassionately and impartially that the momentary gain—say, some psychological thrill—from submitting to slavery could be reasonably balanced against the value *to the individual* of independence permanently lost. This differs significantly from 'slavery' in sex play where the thrill to the 'slave' lies in continuous voluntary submission. To imagine the pure case, however, is as hard as trying to imagine (Mishima aside) someone seeing suicide as the culmination and chief organizing principle of his life rather than as an exit from a life that has become incapable of significance.

SEX AND LIFE

However an impartial examination of the role of sex in an individual's life would show that, far from having any imaginable value or at most a trifling one, sex, like health, is in general a central personal concern, and that for those people with a sex drive, addressing sex as central and appropriating it to oneself in some way or another is probably necessary to meaningful life. Or at least the lives of those like priests and nuns who renounce it altogether would support a belief that one's sexual choices are as central as any aspect of one's life. For vows of chastity are as central to their religious life—their most meaningful life—as any vows they take.

The centrality of sex as a value is indicated by the very vocabulary, or *lack* of it that surrounds sex. Sex used to seem so central and yet seemingly frightening that for centuries, as Murray S. Davis has noted, only theologians and pornographers could discuss it.[16] Only the power of considerable and complex institutions was strong enough to preserve this gap in discourse and thought, a power so pervasive as to appear invisible. Thus when one looks at a newspaper's cavalcade of engagement and wedding photos, it never even crosses one's mind to think 'gosh, what a slew of heterosexuals.' When discourse about sex simply could not be avoided, the institutions were strong enough to fill the void with euphemisms so automatic and arcane as not to suggest a present presence—the language of 'to have and to hold' and 'blessed events'. Even so, some 'things' were so powerful and frightening that they had to remain unnamed and unmentionable, to be dealt with not by appeal to and through institutional arrangements but only by extraordinary direct appeal to some allegedly preinstitutional fundament.

When now sex is discussed forthrightly, the terms are not merely those of desire but also those of need, and correctly so for two reasons. First, though sexual activity is not necessary to the continued biological existence of the individual as are some things that are called natural needs, it is a desire (unlike addictions) that is recurrent independently of its satisfaction—a natural object, not a product. Second, (like addictions and desires for the prerequisites of continued biological existence) its frustration tends to sponsor aggression. The pleasures of sex are not mere forgoable pleasures like the quest for sugar. To forgo them would itself have to be a major life commitment.

The centrality of sex to life means that it may have to be balanced with the value of continued independence—all the more so if independence is chiefly, like health, a generalized means to individuals' ends rather than an end in itself. Independence is not the only value of life, nor one prior to all other values. Further, central values are not equally central for all—some people indeed do not find sex very important and yet do not seem repressed. These people seem to be missing something, not to be morally lesser beings but somehow, like Gertrude Stein's Oakland, to have

[16] Davis, Murray S. 1983. *Smut: Erotic Reality/Obscene Ideology*, Chicago, University of Chicago Press, p. *xx*. Davis' book offers an excellent phenomenology of sex acts and an intriguing account of the conservative mind on matters sexual.

less there there. It would be silly for them to take high sexual risks, for the balance for them is so clearly tilted in one direction, and little would be lost if the state nudged them that way. But this tilt will in general not be so clear. The balancing in cases of conflicting personally-affecting values is not a decision that the state could reasonably make across the board for all. The state is not capable of the probings of the soul that would be necessary for such a decision. Individuals, not the state, must make the difficult choices where values centrally affecting the self come in conflict.

That such choice falls to the individual is generally recognized where religious commitment and health come in conflict. The state cannot legitimately make the trade-offs that an informed adult will make between religious values and health by, say, coercing a person—for the sake of preserving his own independence—to have a blood transfusion against his belief that a transfusion, even a coerced one, will damn him for all eternity. Sexual attitudes and acts in accord with them are at least as central to a person as religious beliefs and acts, and so they too are not fit subjects of state coercion for the individual's own good, even when that good is the continued ability to make choices.

Governments that have written off the value of gay sex altogether by having made it illegal, largely on religious or other grounds that do not appeal to the causing of harms to others, should be viewed as especially suspect when they make paternalistic arguments on behalf of gays. For they have already clearly shown that they do not respect gays as independent beings.

PUBLIC HEALTH AND TOTALITARIANISM

Arguments offered so far by the medical community against quarantines and bathhouse closings have largely adopted the terms of mere practicality, appealing to such facts as the large number of people involved, the permanence of the virus in those exposed, and the possibility that the sexual arena may simply shift away from bathhouses where some educational efforts may be possible.[17] I have suggested to the contrary that quarantines and closings should be opposed, not because they are impractical (though they may be), but because they are immoral.

Doctors tend to hold their unrefined view that health policy is merely a matter of strategy because they, not surprisingly, tend to see health itself as a trumping good, second to none in importance.

[17] For examples, see Mayer, Kenneth H. 'The Epidemiological Investigation of AIDS'. *Special Supplement* (see n. 4 above), p. 15 (against both quarantines and bath closings) and Silverman and Silverman, p. 21(against quarantines).

This is a dangerous view, especially when coupled with their idea that health is an undifferentiated good. They fail to distinguish between my harming my health and my harming your health. Behind this oversight lies the further (sometimes unarticulated) presumption that you and I both are absorbed into and subordinated under something called the public health—a concept that tends to be analyzed in inverse proportion to the frequency with which it is used when trying to justify coercive acts.[18]

No literal sense exists in which there could be such thing as a public health. To say the public has a health is like saying the number seven has a color: such a thing cannot have such a property. You have health or you lack it and I have health or lack it, because we each have a body with organs that function or do not function. But the public, an aggregate of persons similarly disposed as persons, has no such body of organs with functions which work or fail. There are, however, two frequently used metaphoric senses of public health that do have a reference: one, is a legitimate use but largely inapplicable to the AIDS crisis; the other, when used normatively, is the pathway to totalitarianism.

The legitimate sense places public health in the same conceptual scheme as national defense and water purification. These are types of public goods in a technical sense—not what most people want and thus what democratic governments give them nor what tend to maximize by state means some type of good (pleasure, happiness, beauty), but what everyone wants but cannot get or get efficiently through voluntary arrangements and which thus require coercive coordinations from the state, so that *each* person gets what he wants. Thus, the private or voluntary arrangements of the market system do not seem likely to provide adequate national security, because a defense system that protects those who pay for it will also protect those who do not; everyone (reasonably enough) will tend to wait for someone else to pay for it, so that national security ends up not being purchased at all, or at least far less of it is purchased than everyone would agree to pay for if there were some means to manifest that agreement. The coercive actions of the state through taxation are then required to achieve the public good of national defense.

[18] For a signal example, see 'Additional Recommendations to Reduce Sexual and Drug Abuse-Related Transmission of HTLV-III/LAV,' *MMWR*, 14 March 1986, 35:10, 154, recommending the closing of bathhouses 'on public health grounds'. No definition, elaboration or analysis is offered of the notion 'public health'. The recommendation stands in marked contrast to the CDC's employment recommendations (see n. 2 above), for which elaborate analysis and argumentation are offered.

For exactly the same reason, the state is warranted in using coercive measures to drain swamps and provide vaccines against air-borne viruses. But the state is not warranted by appeal to the public good in coercing people to take the vaccine once it is freely available, for then *each* person is capable on his own—without further state coercion—of getting the protection from the disease he wants.[19] The mode of AIDS contagion makes it relevantly like this latter case. Each person on his own—without state coercion—can get the protection from the disease that he wants through his own actions, and indeed can get it by doing himself what he might be tempted to try to get the state to force upon others, say, avoiding bathhouses. As far as the good of protection is concerned, it can be achieved with no state coercion.

Is there a public good involved simply in reducing the size of the pool of AIDS-exposed people? I see just one, the one I argued for—the ability to have a robust sex life, without fear of death. But this good does not permit every form of state coercion. Not every public good motivates every form of coercion. The public goods mentioned so far could all be achieved by *equitable* coercion (e.g., universal conscription, taxation, compensated taking of property). When equitable coercion is the means, the public good can be quite slight and still be justified (as in government support for the arts). But when the coercion is inequitably dispersed, the public good served must be considerably more compelling than the means are intrusive. Thus, dispersed coercion against select individuals that involves restricted motion and physical suffering is warranted only by unqualifiedly necessary ends: when the individuals coerced have harmed others (as in punishment) or when it is necessary to the very existence of the country (as a partial military draft may be for a nation at defensive war). And thus too, the substantial good of civil rights protections is advanced only through the considerably weak intrusion of barring the desire of employers to indulge in whimsical and arbitrary hiring practices. The public good of an unencumbered sex life however fails this weighted ends-to-means test if the means are a dispersedly coerced sex life. For the intrusion and the good are on a par—on the one

[19] The Supreme Court's leading medical case, *Jacobson* v. *Massachusetts*, 197 US 11 (1905) (upholding criminal penalties—a five dollar fine—for refusing a free vaccination), because it leaves the notion public health wholly unanalyzed, contradicts its own declaration that the principle of independence is overridden only by public goods on a par with national defense. The upheld law's resort to criminal penalties for a person refusing the vaccine rather than to coercing directly the taking of the vaccine shows that the law is incoherent as a measure aimed to protect against indiscriminate harms.

hand encumbered sex, on the other unencumbered sex. And so it appears that only equitably coercive means are available to achieve the end of reducing the pool of AIDS-exposures—taxation for preventive measures like vaccine development, but not coercive measures that effect some but not others, like closing bathhouses or banning or regulating sex practices selectively.

Those who do not find the possibility of carefree sex a public good—probably the bulk of those actually calling for state coercion—will find no legitimate help in the notion of public health for state coercion here. Those who do will find it justifies only equitable measures.

The other metaphoric sense of public health takes the medical model of the healthy body and unwittingly transfers it to society—the body politic. But this transfer (when it has any content at all) bears hidden and extremely dangerous assumptions. Plato in the *Republic* was the first thinker systematically to press the analogy of the good society to the healthy body. The state stands to the citizenry and its good, as a doctor stands to the body and its health. Society, so it is claimed, is an organism in which people are mere functional parts, ones that are morally good and emotionally well-off only insofar as they act for the sake of the organism. The analogy is alive and well today and calling out for extreme measures now: 'Much as a physician treating one organ must consider the effects on the entire organism, a public official has the community as the patient and must attend to all factors in seeking the greatest overall good' (Silverman and Silverman, p. 22). On this view, the individual however harmed cannot fulfill his role. A damaged organ, the spleen for example, can be, to continue the analogy, simply cut out. By comparison, quarantines and coerced sex lives might appear as mild remedies on this analogy. But something has been lost here—persons.

The medical model of society is the conceptual engine of totalitarianism. It presumes not that the goods of individuals are final goods but that individuals are good only as they serve some good beyond themselves, that of the state or body politic. The state exists not for the sake of individuals—to protect and enhance their prospects as rational agents—but rather individuals exist for the state and are subordinated to society as a whole, the worth of which is to be determined only from the perspective of the whole. The individual, thus, is not an end in himself but exists for some social good—whether that good be some hoped-for overall happiness or some social ideal—like, purity, wholesomeness, decency, or 'traditional values'. Unconscious obedient servicing is dressed up as virtue.

The worst political consequence of the AIDS crisis would not be simply the further degradation of gays. Gay internments would not be anything new to this century. In the European internment camps of World War II, gypsies wore brown triangle identifying badges, Jehovah's Witnesses purple, political prisoners red, race defilers black, and gays pink triangles. Worse than the further degradation of gays in America would be a general, and not easily reversed, shift in the nation's center of gravity toward the medical model and away from the position, acknowledged in America's Constitutional tradition, that individuals have broad yet determinate claims against both general welfare and social ideals. The consequence of such a shift would be that people would come to be treated essentially as resources, sometimes expendable—a determination no less frightening when made by a combined father, colonel, and doctor than by a fearful mob.

The Department of Philosophy
University of Illinois, Urbana.

Gender-Transposition Theory and Homosexual Genesis

John Money, PhD

The genesis of homosexuality, and therefore of heterosexuality also, has traditionally been argued as either wholly biological or wholly social-environmental. The theory of gender transposition integrates findings regarding both prenatal hormonal programming of the sexual brain, and postnatal social programming.

Definition

Gender transposition is a generic term that characterizes divers degrees of male/female crossover, especially in erotic and sexual practice and/or imagery of the type conventionally classified as either masculine or feminine according to the criterion of procreation in two-sexed species. It includes the simple and sometimes time-limited phenomenon of having a partner of the same genital morphology as the self, with or without being pairbonded. It includes also the more extensive transpositions exemplified in the syndromes of transexualism and transvestism.

Role Inconstancy

In attributing cognitive order and system to their existence in a social environment of selectively withheld sexual learning, some children are more, and some less, versatile than others at dramatic play-acting and theatrical make-believe in gender-inconsistant roles and strategies.[1] Those who are more versatile constitute a population at risk for gender inconstancy and possible gender transposition, if they are born of parents whose reciprocal compatibilities and incompatibilities, in their careers as mother and father, and in their sex lives as husband and

---

John Money, PhD, is at the Department of Psychiatry and Behavioral Sciences and Department of Pediatrics, The Johns Hopkins University and Hospital, Baltimore, MD 21205. Supported by USPHS Grant #HD 00325 and Grant #83086900, The William T. Grant, Jr., Foundation.

Journal of Sex & Marital Therapy, Vol. 10, No. 2, 1984, ©Brunner/Mazel, Inc.

wife, remain perpetually unreconcilable. In this formulation, the key concept is that of versatility. If one defines gender transposition as pathology, then the concept is not versatility, but vulnerability to gender inconstancy and transposition.

The development of gender inconstancy and transposition can be observed, and has been documented in children as young as three to four years of age. It is either more exaggerated and frequent in boys than in girls, or else it generates more alarm in those adults who take action toward changing it. In our society today, sissy boys are severely stigmatized. Tomboyish girls are not.

In boys, gender transposition expresses itself in playing with girls' toys and associating with girls instead of boys, in wearing clothing and accessories of feminine style as often as possible, and in expressly wanting to be a girl. In the early stages of gender transposition, a child is able to walk, talk, and gesture like either a boy or a girl.

Less is known about gender transposition in girls than boys, in part because clinical referrals are far less common. In general, gender transposition is less conspicuously expressed in girls than boys. It is more a matter of repudiating the historical stereotype of the idealized little girl than of impersonating a macho boy, though there are exceptions. In extreme cases, the girl with a gender transposition has a macho alliance with the father, and with the mother a contemptuous, dominating, and abusive relationship.

Father-Son Allegiance

Contrary to established beliefs, the fathers of sissy boys are typically blandly indifferent to the signs of their son's nonconformity to the standard of masculinity in boyhood development. They write it off as something the boy will grow out of.

For years, I did not know what to make of this indifference. I had no hypothesis until a few years ago when a psychiatrist consulted me about his own son, aged five, the younger of two children, both boys. He and his wife excluded the boy from a family appointment, ostensibly to spare him from stigmatizing himself as abnormal. They distanced themselves from one another, spatially and verbally. Their matrimonial relationship was that of wedded adversaries practicing insidiously clever strategies of mutual sabotage. For example, even though he was a professed agnostic, the husband criticized his wife for being religiously too laissez faire. She reacted by becoming a conservative fundamentalist. Family religious observances became a source of unending dispute.

The rift thus created was additionally widened in disputation regarding acoustic sensitivity. For her, loud music was noxious, so he was obliged to pursue his interest in live rock performances without her. In fantasy, he anticipated that his younger son would become his companion in music. The older son, by contrast, already at age eight coerced his reluctant father to share his all-boy interest in fishing and the outdoors.

Professionally trained to be self-analytic, this father was also self-revealing. After soliciting my prognosis of his son's cross-dressing and girlish inclinations, and hearing that it was not necessary to be pessimistic at age five, he asked why he was feeling so angry with me—and angry because of what I had said. My reply was to the effect that perhaps he didn't wholly want his son to stop cross-dressing, and did not want to be robbed of the one member of the family whom he might consider his special escort.

Subsequently I dictated a note "to put on record a new hypothesis or formula regarding the role of the father in the genesis of feminism in a son's G-I/R (gender-identity/role). This is the formula: the father covertly courts his son's allegiance, in place of what he finds missing in his wife, and casts him in the role of a wife substitute, if not for the present, then for the future." The son, for his part, may solicit his father's allegiance as a formula for keeping him in the household, and for preventing a parental separation. If the father has already gone, or even if he had died, the son's gender transposition may serve to solicit his miraculous return.

Within a family, the allocation or reallocation of roles is not necessarily covert. It is more or less inherent in the idea of naming or nicknaming a baby after an ancestor, parent or other relative, also in the wisdom of the kin regarding whom a particular child takes after. Parents have favorite children—mommy's boy, daddy's girl—just as children may favor one parent over the other, or one relative over another.

The young son who becomes self-allocated to the role of daughter, and thereby becomes a bonding agent who keeps the family intact, is likely to keep the role of bonding agent in perpetuity. The evidence of one longitudinal, outcome study[2,3] is that such a son reaches adulthood with not a transexual or transvestite gender status, but a nonparaphilic homosexual one.

Parental Compatibility/Incompatibility

There is now new preliminary evidence, unpublished, that the transpositional course of events may be changed if the child can be relieved of the self-imposed responsibility of keeping his parents together. In one case, that of a three year old, the gravity of the boy's responsibility for keeping the parents together could be measured against the intensity of the father's response when confronted with the possibility of losing a custody battle, in the event of divorce. That was absolutely out of the question, he said, so far as he was concerned, and he hinted darkly at homicide rather than permit it to happen.

The son's change away from girl-imitative behavior ensued with unexpected rapidity in the immediate aftermath of the family's first visit—a marathon five hours of individual evaluations and joint discussions. The change in the boy was concomitant with a change in the parents, as they achieved more focus on their compatibility, and less on their incompatibility.

They were strongly compatible in their professional and domestic lives, and equally incompatible in their sexual and erotic lives. In four years of follow-up, their sexual and erotic incompatibility has remained stubbornly intractable to change. Nonetheless, there was only one brief occasion when it threatened to bring an end to their compatibilities. It was then that a resurgence of effeminacy threatened in the boy. It was transient. It did not, as had been the case in the original diagnostic toy-play sessions, generate dramas of desperation in which members of a toy family became victims of catastrophe, abusive violence and murder.

This boy's play enactments did not include any dramas of explicit erotic or sexual content. Nor was there a history of overtly initiated erotic or sexual conduct other than age-typical masturbation in private, which the parents did not condemn. If the boy experienced erotosexual imagery in dreams and fantasies, their content remained private and undisclosed. Explicit erotosexual fantasies with the father as partner have been retrospectively dated to boyhood by some young adult homosexual men, however.[4]

In a young child's development, gender transposition is a rudimentary and inchoate response to diffusely mixed covert and overt signals that seem to indicate that, by being a girl with a penis, or a boy with a vulva, a child will somehow be more satisfactory to each parent. Thus, the two parents can be retained in or restored to an intact family unit and their continued allegiance to one another mutually ensured. This formulation sounds outrageous and absurd only if it is elevated to the status of being sufficient, instead of only a necessary condition in the genesis of developmental gender transposition.

PRENATAL HORMONALIZATION

Adam/Eve Principle

In gender transposition, the phylogenetic basis of the transposition and its attachment to sex and eroticism is epitomized in the Adam/Eve principle, namely, nature's rudimentary principle of sexual differentiation, which is to differentiate a female and to have to add something to differentiate a male. In gender transposition, the successive phases of differentiation, beginning prenatally and continuing postnatally, do not proceed concordantly in the usual orderly fashion. Discordance may begin prenatally under hormonal influence so that, at birth, a baby is at risk postnatally for a transposed gender status, provided convergent social influences and experiences increase the risk.

Historically, gender transposition of the complete type was explained as hereditary. However, the hereditary attribution has proved too simple and is now anachronistic. The contemporary explanation is hormonal. Like its hereditary predecessor, the hormonal explanation applies to development that takes place before birth. This development is governed not by the genetic code directly, but by sex hormones that program the sexual differentiation of the brain.[5]

According to the Adam/Eve principle, simply stated, if the fetal brain is not hormonalized, it will develop from its early, sexually bipotential stage to be, like Eve, feminine. To be like Adam, it must be hormonalized. The hormone is testosterone or one of its derivative metabolites.

Masculinization/Defeminization

Brain hormonalization is not inevitably an all-or-none affair. It may be a matter of degree. It is possible to be masculinized without being also completely defeminized or, conversely, to be feminized without also remaining completely demasculinized.[6-10] Thus, it is possible for a boy to be born with a brain that is both masculinized and feminized (that is, not defeminized) to some degree—and correspondingly for a girl. At birth, and immediately after (see below), the masculine/defeminine ratio in boys, and the feminine/demasculine ratio in girls is potentially widely variable.

The source of variability could be spontaneous. It might be secondary to stress that changes the pregnant mother's own hormone levels, which then affect the fetus. It might also be induced within the intrauterine environment or through the placenta by substances breathed, swallowed or otherwise absorbed by the mother. For example, it is known that barbiturates may have a demasculinizing effect on a fetus; and that in the last half century literally millions of pregnant women have taken sleeping pills and other medications containing barbiturates.[11]

In most instances of gender transposition, regardless of degree, it is impossible to reconstruct the prenatal sex-hormonal history in retrospect. Ethically, it is not possible to conduct experiments on pregnant women in order to find out everything that needs to be known about the causes and the timing of prenatal masculinization and defeminization of the sexual brain in boys, and of its prenatal feminization and demasculinization in girls. Therefore, it is necessary to garner whatever evidence one can from spontaneously occurring clinical syndromes or so-called experiments of nature.

Clinical Syndromes

The relevant syndromes are those in which the prenatal sex-hormonal history is known to have been atypical because the baby is born with a sex-hormonally generated hermaphroditic (or intersexual) ambiguity of the reproductive organs. There are also syndromes in which the postnatal hormonal history is atypical, for example in adolescent gynecomastia, but in which the prenatal hormonal history has not yet been spelled out, though it too may be presumed to have been atypical.

In order to make an inference regarding the prenatal influence of sex hormones on the sexual differentiation of the brain, it is necessary to follow a patient clinically into teenage and young adulthood when masculine and feminine sexuoerotic behavior and imagery may be expected to be fully expressed.[12-16]

The evidence from clinical studies supports the hypothesis that there is in human prenatal development a sex-hormonal effect on sexual brain differentiation, but that it does not have a hormonal-robot effect of the type described for sheep and other subprimate mammals. Rather, the effect is one of laying down a threshold so that behavior that is generally defined as masculine or feminine, respectively, is expressed either rapidly or unhindered, or only after surmounting a barrier. The only irreducible sex difference is that men impregnate, and women menstruate, gestate and lactate. Other behavior that is commonly regarded as sex different, including aggression, is actually sex shared. It is the threshold for its elicitation and expression that distinguishes most men from most women.

POSTNATAL GENDER DIFFERENTIATION

Identification/Complementation

Whereas sex hormones are responsible, prenatally, for programming individual variation in the sex-divergent thresholds of sex-shared behavior, postnatally the sex-hormonal influence goes into a period of dormancy. In girls, sex-hormonal dormancy begins at birth. In boys, by contrast, there is a great surge of testosterone beginning at about two weeks of age. It becomes spent by age three months and remains so until the onset of puberty.[17] The effect of this testosterone surge remains to be ascertained. It could be the grand finale of sexual brain differentiation, according to David Abramovich in Aberdeen (personal communication).

When the sex hormones flow again at puberty, they activate male/female erotosexual programs or schemas already differentiated in the brain. Contrary to popular assumption, they do not cause behavior to be masculine instead of feminine, or vice versa.[18-20] That is why, among other things, it is not possible to change heterosexuality into homosexuality, or the other way round, by giving injections of sex hormones.

During the period between birth and puberty, when male/female erotosexual programming of the brain is no longer affected by sex hormones, the special senses take over. The eyes, the ears and the skin senses, more than the senses of smell and taste, are the brain's gateways to information about the gender status and erotosexual programming of the people among whom the child grows up. Gender related information, like information about native language, is assimilated through usage and experience, and not simply as a product of training and indoctrination.

Listening and being heard together are imperative for the brain to be successful in allowing a native language to take up residence within it. Likewise, copying and practicing gender-divergent behavior together are imperative to the establishment of one's gender status within the brain. Gender copying is conventionally referred to as identification with persons assigned the same gender status as oneself. The converse, gender practicing, only recently has been referred to as complementation or reciprocation.[21] That which is assimilated and learned by way of identification is put into practice with persons not assigned the same gender as oneself. To illustrate, the little girl learns to dance by identifying with her mother or sister and copying them, but she dances with her father or brother, complementing them. The same two principles apply across the entire spectrum of gender divergent status, sexuoerotic rehearsal play included. Age mates have exceptional authority in transmitting gender dimorphic standards and stereotypes.

Sexuoerotic Rehearsal Play

Rehearsal of the positions of presenting and mounting is widespread in the agemate play of early childhood primates. It has been most intensively investigated in rhesus monkeys (Goldfoot et al.,[22] and personal communication). Monkeys deprived of play grow up unable to copulate and breed. Restricting play to as little as a half-hour a day allows one out of three young ones to achieve the correct copulatory position, but a year or more too late. They grow up able to copulate, but their breeding rate is subnormal.

Monkeys allowed unrestricted play time, but only in all male or all female groups. engage in presenting and mounting play with one another when they become adolescent. Although normally reared partners of the opposite sex find them sexually attractive, they cower and are scared. A male does not mount a female, even though he inspects and touches her genitalia with curiosity. A female resists the approach of a male partner, who succeeds in copulating only if he is exceptionally gentle and skilled at not making her more scared. When back with their same-sexed friends with whom they played as juveniles, males continue to mount males, and females to mount females with a frequency unrecorded in males and females that grew up and engaged in sexual rehearsal play together as juveniles (David Goldfoot, personal communication, January 7, 1984).

TABLE 1

Gender Transpositions

	Total	Partial*	Adventitious
CHRONIC	Transexualism	Gynemimesis andromimesis, male androphilia, female gynophilia	Androgeny of gender-coded education, work legal status
EPISODIC	Transvestism	Androgynophilia (bisexualism)	Androgeny of gender-coded play, body-language, grooming, ornament

**Gynemimesis* and *andromimesis* mean impersonating a female and a male, respectively, on a full-time basis.[24] *Male androphilia* means erotosexual attraction between men, and *female gynophilia* between women. *Androgynophilia* means erotosexual attraction, to some degree, to men and women.

Among human beings, the hallowed social policy of prohibiting, preventing and punishing erotosexual rehearsal play in late infancy and the juvenile years may interfere with the genital component of identification and complementation to a degree as yet barely suspected. Social failure to endorse healthy masculinity and femininity in erotosexual rehearsal play may very well permit this aspect of development to become permanently and irrevocably stunted—misrepresented or transposed in the brain.

BRAIN SCHEMAS

Identification and complementation each have their representation or schema implanted in the brain. One is the schema of one's own gender status. The other is the schema of the other gender status to which one must complement one's own. On the basis of actuarial statistics, one expects that the identification schema will differentiate to be concordant with the morphology of the genitalia of the self, whereas the complementation schema will be concordant with the morphology of the genitalia of the other sex. It is when this expectation is not realized that one has a gender transposition. The degree of transposition is variable, from total or obligative to trivial or adventitious. A total, but episodic transposition is evident in cases of two names, two wardrobes, and two personalities—one male, and one female, each alternating with the other and having a different lifestyle and personality.

Table 1 shows a 2 × 3 classification of gender transposition on the criteria of duration and degree of pervasiveness. By itself alone, a transposition is neither an asset nor a debit. It becomes one or the other on the basis of the value judgments, both informal and official, of other people.

REFERENCES

1. Green R, Money J: Stage-acting, role-taking, and effeminate impersonation during boyhood. *Arch Gen Psych 15*:535–538, 1966.
2. Money J, Russo AJ: Homosexual outcome of discordant gender-identity/role in childhood: Longitudinal follow-up. *J Pediat Psychol 4*:29–31, 1979.

3. Money J, Russo AJ: Homosexual vs. transvestite or transexual gender-identity/role: Outcome study in boys. *Int J Fam Psychiat 2*:139–145, 1981.
4. Silverstein C: *Man to Man: Gay Couples in America.* New York: Morrow, 1981.
5. Money J: The development of sexuality and eroticism in humankind. *Q Rev Biol 56*:379–404, 1981.
6. Baum MJ: Differentiation of coital behavior in mammals: A comparative analysis. *Neurosci Biobehav Rev 3*:265–284, 1979.
7. Baum MJ, Gallagher CA, Martin JT, Damassa DA: Effects of testosterone, dihydrotestosterone, or estradiol administered neonatally on sexual behavior of female ferrets. *Endocrin 111*:773–780, 1982.
8. Nordeen EJ, Yahr P: Hemispheric asymmetries in the behavioral and hormonal effects of sexually differentiating mammalian brain. *Science 218*:391–393, 1982.
9. Ward IL: Prenatal stress feminizes and demasculinizes the behavior of males. *Science 175*:82–84, 1972.
10. Ward IL, Weisz J: Maternal stress alters plasma testosterone in fetal males. *Science 207*:328–329, 1980.
11. Reinisch JM, Sanders SA: Early barbiturate exposure: The brain, sexually dimorphic behavior and learning. *Neurosci Biobehav Rev 6*:311–319, 1982.
12. Lewis VG, Money J: Gender-identity/role: G-I/R Part A: XY (androgen-insensitivity) syndrome and XX (Rokitansky) syndrome of vaginal atresia compared. In L Dennerstein, G Burrows (eds), *Handbook of Psychomatic Obstetrics and Gynecology.* Amsterdam-New York-Oxford, Elsevier Biomedical, 1983.
13. Money J, Daléry J: Iatrogenic homosexuality: Gender identity in seven 46,XX chromosomal females with hyperadreocortical hermaphroditism born with a penis, three reared as boys, four reared as girls. *J Homosex 1*:357–371, 1976.
14. Money J, Lewis VG: Homosexual/heterosexual status in boys at puberty: Idiopathic adolescent gynecomastia and congenital virilizing adrenocorticism compared. *Psychoneuroendocrin 7*:339–346, 1982.
15. Money J, Mathews D: Prenatal exposure to virilizing progestins: An adult follow-up study of twelve women. *Arch Sex Beh 11*:73–83, 1982.
16. Money J, Schwartz M, Lewis VG: Adult erotosexual status and fetal hormonal masculinization and demasculinization: 46,XX congenital virilizing adrenal hyperplasia (CVAH) and 46, XY androgen-insensitivity syndrome (AIS) compared. *Psychoneuroendocrinology*, 1984.
17. Migeon CJ, Forest MG: Androgens in biological fluids. In B Rothfeld (ed), *Nuclear Medicine in Vitro,* 2nd ed. Philadelphia, Lippincott, 1983.
18. Parks GA, Korth-Schultz S, Penny R, Hilding RF, Dumars KW, Frasier SD, New MI: Variation in pituitary-gonadal function in adolescent male homosexuals and heterosexuals. *J Clin Endocrin Metab 39*:796–801, 1974.
19. Sanders RM, Langevin R, Bain J: Hormones and human sexuality. *Neuroendocrinol Letters 5*:129, 1983.
20. Sanders RM, Bain J, Langevin R: Peripheral sex hormones, homosexuality, and gender identity. In R Langevin (ed), *Erotic Preference, Gender Identity, and Aggression in Men.* Hillsdale, NJ, Erlbaum, 1984.
21. Money J: Identification and complementation in the differentiation of gender identity. *Dan Med J 19*:256–268, 1972.
22. Goldfoot DA, Goy RW, Neff DA, Wallen K, McBrair MC: Social influences upon the display of sexually dimorphic behavior in rhesus monkeys: Isosexual rearing. *Arch Sex Beh* in press.
23. Money J: Two names, two wardrobes, and two personalities. *J Homosex 1*:65–70, 1974.
24. Money J, Lamacz M: Gynemimesis and gynemimetophilia: Individual and cross-cultural manifestations of a gender coping strategy hitherto unnamed. *Compr Psychiat* in press.

Medical Policy without Scientific Evidence:

The Promiscuity Paradigm and AIDS

Stephen O. Murray and Kenneth W. Payne

El Instituto Obregón
1360 De Haro
San Francisco, CA 94107–3239

Abstract

The inability to cure or even explain the aetiology and transmission of a disease potentially threatens the high status of medicine in U.S. society. Without any technological fix available, medical practitioners tend to blame disease victims' personalities, lifestyles, and/or "non-compliance" to physicians' recommendations of traditional morality. The original identification of a syndrome of opportunistic infections, suggesting impaired immune functioning among gay men during the early 1980s, fit into the dominant medical view of sexually transmitted diseases, and all but foreclosed other kinds of research. The removal of a "recent Haitian immigrant" risk group for acquired immune deficiency syndrome provides a clear case study of nonscientific influence on public health classification. The need to legitimate medical power and expertise created great pressure to "do something" once segments of the public conceived the threat of

* *Earlier versions of portions of this paper were presented at the 1985 and 1986 meetings of the Society for the Study of Social Problems, and the 1987 meeting of the Kroeber Anthropological Society. The authors wish to acknowledge encouragement and helpful criticisms given by Barry Adam, Edward Albert, Dianne Beeson, Ralph Bolton, Wayne Dynes, Peter Goldblum, Keelung Hong, Philip Kayal, John Kitsuse, Martin Levine, Richard Mohr, Steven Nachman, Peter Nardi, James Orcutt, and anonymous referees.*

an epidemic ofAIDS in the mid-1980s. The something done did not need to be medically efficacious, but the symbolic politics of public health require rationalizations in terms of "scientific" evidence. Traditional moralism better explains the public health policy initiatives taken and not taken regarding the incurable disease AIDS than does existing scientific evidence. Actions taken against gay bathhouses and heterosexual prostitutes, attempts to prescribe routine HIV-antibody testing, and recurrent political obstacles to "promoting immorality" by making prophlyactics more available are reviewed.

The great successes in finding cures or means to eradicate infectious diseases in industrialized societies from the era of Koch and Pasteur to that of antibiotics enormously increased the prestige of medicine within industrialized societies, and increased expectations of technological "fixes" ("magic bullets") far beyond the important advances which had been made (McKinley and McKinley 1977). The high status and concomitant rewards of medical professions rest on expectations of cures. This produces a strain between recognizing the limitations of scientific medical competence (Stelling and Bucher 1973; Fox and Swazey 1978; Bosk 1979), and wanting prestige and rewards to be maintained, or (preferably) enhanced. Such strain—which is probably a universal attribute of the healer role—leads to claiming more understanding of illness and what to do about it than scientific knowledge and therapeutic art can support.

Credibility crises are generally avoided only because the hopes of clients[1] complement practitioners' pretensions. When the miracle workers can do nothing at all, anxiety—profession-wide and individual—mounts. Frustrations of health practitioners are compounded by clients' perception of the inability to work more miracles. The pressures and temptation to blame the patient or some other scapegoat increase when a failure becomes common knowledge throughout a society. "We don't know" is a difficult answer for healers (of any sort) to give to the question "What should we do?" (see Kleinman 1980).

There is a push from within medical organizations and professions to increase the domain of medicine in order to achieve still higher status for medicine. There is also a pull from policymakers, as well as from patients, to apply medical knowledge. This pull does not wait for a knowledge base to develop. Individuals terrified with what is going wrong with their bodies want immediate reassurance that someone knows what to do, and is undertaking to do it. Public health bureaucrats also want to be able to say that everything possible is being done to protect the public and cure the sick.

The legitimacy of the high status and ever-increasing share of resources accorded scientific medicine in the USA is best supported by visible efficacy in dealing with dramatic physiological crises. If such efficacy is not demonstrable, the reputation and influence of scientific medicine are endangered.[2] Any such occasion triggers something of a vested interest in attacking those who manifest inconveniently incurable or chronic diseases not amenable to displays of capital-intensive medical virtuosity. If no high-tech cure or management of the disease is available, resort to explanations in terms of patient "non-compliance," lifestyle, or personality is likely (see Sontag 1978; Brandt 1985). Blaming the victim is more likely than reconsideration of the basic conceptual and clinical organizations of disease and of medicine.

Moreover, as social control increasingly operates under a medical guise in industrialized societies (Zola 1972; Kitsuse and Spector 1973; Bullough 1974; Conrad and Schneider 1980; Foucault 1980), categories from the discourse of scientific medicine become the basis for public policy. Expert opinion on how to safeguard public health is sometimes pressed, sometimes sought, but rarely is it presented as heuristic and hypothetical rather than as established fact (Murray 1980a; Goodfield 1982)—not even when it interferes considerably with the lifeways and life chances of various populations. In their own view, as well as in that of many others, doctors know best. Saving lives is what doctors (and other health professionals) seek to do—without asking questions about the quality of life after salvation, and usually with expectations of not having this absolute value questioned. They are accustomed to violating the bodily integrity of their patients with little question or challenge to the legitimacy, rationality or effectiveness of what they do.

Clinical experience of overriding personal autonomy tends to be generalized from doctoring to individuals to doctoring to communities. At both levels of practice, there are many doctors who do not distinguish between trying their clinical guesses and applying a widely accepted scientific consensus. In their view, no one should question them, so long as their intentions are therapeutic. At both the level of treating individuals and that of intervening in the name of "the public," medical professionals take any second-guessing of their prescriptions as non-compliance, irrational resistance, or mental illness. It is genuinely difficult for those dedicated to medicine to conceive that health may not be everyone's highest value. Hence, medical professionals are generally insensitive to quality of life and individual liberties issues. As Mohr (1987a: 46) noted, "Doctors tend to hold their unrefined view that health policy is merely a matter of strategy because they tend to see health itself as a trumping good, second to none in importance."

In analyzing the challenge to the psychiatric medicalization of traditional Western condemnation of male homosexuality, Conrad and Schneider (1980: 211) predicted, "If a behavior is demedicalized but not vindicated (absolved of immorality), it becomes more vulnerable to moral attack." Besides showing the competition among would-be agents of social control, Conrad and Schneider suggested the possibility of remedicalization following demedicalization. Soon after their book was published, a new cycle began with the discovery of a new medical basis for proscribing male homosexual behavior. Just as with the psychiatric proscription, medical claims far outstripped the scientific evidence which was plastered onto traditional Judaeo-Christian intolerance of male homosexuality. Also repeating the history of the psychiatric colonial expeditions into male homosexuality, there have been struggles over territory between different medical specialties and organizations (most visibly between the National Cancer Institute and the Centers for Disease Control within the federal Department of Health Services), and the new medical model of why male homosexuality is unhealthy does not include any cure (cf. Conrad and Schneider 1980: 207).

We shall show how the original identification of a syndrome of opportunistic infections in gay men living in the most institutionally elaborated gay communities (Murray 1979, 1988a) made it a "gay plague" and therefore sexually transmitted, and how such identification constrained conceptualization and research subsequent to the initial "explanation" of "gay promiscuity."[3] The "discovery" of cases in populations with less access to medical facilities (viz., heterosexual Haitians, central Africans, and American intravenous drug users) was not merely delayed, but was muted for several years by attempts to fit such cases into the promiscuous male homosexuality etiology.[4] We shall also suggest that public health intervention has been inhibited by moralistic pressures so that tactics of high cost to individual liberties and little likely benefit to preventing cases of AIDS have been adopted, while those which would be challenged by moralistic Christians as "condoning immorality" have been avoided despite their greater likely benefit and lower cost (see Crimp 1988:259–65).

Paradigms

> As new medical terms become known in a society, they find their way into existing semantic networks. While new explanatory models may be introduced, changes in medical rationality seldom follow quickly. —Good (1977: 54)

Not just medical practitioners (see Roth 1957; Lipton and Hershaft 1985), but medical researchers apparently accept "scientific" claims without any empirical evidence, if they fit with prejudices (whether these are theoretical and/or religious). Indeed, in borrowing the term "paradigm" from linguistics, Kuhn (1962, 1977) argued that not just the "folk," but also scientists think along lines constrained by the terms of particular theories, sometimes failing to see what does not fit into the terms or within the theory, sometimes seeing what doesn't exist (archetypally, phlogiston). **Conceptions shape perceptions, even if they do not entirely determine them.** In particular, paradigms channel inquiries along established routes. Before scientists draws a new map, they are likely to proceed along well-mapped and -travelled roads which have led to payoffs in the past.

Within the dominant paradigm of western "scientific" medicine, chronic illness is barely recognized, let alone understood (Strauss et al. 1985). Chronic illness leading to the death of men in their twenties and thirties is hard to accept (for clinicians as well as for theorists and researchers; see Lessor and Jurich 1985). The clinical entity conceived in the early 1980s within Western scientific medicine as Acquired Immune Deficiency Syndrome was forced into the theoretical procrustean bed of an acute, discrete sexually transmitted disease rather than being conceived as a a chronic illness (triggered by introduction of a virus into the bloodstream).

Labeling a syndrome

In the first reports in 1981, there was no single label for a mysterious outbreak of Kaposi's sarcoma and pneumocystis pneumonia among previously healthy gay men (Centers for Disease Control 1981a,b). By the end of 1981, "gay compromise syndrome" (GCS) seemed to be emerging as a consensus in medical reporting, and GRID (gay-related immunodeficiency) in the gay press.[5] As Albert (1984: 12) observed, "The major source for early information on AIDS was the CDC [Centers for Disease Control] in Atlanta. CDC reports tended to emphasize who got sick rather than the nature of the disease itself." The first mass media attention in the summer of 1982 presaged the media onslaught of the first months of 1983 by focusing on "hotbeds of homosexual promiscuity", "living playgrounds for infectious agents" (*Newsweek* 9/6/82; see Albert's Table One; Murray and Payne 1985).[6] The leader of the CDC task force, James Curran, was quoted (in Astor 1983: 56) as recognizing a predisposition, which we would extend to CDC epidemiologists: "You get heterosexual doctors examining gays, and they jump on the first possible hypothesis, that it must be due to the sexual behavior of gays."

It was almost a year into CDC reports in the *Morbidity and Mortality Weekly Reports* (MMWR), in June 1982, that it was mentioned that almost twenty percent of the first 355 U.S. cases were heterosexual male and female intravenous drug users (and another three years before official notice of homosexual IV drug users was taken; see below). By the end of the year, AIDS in heterosexual hemophiliacs was also recognized, and in the 4 March 1983 report transfusion of blood was acknowledged as a vector for the same unexpected infections.

During this same period, a label crystallized. In the 24 September 1982 *MMWR* "AIDS" replaced the previous "Kaposi Sarcoma and Opportunistic Infections in Previously Healthy Persons." The new label was already current in *Science* (though not in medical journals) a month earlier. Although no longer containing "gay" as a preface, as in GCS and GRID, AIDS was already indelibly stamped as a "gay disease," a "gay plague" as some sensationalized it. Because early cases were urban gay men, the syndrome from the beginning was presumed to be a "sexually transmitted disease," an already trendy classification in the *zeitgeist* of "sexual counter-revolution":

> Once a disease is classified as being transmitted sexually, the disease and its spread arouse strong negative emotional reactions of a kind not aroused by waterborne or airborne diseases or those carried by insects. The emotional reactions are often as marked in doctors and scientists as they are in other people, and like any powerful emotion, they are liable to impair clear thought. The recent classification of many diseases as venereal has been accepted very uncritically... Because of the emotional overtones, once doctors are convinced that a disease is transmitted through sexual contact, many assume that any patient with the disease must have acquired it by promiscuous sexual activity. Those afflicted are assumed to be guilty till they can prove their innocence. This medical attitude is not only arrogant, but potentially dangerous, because other means of transmission will inevitably be overlooked (Seale 1985: 38; on the original construction of a sexual-transmission paradigm to replace astrological and metallurgical explanations of syphilis see Fleck 1979[1935]).

The initial epidemiological discourse focused on sexual promiscuity. The word "promiscuity" itself was not used in CDC publications, but the number of (self-reported) sexual partners over varying durations of time was the datum most frequently gathered and analyzed in epidemiological work, and the CDC's semantic ascetism in eschewing the heavily-loaded and imprecise term "promiscuity" was not practiced by others.

Urban public health officials and CDC epidemiologists were familiar with endemic gonorrhea and hepatitis and with epidemic amebiasis among sexually active urban gay men. For those diseases there were identified etiological agents. Their ultimate causes were not sexual practices, although the proximate cause of transmission of the agents was often sexual practices.

The simultaneous occurrence of relatively high rates of diverse ailments, many of them induced by parasites, had given rise to a clinical concept, "gay bowel syndrome" (GBS) in the late 1970s. Parasites thought to be the province of tropical medicine became a new focus of healthcare for gay men. Young American men were not supposed to turn up with such parasites, just as they were not expected to present Kaposi's sarcoma (KS) or pneumocystis carinii pneumonia (PCP). Although KS and PCP were not directly added to the inventory of GBS, this model of a syndrome of exotic (for middle-class Americans) diseases was an analog.

Work developing a vaccine for hepatitis-B also familiarized some medical scientists with the anal sexual practices and high number of sexual partners of the gay men whose bodies were culturing antibodies to be used in the vaccine — the *in vivo* factories as well as test site for manufacturing it.

A predisposition existed to equate an outbreak of unexpected diseases among gay men with anal transmission;[7] and hepatitis-B remains, even now, as the favorite analog of the epidemiology of AIDS-risk, despite differences in contagiousness between the two.[8] So satisfied with anal intercourse as an explanation for AIDS were American health officials that a 1984 New York State Department of Health AIDS information pamphlet attributed heterosexual African cases to it without any evidence of actual sexual practices in central Africa (Lieberson 1986: 44). Similarly, CDC researchers attempted to persuade those with AIDS in Belle Glade, Florida (where the per capita rate of cases is the highest in the United States) that they must be homosexual or intravenous drug-users (Fettner 1986; Norman 1986).

Most of the epidemiological data gathered from Africa (or even from North American gay communities) have not been published (as of late 1988), except for self-reported number of partners and sexual practices. Despite the relative difficulty of female-to-male transmission of the virus supposed to trigger AIDS, the equal sex ratio of African AIDS cases has not been conceived as an anomaly to sexual transmission. Instead, various hypotheses about anal sex (and genital ulcers) in Africa have been advanced without being evidence of prevalence. For instance, female circumcision (which occurs in areas to the north of the central African societies beset with AIDS) was supposed to lead to substituting anal for vaginal sex, though this still does not explain male cases. Unacknowledged bisexuality has been presumed despite invariant denial by Africans (and Haitians) with AIDS (Murray and Payne 1988; Murray 1988b).

The need for a virus

The "organized skepticism" of science expected by some (Merton 1968: 614–615) seems to have been overpowered by the need of at least an explanation for AIDS, pending any effective remedies, a cure, or a vaccine. An explanation in terms of stigmatized behavior (anal sexuality, heroin injection) among stigmatized populations (gay men, black heroin users, and Haitians) was comforting to many white heterosexuals, including medical researchers, and also federal bureaucrats attempting to minimize the need for federal health initiatives and to further privatize health care in the USA. In particular, in 1984 the Reagan administration's Department of Health and Human Services was under mounting pressure to show that it was doing something and making progress in controlling what was nominally its first health priority—without seeking additional funding.[9]

Statistically, if not morally, receiving blood transfusions is abnormal. Unlike homosexual behavior, it is a recent innovation, it does not occur "in nature," and it is viewed, at least by Christian Scientists, as "unnatural," indeed "contrary to nature." After the link between the opportunistic infections associated with AIDS and earlier transfusions was reluctantly made in 1983, "deviant lifestyle" lost some of its comforting explanatory power for those not particularly perturbed to have gay men and IVDUs dying. The syndrome was "acquired" just as unknowingly as it was among gay men, and everyone knows that surgery is dangerous, yet no one (to my knowledge) mobilized the rhetoric of "trying to fool Mother Nature and reaping the penalty." Although members of the president's generation and political leanings, such as Paul Gann, who were infected with HIV could focus on finding the "deviant" who had infected them by donating blood that no one at the time knew was "contaminated," recognition of transfusion cases greatly increased the pressure to find a microbe — and a means of neutralizing any danger to "the general public."

The American "discovery" of a putative aetiological agent, labeled HTLV-III, within the National Cancer Institute was announced in a press conference by HHS Secretary Margaret Heckler, who at that time predicted development of a vaccine within six months. So eager was that National Institute of Cancer laboratory headed by Robert Gallo to assimilate a virus already linked to AIDS by Institut Pasteur researchers (Barre-Sinoussi et al. 1983) to the series of retroviruses that Gallo had been studying, that they retained their HTLV acronym, which had stood for Human T-cell Leukemia Virus in HTLV-I and HTLV-II, to Human T-Lymphotropic Virus in HTLV-III (see Connor and Kingman 1988 on the involved political history of credit for discovering what is now labeled the Human Immunodeficiency Virus). Similarly, so eager to claim progress, a causal model, and a potential marker with which to protect the nation's blood supply were HHS administrators and scientists, that this putative causal agent was not assessed using Koch's postulates, the usual standards for evaluating causal models for diseases:

> To establish a microorganism as the cause of a disease (a) it must be found in all cases of the disease; (b) it must be isolated from the host and grown in pure culture; (c) it must reproduce the original disease when introduced into a susceptible host; and (d) it must be found present in the

> experimental host so infected (Duesberg 1987; see Koch 1890; Duesberg 1988).

In particular, the third postulate of sufficiency has not been met, since many persons with evidence of exposure to the virus do not show suppressed immune systems.[10] The first postulate of necessity remains dubious with about ten percent of the AIDS cases written off as "measurement error" by NCI scientists. The existing correlations between AIDS and HIV do not prove causation, for "correlations without evidence for biochemical activity are not sufficient to prove 'etiology'... It is necessary to demonstrate some HIV-speficic biochemical activity at the onset of AIDS to prove that HIV causes AIDS" (Duesberg 1988:516). Although there are viruses which become pathogenic after evidence of immunity appears (including hepatitis viruses, and herpes zoster virus), they are "very active when they cause fatal, degnerative diseases," as HIV is not (Ibid.). Moreover, Duesberg (1987, 1988) called attention to the logical impossibility of the Gallo model of a virus which is supposed to kill the few cells it infects yet survives in cells for eight or more years before the onset of AIDS.[11]

Once the challenge to the basic HTLV/HIV causal model was finally made in the spring of 1987 (Duesberg 1987:1211–15), the Centers for Disease Control suggested that cases falling outside its postulated risk groups and testing negative for the presence of HIV antibodies not be reported as AIDS cases, even if the cause of death was one of the opportunistic diseases in the official CDC definition. Such a tactic preserves the model of risk and causation from empirical counter-evidence. Given the stake the federal government has in the profits of marketing HIV tests, such paradigm maintenance strikingly departs from the norm of disinterestedness (Merton 1968: 612–14), as well as that of organized skepticism. At the level of clinical practice, gay patients without the opportunistic infections of the CDS definition were being reported as AIDS cases, and non-gay patients with the infections were not being reported all along (McCombie 1986).

If the stigmatizing diagnosis of AIDS is applied disproportionately (or only) to those belonging to already stigmatized groups and withheld from other persons, the patterning of cases becomes distorted. The schema of categorizing "risk groups" becomes tautological, confirmed by recognizing cases from "risk groups" and refusing to recognize other cases.

Risk factors

The identification of AIDS as a "gay disease" was continuously reinforced by the CDC's classification system. Rather than report all cases with each characteristic, AIDS reports in *MMWR* suppressed interaction effects, e.g., a gay IV drug user was categorized as a gay case, a Haitian IV drug user as an IV drug user, etc. Such tidy classification precluded independent judgment of the relative weight of risk factors and of their prevalence in the population at risk. As early as late 1982 a CDC report found that 58 percent of AIDS cases classified as "gay" rather than as "drug user" used five or more different street drugs; 68 percent had used amphetamines with a median of 120 times (Lauritsen 1985:7; Krieger and Caceres 1985: 53).[12] Although these data seemed far more exceptional to observers of urban gay subcultures than the number of lifetime sexual partners reported, the presumption of sexual transmission has guided data collection and reporting. Although a gay/bisexual IV drug user category was eventually added to the hierarchy, most behavioral data gathered by epidemiologists dealing with anything other than sexual behavior and needle use have gone unpublished.[13]

Published analyses been strikingly univariate in an age when sophisticated multivariate analysis is the norm in social, biological, and medical science, and when multifactorial disease models are supposedly paradigmatic within the profession of epidemiology (Oppenheimer 1988:269). As Lauritsen (1985:7) concluded, CDC hierarchical presentation of risk factors along with confining "drug use" to intravenous injection "de-emphasizes and under-represents every patient characteristic **except** homosexuality. One cannot help but suspect a theological mindset behind this statistical misrepresentation of reality: that which is most 'sinful' is presumed to be most dangerous." As Conrad and Schneider (1980) noted of the dialectic of medicalization, the scientistic veneer over traditional Judaeo-Christian condemnation of homosexuality is very thin.

That risk factor classification is subject to extra-scientific consideration is perhaps even better demonstrated by the 1983 removal of "Haitian immigrant" from the CDC's hierarchical list of risk groups in 1983. That there was direct political pressure is indisputable. The minister of health for Haiti, Dr. Ary Bordes, ordered re-evaluation of results (reported in *Medical World News* 9/26/83), already having announced what results should be found via *The New Republic* (8/1/83). The Haitian ambassador to the United States decried linking AIDS and Haiti in a letter to *Newsweek* and to the *New England Journal of Medicine* in September 1983, although the CDC had moved Haitian AIDS cases in the U.S. from a separate risk group into the category "other" a month earlier (8/9/83 *MMWR*), following New York City Health Department's removal 28 July (Altman 1983). In June of 1983 the Groupe Haitien d'Etude du Sarcome de Kaposi et des Infections Opportunistes (GHESKIO) complained that Vieira et al. (1983) had proposed the transmission of AIDS from Haiti to the United States "without any scientific basis" and countered with a hypothesis that AIDS was introduced to Haiti by vacationing U.S. homosexuals (Boncy et al. 1983: 1419). This complaint was the prototype of defenses of Haiti's "national honor" (and tourism revenue). The Haitian government's interest in explaining away Haitian cases with homosexuality dovetailed with the U.S. government paradigm's inability to explain heterosexual cases in Haiti or among Haitian-Americans.

Later in 1983, a more direct attempt to maintain AIDS as a "homosexual disease" rather than a "Haitian disease" was made under the title "Only Homosexual Haitians, Not All Haitians." Altema and Bright (1983: 878) were either uninformed about or oblivious to the fact that the CDC AIDS risk factor classification methodology would not include anyone who could be labeled "homosexual" in any other risk category. They claimed, "Over the past several years there have been many gay clubs in Haiti, usually frequented by young, poor Haitian male prostitutes and vacationing gays," although they did not present any evidence linking AIDS cases in either Haiti or the United States to such clubs, or, for that matter, to homosexual behavior. Instead, they concluded, "The controversy hinges on most men denying homosexual behavior. The truth of the matter is that normally a Haitian homosexual disclaims his tendency to a heterosexual."

The truth is that in most cultures — including even in the half of the states of the United States where, like Haiti, there are no laws against sodomy — most people who have been involved in homosexual behavior and even most of those with a gay identity frequently disclaim the "tendency" to many people, including doctors (Ross 1984). Such denial is not unique to Haiti by any means, any more than is the existence of prostitution or of gay clubs. Although for a former (quasi-)colony, Haiti has received relatively little attention from American social scientists, those who studied rural Haiti were able to elicit information about attitudes towards local homosexuals (Herskovits 1937a,b; Simpson 1942). The reported attitude of bemused denigration and the lack of any attempts to extirpate homosexual behavior do not differ from those reported throughout Latin America (Carrier 1975,1976; Murray 1980b,1987). If anything, less prominent machismo in Haiti connects with greater toleration of homosexuals—especially in such indigenous niches as *rara* bands (Davis 1986) and *voudou(n)* nations (Bourguignon 1976)—than is imaginable in any Spanish-speaking Latin American societies. Bahia, which was similarly populated from the West Coast of Africa, is the closest cultural analog, and there, cross-gender possession and homosexuality are prominent parts of Sango cults (Landes 1940; Fry 1987). The particularly notable taboo on homosexuality is not reported in pre-AIDS ethnographic literature about Haiti. Instead, in the folk religion, which was cultivated by the Duvalier regime (see Davis 1986; Fettner 1986), explicit gender non-conformity was notable. There is not any evidence in earlier literature on Haiti of a taboo on **mentioning** homosexuality.

Certainly, any serious assertion that it is particularly difficult to elicit information about homosexuality from Haitians must be comparative, but no one has compared elicitation in Haiti to elicitation in the Dominican Republic, Bahia, or any other point for comparison. In the United States itself, "except for three cases of AIDS in admittedly homosexual Haitians, none of the other cases reported have admitted to homosexual activity despite intensive questioning in both French and Creole by both American physicians and by Haitians" (Landesman 1983: 33). Taking all the 1983 reports of AIDS linked to Haiti in *Lancet* and the U.S. and Canadian medical literature, there were 53 female cases and 69 male cases. Twenty of the latter were linked to homosexuality/ bisexuality. In addition, Landesman (1983) reported three of seventy cases of Haitian immigrants to the U.S. identified as homosexual. By the end of 1983, 23 of 266 (8.6 percent) AIDS cases born in Haiti had been linked to homosexual activity.[14]

The popularity of Haiti as a vacation spot for gay Americans suggested in GHESKIO communiques was unaccompanied by even anecdotal evidence. Examination of official U.S./Caribbean air travel statistics for the years preceding the recognition of AIDS shows that while travel to Haiti was increasing, both the absolute magnitude of travel and the rate of increase were greater for other Caribbean countries than for Haiti. Insofar as gay travel can be estimated from gay guidebooks,[15] Haiti was once of the least-favored destinations in the Caribbean for gay travelers during the 1970s and the less-favored half of the island of Hispaniola (Murray 1988). Epidemiological data published through late 1988 does not include data on

Haitian travel of American AIDS cases ("gay" or other).[16] At the Haitian end of the hypothesized transmission vector, Dr. Jean-Michel Guerin of GHESKIO told d'Adesky (1986: 16) that "all his patients—without exception—had denied having sex with tourists." He flatly stated, "AIDS in Haiti is not a homosexual disease" (*Ibid.*). Warren Johnson, a Cornell epidemiologist working with GHESKIO, was quoted by Norman (1986: 415) as saying that only eleven percent of AIDS cases in Haiti could be linked to homosexual sex, blood transfusions, or intravenous drug abuse. It should be noted that these statements were made after the fall of the Duvalier dynasty in 1986.

From special methods to special logic

Although the director of the Centers for Infectious Diseases, Walter Dowdle, justified dropping the Haitian risk factor on the basis it was "the only risk group identified because of who they were rather than what they did" (*American Medical News*, 19 April 1985, p. 11), it is in fact the risk factor most difficult to understand by behaviors thought to transmit the AIDS virus. The non-Haitian risk factors are all kinds of people: drug users/abusers/addicts, homosexuals, bisexuals, hemophiliacs, even recipients of blood transfusions. All these classifications can be resolved into behavior proposed to be means of transmission: sharing needles, passive anal intercourse without condoms, injecting clotting factor or blood containing the virus. The sharing of needles, which differentiates U.S. from Canadian case patterns, may also be a risk factor for Haitians (and Africans, as well). Especially after the introduction ot tests for exposure to HIV, there was no logical/scientific reason to continue to speak of "risk groups," especially since as early as the 4 March 1983 MMWR, there was CDC cognizance that "each group contains many persons who probably have little risk of acquiring AIDS."

The logic of Dowdle's "what they do"/"who they are" dichotomy of AIDS risk groups could easily be extended to the "homosexual/bisexual" (who they are) risk category, making the risk male-male anal intercourse (what they do). Instead, the facile CDC equation of homosexual behavior and "homosexuals" ignores the large literature about the problematic link between homosexual behavior and identity. Fischl and Dickinson (1984: 331) claim, "Haitian men who are the passive partner or homosexual prostitutes generally will not consider themselves homosexual." The same could be—and frequently has been—said about North American hustlers and about many other active partners in homosexual relations outside contemporary gay communities, as well. Not every man in the United States or in Haiti whose behavioral repertoire includes passive anal intercourse without condoms classifies himself or is classified in his social circle within the risk category "homosexual and bisexual men," whereas many men who consider themselves gay do not engage in that behavior, and some others who consider themselves gay do not engage in any homosexual behavior (Reiss 1961; Bell and Weinberg 1978; Weinberg 1978; Humphreys 1975; Murray 1987a).

Doing Something

> Experience should teach us to be most on our guard to protect liberty when the Government's purposes are beneficent. Men born to freedom are naturally alert to repel invasion of their liberty by evil-minded rulers. The greatest dangers to liberty lurk in insidious encroachment by men of zeal, well-meaning but without understanding. —Justice Louis Brandeis in *Olmstead* vs. *U.S.*

The role of symbolic politics in the identification of an aetiological agent of AIDS and assignment of risk factors was considerable. AIDS was fit into the pardigm of consequences of "promiscuity," with drug use as well as stigmatized sexual behavior included within "promiscuity." This mindset led directly into paternalistic and punitive policy initiatives. The "application" of AIDS science to public health has been driven by the symbolic politics of conventional "morality" even more obviously than were the "scientific" classifications of the disease, its aetiology, and "risk groups." Blaming victims is a leitmotif of public discussion of AIDS, derived directly from the view that "promiscuity" is an invariant, defining characteristic of gay men. In media coverage and the cosmologies of many, gay men exposed to the virus in the late 1970s or early 1980s before AIDS appeared are viewed by many as less "innocent victims" than those who received blood transfusions during the same time, before anyone knew there was a risk of a yet-to-be-identified disease.

Protecting the nation's blood supply—and thereby removing exclusively heterosexual white males other than those who received blood transfusions between the mid-1970s and March 1985 from all but the remotest risk of AIDS—was quickly accomplished. In March 1985 the Food and Drug Administration licensed the ELISA test to detect HIV antibodies (with an explicit statement that the test was to screen blood and was not a diagnostic test to predict acquisition of immunodeficiency). Tactics based on making behaviors found immoral by some safer, on the other hand, have been obstructed or blocked by moralists. They have been more intent on avoiding any appearance of state "condoning of immorality" than with concern about saving lives (or liberties) of those they regard as "immoral." Promoting safer sex is too controversial for U.S. public health departments. Politicized religious pressure presses pre- and extra-marital chastity as the only legitimate goal. At least annually, the U.S. Senate bans funding for any educational material that represents safe homosexual sex. In American public health during the 1980s, empiricism, realism, common sense, and rational weighing of costs and either benefits or dangers must oppose a flood of moralistic doublespeak, transparently specious rationalizations, and feverish anxiety about sex and disease.

In the following section the lack of scientific/statistical basis for some public health "applications" of knowledge/misinformation about AIDS will be outlined. Special attention will be devoted to an early action by what is generally conceived to be the most enlightened and liberal American city health department (see Altman 1986). If the ideology of the sexual counter-revolution can force the kind of symbolic politics that upholds "traditional morality" however slight the likelihood is that they effect AIDS transmission in San Francisco, it can drive health policy anywhere in the United States. Personal privacy is more cherished in California than in many other states, as evidenced both in initiative balloting and in state constitutional decisions. Yet, freedom of assembly was overridden without any demonstration of countervailing medical necessity in a city with a widely known history of tolerance for diversity—a diversity which includes four gay political clubs. The case is further deserving of special attention because of the dangers of well-meaning interference with liberty warned against by Justice Brandeis in the epigram to this section and because a best-selling historical novel (Shilts 1987) by one participant is taken, even by sociologists, as factual reportage.[17]

Closing gay baths

Until 1984, resisting pressure from San Francisco Mayor Dianne Feinstein (whose distaste for gay male "promiscuity" was a matter of public record prior to the identification of AIDS, and who is viewed by local civil libertarians as extraordinarily insensitive to civil liberties issues in general) and from others, Dr. Mervyn Silverman, director of public health, had refused to close down bathhouses and private sex clubs in the county, maintaining that it was behavior rather than its locale which mattered in risking AIDS. The formula for the alternative was "Out of the tubs, into the shrubs." Bayer (1989:32–33) quotes 1983 letters from Silverman asserting, "Because the facilities of most bathhouses do not present a public health hazard I feel it would be inappropriate and in fact illegal for me to close down all bathhouses and other such places that are used for anonymous and multiple sex contacts" (10 May 1983) and "I do not share your impression that the subculture who use bathhouses would not immediately switch to other locations where we would have less access to post warnings and provide some education" (12 September 1983). Public health warnings and guidelines were distributed in the baths, whereas no education campaign was feasible in locales of "public sex" such as the parks. Silverman also stressed that those engaging in homosexual sex in the baths, tearooms, and parks were not necessarily gay-identified (see Humphreys 1975; Bell and Weinberg 1978; Murray 1984), and, therefore, could not be reached with information via the gay press.

Silverman could have rationalized continuing not to interfere with the (federally recognized) right of assembly and the (state-recognized) right of privacy for adult consensual sex by citing the indicators of behavioral change, viz., the drop in rectal gonorrhea from 1,700 cases in the second quarter of 1982 to 400 cases in the second quarter of 1984 (see Figure One),[18] and a still unreleased CDC study of bathgoing which failed to establish bathgoing as an AIDS risk factor.[19]

However, two gay San Franciscans took it upon themselves to force closure of the baths. Randy Shilts, a *San Francisco Chronicle* writer, who viewed constitutional rights of privacy and freedom of assembly as "let[ting] gay businessmen murder gay people" (quoted by Hippler 1989:130), was the most peripatetic. His first tactic was to supply a *California Magazine* attack on the San Francisco Department of Public Health for minimizing the threat of AIDS to the wider community (this venture is not mentioned in Shilts 1987). At the height of general paranoia about blood banks and the safety of living in the same city as gay men, this was in itself a signal contribution to enhancing homophobia. At the same time it was a means of waging a new offensive in the interminable internecine struggle between San Francisco's two largest gay Democratic clubs (politics far too complex to explicate here, although the Department of Public Health's gay and lesbian liaison, Pat Norman, associated with the Alice B. Toklas Gay Democratic Club, was preparing to run for the Board of Supervisors, where Harry Britt, a former president of the Harvey Milk Gay Democratic Club, was running for re-election to one of six at-large slots).

Shilts' second offensive (*Chronicle*, 2 Feb. 1984) was to seize on a miniscule fluctuation in the trend of decreasing incidence of rectal gonorrhea as evidence that San Francisco gay men were resuming unsafe sexual practices. The rates of rectal gonorrhea are taken to be indicators of the amount of receptive anal intercourse with strangers. Since the latter is the major means of transmitting AIDS among gay men, the rates are taken as indicators of future AIDS rates (the time lag being due to the hypothesized incubation period of the posited virus, 11.8 years in the current best estimate of Lemp et al. 1990:1499). If this indicator is accepted, obviously its trend is important, so that prediction must depend not on differences from one quarter to another but a trend line. However, Shilts sensationalized a small fluctuation, ignored the trend, and, when the rate dropped the following quarter more than it had increased in the quarter he chose to publicize, he did not bother to report it at all. Indeed, Shilts (1987:415–16) again reported the fluctuation as if it were a change in the trend line.

The other offensive by a San Francisco gay man in 1984, the real "triggering event" (see Galliher and Cross 1983), was undertaken by Larry Littlejohn, a gay deputy sheriff later shown to be engaged in competition with bathhouses—he was dismissed in 1987 after being charged with pandering for young male prostitutes.[20] Littlejohn did not attempt to organize a gay response, such as picketing the establishments. After meeting with Shilts and Leonard Matlovich (Hippler 1989:122), Littlejohn's first resort was to seek state intervention. He began seeking signatures for a city initiative closing the baths in the spring of 1984, arguing, "We must not fool ourselves. There are no educational programs that will effectively change high risk for AIDS sex habits of bathhouse patrons to safe sex" (*California Voice*, 5 April 1984, p. 2). Matlovich explained,

> Some people argued that they were a place to educate. But I thought it was a far better strategy to close the places down first and then to educate, because people wouldn't have paid attention otherwise. Furthermore, I thought it was very foolish for our community to start drawing battlelines at the bathhouses (quoted by Hippler 1989:123).[21]

Under pressure from Mayor Dianne Feinstein (*Chronicle* 28 March 1984, p. 20), and supported by some leaders of the Harvey Milk Gay Democratic Club and eager both to close the baths and to avert a plebiscite on the baths by San Francisco voters,[22] Silverman assembled a group of gay medical and political leaders to discuss closing the baths as a menace to public health. Reportedly the orchestrated gay demand to close the baths to protect gay bathgoers from themselves was more dissonant than expected. The Bay

Area Physicians for Human Rights, a group of doctors concerned with gay health concerns and recognized for special expertise about diseases affecting gay men, refused to endorse any governmental action to close bathhouses. The National Gay Task Force stated its opposition in traditional civil liberties terms:

> NGTF feels most strongly that personal behavior should not be regulated by the state, which historically has been an instrument of our oppression. Furthermore, state closure of such establishments would be largely symbolic, a largely symbolic gesture that would provide a false sense of security that the AIDS epidemic had somehow been contained (*NGTF Update*, 28 March 1984).

The consensus of gay community leaders for bath closure, which the Milk Club leaders assured Silverman existed, was far from evident at a 29 March meeting. The next day, at the news conference scheduled for announcing closure of the baths, Dr. Silverman merely announced that no decision had been reached pending determination of the legality of various courses under consideration. Although there can be no doubt that Mayor Feinstein continued to press for bath closure, gay doctors and their organizations did not support state intervention. For instance, the president of the American Association of Physicians for Human Rights wrote Silverman,

> The closing of businesses to protect people from themselves cannot be accepted. . . There should be no understanding. AAPHR strongly discourages sexual contact with multiple anonymous partners. But we cannot and will not support any effort to enforce that viewpoint (2 April 1984 letter quoted by Bayer 1989:37).

From New York City, where the preponderance of AIDS cases were, both the Commissioner of Health and the director of New York City's Office of Gay and Lesbian Health stated that they would not act to close private clubs, the latter stressing that "there is no science to support the closing of the bathhouses" (quoted in the April 1984 *Coming Up!*, p. 9).

Bayer (1989:38) asserts that "action against the baths was inevitable" in San Francisco. In his retrospective accounts of his pacing of bathhouse closure (to Fitzgerald, to Bayer, and in Silverman [1986]), Dr. Silverman has contended that in addition to waiting for opinions about the legality of various actions he could take (including quarantine), he was waiting for gay leaders, or at least gay physicians with experience of the ravages of AIDS, to orchestrate closure of private clubs in which anonymous sexual interaction with multiple partners continued, or at least to mobilize support for action by the Department of Public Health. The scientific literature available to him was the same as that available to directors of public health in other jurisdictions. If there was any evidence that the locale of multiple sexual encounters could be differentiated as a risk factor for AIDS, it would surely have been available in the other epicenters of the disease. If scientific evidence (new or not so new) suggested a course of action, let alone demonstrated the need for this particular one, it would be very remarkable that public officials elsewhere, particularly in places without vociferous and organized gay rights organizations, did not draw the conclusions Silverman did.

Bayer (1989:38–9) reports that there was a long meeting of health officials on 3 April at which the tactic of regulating rather than closing private sex clubs was agreed upon. Such a meeting was not reported at the time, and would almost certainly violate California laws requiring meetings at which public policy are determined to be open to the public. Whatever the truth and source reporting a meeting on the third, it is certain that on the ninth of April Silverman held another press conference and announced a ban on sex between individuals in "public facilities."[23] Behind him were twenty-four of those with whom he had discussed what to do. Within a few days eleven of this group publicly rejected the policy (*Bay Area Reporter* 19 April 1984, p. 8).

Banning sex rather than closing the baths outright was a compromise sufficient for Littlejohn to halt collecting signatures for his initiative petitions. All sex, not just the kinds of sex the official policy and educational literature of the Department of Public Health had urged curbing until then, was proscribed in the baths and other kinds of private membership clubs licensed by the city and county of San Francisco. Mayor Feinstein was not satisfied that this action was sufficient. Although the Department of Public Health was supposed to enforce the edict, and also to monitor threats to the public health, some weeks after the promulgation of the bath sex ban, the mayor sent policemen (presumably in towels) to report on what was going on in the baths post-sex-ban. She refused to release the report even to the Board of Supervisors, but there is no doubt that the report indicated that sex continued to occur in the baths and clubs. No arrests for violating the sex ban were made, nor were any licenses to operate clubs or baths revoked, so there has not been a court test of whether Dr. Silverman had the legal authority to override the state's consensual sex-in-private law. Toronto police got around the problem of how to accuse men in locked cubicles in Toronto baths of having sexual relations in public: tearing down the doors. San Francisco public health regulation aimed to accomplish the same end without such clumsy force: Silverman's draft revision of Section 263 of the San Francisco Police Code (under which the baths are licensed) banned doors on cubicles.

Surveillance by private investigators reported continued (primarily oral or manual) sex in various places. On the morning of 9 October 1984, Dr. Silverman decreed that the operation of three bookstores, two theaters, and nine private clubs,

> contributed to the spread of the virus that causes AIDS; accordingly, the Director of Public Health has determined that the continued operation of the above designated businesses constitutes a hazard and menace to the public health; then by virtue of the power yielded in him by the law of the State of California, the Charter of the City and County of San Francisco, the Director of Public Health for the City and County of San Francisco hereby orders the

above designated businesses to close no later than 12:00 noon (notice posted on doors of closed businesses).

His press statement elaborated:

> The places I have ordered closed today have continued in the face of this epidemic to provide an environment that encourages and facilitates multiple unsafe sexual contacts, which are an important contributory factor in the spread of this deadly disease. When activities are proven to be dangerous to the public and continue to take place in commercial settings, the Health Department has the duty to intercede and halt the operation of such establishment.[24]

Because the order was delivered by armed policemen and alluded to power vested by state law, the order was initially perceived to be a quarantine. However, the power invoked was that of "abating a public nuisance" (i.e., local rather than state grant of authority to the county Director of Public Health). Once this was learned, six of the businesses reopened to challenge the authority of public nuisance regulation (*Bay Area Reporter*, 11 October 1984). Within a week, San Francisco Superior Court Judge William Mullins signed a temporary restraining order that reclosed the clubs (but left theaters and bookstores open out of First Amendment considerations), pending a 30 October hearing on the city's petition to close them indefinitely. In the request for a temporary restraining order Silverman again equated commercial with public, contending that "altering sexual activity is a matter of individual privacy; when that sexual activity takes place in a commercial setting, this government has the prerogative and duty to intercede," and emphasizing that his professional judgement as a public health officer was that it was necessary to "bring to an end commercial enterprises that involve exploitation for profit of an individual's willingness to engage in potentially lethal forms of recreation" (*People of the State of California v. Ima Jean Owen et al.* memorandum from Mervyn Silverman). As Bayer (1989:48) noted, "Perhaps most remarkable in the city's [actually county's] well-prepared case was the failure to obtain a clear declaration of support for closure from any nationally known epidemiologist involved in the study of AIDS and the patterns of sexual behavior among gay men."

The response for the defendants cited the lack of scientific evidence that bathgoing was a risk factor for AIDS, challenged the unsafeness of the sex reported by private investigators, and rejected Silverman's equation of "commercial" and "public," arguing, "There is simply no legal basis to distinguish the right to engage in consensual sexual activity in defendants' premises from the right to engage in consensual sexual activity in hotels or private home, no difference between someone who rents a cubicle in a bathouse and someone who makes a mortgage payment on his house." They contended that the burden of proof that closure "will be sufficiently effective to justify the obviously serious intrusion on property rights, privacy rights, and associational rights" should rest on the county health department. They were also able to do what San Francisco officials had not been able to do, present briefs from experts outside the county government (specifically, public health officials from Los Angeles and New York) to argue that the proposed closures could not be expected to have any reasonable likelihood of affecting the rate of AIDS cases.

Judicial review in late November by Superior Court Judge Roy Wonder rejected the county's case for closure. On 28 November, Wonder ruled that the clubs could reopen, but ordered them to remove private rooms, to hire monitors (one for every twenty patrons) to survey the premises every ten minutes to ensure that no unsafe sex acts were occurring, and to expel patrons observed to be engaging in "unsafe sex practices." To the amazement of almost everyone, the delineation of "unsafe sex" was initially assigned to the San Francisco AIDS Foundation rather than to the County Department of Public Health (to which the definitional power was later reassigned along with other "technical" clarifications 21 December 1984).

The weekend after the bath closure in San Francisco, an Oakland bathhouse owner reported that his business increased 142 percent, repeating the pattern from 1950s crackdowns on San Francisco gay bars, when patrons also relocated their cruising across the bay (Bérubé 1984: 18). The decision was not appealed, and over the course of the intervening years owners have closed all the San Francisco bathhouses open in 1984. Commercial venues for safe sex (mutual masturbation) operate in the county, and facilities with private rooms for unregulated sex continue to operate in nearby counties.

Other jurisdictions

In late 1985 in New York City, where most of the diagnosed U.S. AIDS cases were, parallel moves to close several gay bathhouses on the basis of private investigator reports of unsafe sex (mostly fellatio) occurred. As in San Francisco, the reversal of policy about bathhouse closure can be directly related to pressure from above, viz. New York Governor Mario Cuomo, who like Mayor Feinstein had a track record of insensitivity to gay civil rights and what civil libertarians label "statism" in regulating conduct. Also as in San Francisco, the New York City health department was bypassed and surveillance of activity in clubs was conducted by investigators from another department. Also, as in San Francisco, they observed and reported practically no anal sex. In New York City the most visible and gay-owned establishments (the Mineshaft and New St. Mark's) were targeted; less visible, allegedly Mafia-owned establishments remain open.

The major difference (other than a lag in timing) between the New York and San Francisco actions is that the New York judge (Richard Wallach) did not devise a policy of his own for regulating sex clubs. In *City of New York v. St. Marks Baths* the judge deferred to the health department and did not evaluate the evidence about sex clubs as a risk factor. In May 1986 in upstate New York in *Commissioner of Health of the County of Erie v. Morgan Inc., et al* closure was rejected because the county did not sustain the burden of proof of dangerous behavior occurring. Los Angeles County Department of Public Health sex club orders were overturned in the summer of 1986, again because the county failed to establish any likelihood that its regulations would reduce the spread of AIDS. Also during the summer of 1986, the San José Water Garden, the largest and plushest gay bathhouse in northern California, was given special recognition for its contribution to AIDS education by the Santa Clara Department of Public Health.

Just as public officials elsewhere did not rally to Dr. Silverman's side in 1984, Dianne Feinstien, who was chair of the U. S. Conference of Mayors, failed to enlist support from her peers for a resolution urging closure of sex clubs (Bayer 1989:69). In August of 1988 the state assembly and senate passed the Bradley Act to assist San Diego County efforts to shut down bathhouses there under the guise of nuisance abatement. However, as of mid-1990, gay bathhouses in Berkeley and San José continue to operate, and some unknown number of gay San Franciscans go to them. California county public health directors' quarantine power has yet to be used in regards to AIDS.

The "scientific evidence"

There was (and is) no evidence showing bathgoing to constitute a risk factor for AIDS. As mentioned in the chronology above, 1984 CDC data still unpublished in 1989 found bathgoing to have no statistically significant effects. The more or less simultaneous report of an ongoing monitoring of changed sexual behavior among San Francisco gay men, which was funded by the Department of Public Health, appears to have been influenced by the policy of closing bathhouses more than it could have contributed to the policy. At least, its authors showed more interest in contrasting bathgoers with other gay men in the report than in their data collection: McKusick et al. (1984) compared only two self-reported behaviors for bathgoers and bar-goers. To the surprise of many (and no doubt the consternation of some moral entrepreneurs), they found that those in their bathgoer sample were no more likely to have received anal intercourse with new or secondary partners five or more times during the previous month than their bar-going sample. Furthermore, 56 percent of the bath sample in contrast to 50 percent of the bar sample reported none.[25]

Considering that only two of the reports of behavior contrasted the bath subsample to the other subsamples, both the abstract and the conclusions of McKusick et al's 1984 report (abridged and published in 1985) gave inordinate attention to bathgoers, whom they characterized as more rigid and more compulsive than other gay men, although the evidence for these psychological characterizations is nowhere in the report. Similarly, the following indictment seems to have been pulled from the air or from officials' prejudices rather than from any data reported in the study (or in other literature on the baths, such as Lee 1978; Styles 1979; Weinberg and Williams 1975):

> It is apparent that the identities of men in the bathhouses are more attached to sexual behavior than men in other groups and that these men as a group are the most rigid and inflexible in their sexual response patterns. There may also exist in certain members of the bathhouse group a type of fatalism that is not subject to the influence of information, since they may already believe that they have come in contact with the hypothetical transmission agents (McKusick et al. 1984:29).

If it was apparent, it is on the basis of evidence other than that presented in their reports. In neither study did McKusick et al. (1983, 1984) attempt to determine whether bathgoers have more sex or are more "addicted" to sex than any other human group (see Levine and Troiden 1988), nor did they use any psychological scales for rigidity. Unless they asked their respondents why they did not stop more high-risk behaviors, belief by a regular bathgoer that he has already come in contact with the mysterious AIDS agent, and so has either survived exposure or is incubating it, can be considered a success of the dissemination of the scientific consensus, in this case the posited long incubation period and low contagiousness of the searched-for virus.[26]

Moreover, their assertion, "The efforts of the Public Health Department have been ineffective in influencing sexual activity at the bathhouses"(McKusick et al. 1984:2) was misleading. According to their own data, more of those in the bath sample than those in the bar or couple sample listed "public information brochures or posters" as a source of information about AIDS (p. 13). They also showed that "knowledge of the disease process and the risk reduction guidelines closely parallels opinion of experts and is well disseminated across subgroups" (1984:13). That is, for transmitting information, the public education efforts of the gay press (the main source of information for most sampled gay men), public health authorities, and others were successful prior to Silverman's attempts to regulate or close gay clubs.

Sixty-five percent of the bar and bath samples, 88 percent of the coupled sample, and 85 percent of the volunteer sample indicated they had already made the changes in their lives needed to adapt to AIDS (for most this was something, because 84 percent reported AIDS had had an impact upon the behavior), so the informational diffusion could be viewed as quite widespread, presuming the McKusick et al. studies were valid. Whether the behavioral changes were sufficient was, of course, subject to interpretation. Longitudinal data from a random sample of single men in the nineteen San Francisco census tracts with the most AIDS cases in 1984 show HIV seropositivity to have been very high by the beginning of 1984 (48.6 percent), and to have increased only slightly since then (to 49.3 percent; Winkelstein et al. (1987a, 1988). Hessol et al. (1987), analyzing blood stored from gay volunteers attending San Francisco's STD Clinic in the mid-1970s and participating in a hepatitis-B study, found most of the seroconversion occurred between 1979 (when five percent were already infected) and the beginning of 1984 (by which time more than fifty percent had seroconverted).[27]

In Los Angeles County where bathhouses have remained open, Richwald et al. (1988) interviewed 807 men who could speak English leaving bathhouses in 1986. Fifty percent reported that information about AIDS received in bathhouses played a major role in their understanding of AIDS prevention; another 37 percent reported it played a minor role. Ninety-seven percent were familiar with bathhouse information on AIDS prevention. Despite this information, five percent reported receptive anal intercourse without a condom. The ten percent involved in anal intercourse without a condom[28] were significantly more likely than those who did not practice this highest risk sexual activity to be aged less than thirty, to be Hispanic, never to have attended college, to be earning less than $20,000 per year, and to have had five or more male sexual partners in the past month. Unfortunately, no data were obtained from monolingual Spanish-speaking men, who constituted five percent of the sampled population. If one can extrapolate from Los Angeles in 1986 to San Francisco in 1984,[29] it would seem that those who were not heeding the message of condom use were the segments of the population most difficult to reach *outside* the bathhouses. It would also seem that the small minority of bathgoers who continue to receive unprotected anal intercourse with multiple partners from a population which is more than half HIV-antibody positive are already infected, so that closing the baths would not afford them any protection.[30] Whether it would protect their sexual partners (including women for seven percent of those reporting anal intercourse without a condom) or would distribute unsafe sex more widely is not easy to predict or to measure.

Three years after closing the bathhouses and sex clubs, Silverman (1986:34; also see his similar secondary elaborations to Bayer and Fitzgerald) still could not point to any evidence establishing bathgoing as a risk factor. Like any good politician, he could, however, provide folksy non sequiters to make his policy sound plausible: (1) allowing bathhouses to continue to operate was like providing crop subsidies to tobacco growers at the same time public health education funds are spent to stop smoking, (2) "some people would feel that their civil liberties would be violated if we told them they could not have sex in a restaurant or a church" and (3) what gay leader would want to create the institution of the bathhouse if it didn't exist? Obviously, the first is not unthinkable, since it describes policies of the federal government. The second is a peculiar comparison, since banning sex in restaurants and churches would not interfere with the purposes people assemble in those settings. The third non sequiter, the hypothetical question Silverman posed to gay opponents is counter-factual, so the answer is irrelevant to public policy. One could as easily ask, "If there wasn't a bill of rights in the Constitution of the United States, would there be an impetus to amend the Constitution to add it in the 1980s or 90s?" Whatever the original purpose of social institutions, with the passage of time additional meanings attach to them. Gay bathhouses symbolized uncontrolled male promiscuity to some, a haven from violence and homophobia to others (see Weinberg and Williams 1975; Lee 1978; Styles 1979; Bérubé 1984), and the rights to privacy and freedom of assembly to others.[31]

The symbolic politics of Silverman's shifting or evolving policy (and Judge Wonder's modifications of it) attempted to balance competing demands of persons with markedly differing definitions of the situation. Verifiable medical facts were not necessarily of interest to those pressing any of these foci. If there had been compelling medical evidence, the director of public health had and has sweeping quarantine powers (Novick 1985). American courts have shown great reluctance to question official claims of "medical necessity" or "military necessary" (Murray 1987); this is perfectly exemplified by the judge's refusal to question the cogency of the health department case in *City of New York v. St. Marks Baths*).

As was mentioned above, the failure of neighboring counties to follow Silverman's precedent is prima facia evidence that the decision stemmed from local political considerations rather than overwhelming scientific evidence. Yet another indication of the essentially political motivation of the decision is the frequency with which Dr. Silverman referred to a public opinion poll published in the April 8 1984 *San Francisco Chronicle,* in which most respondents favored forcing the baths to close. As Brian Jones (1984: 6) commented, "When a doctor makes a decision because the voters favor it, that doctor is a politician" (see Perlstadt and Holmes 1987).

It is impossible to believe the bath closure was motivated by new scientific evidence rather than by political pressure.[32] There was no new clinical or epidemiological evidence to justify a change of policy, especially since doing so undercut the credibility of the thrust of the education campaign and its most visible proponent until then, Dr. Silverman himself. Even six years later, no link between bath-going and AIDS has been established, and the CDC has not listed bath-going as a risk factor. As for the slight increase of rectal gonorrhea in one quarter sensationalized by Shilts, no serious epidemiologist, statistician, nor experienced public health figure would have staked his or her credibility on so slight an increase indicating a trend back to earlier levels. The Public Health Department's own reports (McKusick et al. 1983, 1984; Werdeger et al. 1987) reported both information about medical opinion and changed behavior, including a 90 percent reduction in the number of gay San Francisco men "practicing receptive anal intercourse with nonsteady partners" between 1978 and 1985. The results could be interpreted as suggesting that more education was not going to lead to more change, although no one has publicly interpreted them that way.

No one knows whether the changes were "enough." Seroconversion had markedly slowed before the bath closure, and no changes in seroconversion trendlines nor in rates of rectal gonorrhea in San Francisco date from April or October 1984. San Francisco County epidemiologists whom I have asked where the effect of bath closure in these data might be have not claimed any.

The Promiscuity Model Extended to Heterosexuality

> If an intervention does not produce results, and yet is supported by officials and the public, one must look to secondary reasons to explain that support. The issue thus becomes not the desire to protect the public from hazard. . . Rather, these activities indicate a transformation from protection to punishment. —Brandt (1988: 165)

Just as AIDS has been used to rationalize traditional attempts to prevent homosexual behavior and close public institutions, it has been seized upon in the latest recurrence in a cyclical attempt to blame prostitutes for medical and/or moral problems of their clients (see Bullough 1976; Pivar 1973; Brandt 1985). The "nature" of prostitutes is to be promiscuous in serving a market, and transmission of sexually transmitted diseases is traditionally blamed on this "nature" rather than on that of their clients. The clients are generally viewed by the law and social opinion as tempted into sin. They are not viewed as being "by nature" promiscuous. Clients of prostitutes may infect their wives, but not the prostitutes — in this often-unconscious cosmology prostitutes are intrinsically diseased, and can never be "innocent victims" of infection by their customers. Given the apparent difficulty of female-male transmission of HIV, or whatever else may cause AIDS, focusing on prostitutes seems to be another instance of blaming the victims and thereby transforming "risk" in the sense of vulnerability to "risk" in the sense of threatening. Prostitutes have been regarded as being risks, not being at risk, although there is no "scientific evidence" implicating handling of money or having sex for money as vectors of AIDS transmission.

Genuinely professional prostitutes tend to protect themselves by using condoms and/or by substituting oral for vaginal intercourse. But it has not been established that even prostitutes who have AIDS or who harbor HIV constitute much of any danger to partners without lesions or cuts on their penises, even through unprotected vaginal intercourse. Moreover, a CDC(1987) study found prostitutes at no higher risk of developing AIDS than are other sexually active women. Similarly, prostitutes' HIV infection rates were comparable to the rates among all heterosexual women in the cities sampled (Barton et al. 1985; Brenky-Fadeux and Fribourg-Blanc 1985).

> Nevada has already tested all of the prostitutes in legal brothels. Over 4,500 tests were conducted on 500 women and not one was seropositive. Needless to say, this did not make the front page of the New York Times (Katy Taylor, Deputy Director of the New York City Commission on Civil Rights in Crimp 1988: 135).

The focus on promiscuity as the essence of prostitution led to overlooking or underplaying intravenous drug use among prostitutes. In San Francisco none of 146 prostitutes who did not use IV drugs tested seropositive (Cohen et al. 1987). Eight of ten seropositive Florida prostitutes were IV drug users (CDC 1985).

Among Africa prostitutes, whose existence has frequently been regarded as the explanation of heterosexual AIDS transmission (Clumeck et al. 1984; Van de Perre et al. 1985), intravenous drug abuse is little known. Kreiss et al. (1986) reported that none of their sample of 90 prostitutes used "recreational" drugs, but that all had a history of intramuscular injections.[33] The combination of popularity of injections for any and all medical problems in Africa and the reuse of often-unsterilized needles needs to be considered before explaining HIV infection among Africa prostitutes as sexually transmitted, especially since reuse of needles in STD clinics would seem to be an especially good way to move a virus from bloodstream to bloodstream of the sexually active—far more efficacious a route than from vaginas to penises.

Similar commitment to the paradigm of sexual transmission is evident in a report dealing with the Caribbean island of Hispaniola: Koenig et al. (1987) reported that "only one of 115 female Dominican prostitutes showed evidence of exposure to HIV. She is an IV drug user..." and ignored the latter factor to reaffirm promiscuity as the danger: "Many of the young people who live near the poverty line accept prostitution as a means of support. Efforts must be made to control this major method of transmission." It would seem that the decision about this "major" danger preceded the data collection and was unchanged either by negative findings (1/115) or by the presence of an alternative source of risk (the needle use of the one).

Interventions that look like "control" or "elimination" of prostitution are politically popular. For public health officials pressed to "do something, anything" about AIDS, prostitutes are inviting targets. In a worldview in which AIDS is caused by promiscuity, actions against prostitutes are easily rationalized. Considerations of statistical analysis, or empirical questions about the actual sexual practices of prostitutes, or due process for stigmatized populations are not as salient to the general public as the wish for demonstrations that the public health is being protected from those who are believed to be willfully endangering it. As generations of politicians both inside and outside public health have known, "crackdowns" on prostitution (and other forms of sexual "immorality") are popular, and are useful for distracting media and/or publics from criticism of officials' other shortcomings. Similarly, both legislation against and publicity about prostitutes who have tested positive in HIV antibody tests and continue to ply their trade fail to distinguish performing safe sex acts from unsafe ones:

> Since sex is not defined in these new laws creating harsher sentences, those who engage in activities such as manual stimulation and fantasy-oriented sex can also be charged with felonies. This scapegoating legislation sets a precedent for criminalizing erotic experience for anyone who is HIV-positive, even if the practices are 100 percent safe (Leigh 1988:181).

Legislation making it illegal for HIV-positive customers to have unprotected vaginal or anal intercourse with prostitutes somehow never follows. Prostitutes are morally contaminated in a way customers of prostitutes (a category which includes more than a few legislators) never are in American demonology. Husbands, sons, and fathers would be pure if it weren't for the corrupting influence of prostitutes, homosexuals, and drug suppliers in this long-running fantasy and American purity crusades are always aimed at the supply rather than at the demand for illicit pleasures (see Pivar 1973). Those who buy drugs or the services of prostitutes are viewed as weak, while those who sell drugs or sex accumulate all the evil to be apportioned.[34]

Moralistic Obstacles to Prevention Strategies

Traditional moralistic politicians seek to ensure that what they see as "sin" is punished on earth. Not just prostitutes and homosexuals, but anyone who ventures from the "path of righteousness" is "asking for trouble" and "deserves whatever they get." To take any public health actions to make it safer to engage in pre- or extra-marital sex or in drug use is opposed as "condoning immorality" and interfering with the "natural punishments" (unwanted pregnancy, sexually transmitted diseases, drug overdoses, hepatitis, AIDS, degradation and, preferably, grisly death) which should deter all right-thinking and -acting people in this "one nation under God."

Condoms

For instance, seeming to condone "sexual immorality" (of which birth control is a significant part in the view of many Americans) is dangerous to careers in the intensely politicized domains of law enforcement and public health. Campaigns to promote greater condom usage by prostitutes (or anyone else) are not politically feasible in the United States. Instead, condoms are routinely confiscated as "physical evidence" when prostitutes are arrested, and no accommodation to the reality of the demand for the service of "the oldest profession" can pass unnoticed by Christian moral entrepreneurs.

Attempts to extirpate any information about condoms—along with censoring any specific acknowledgement of sex outside marriage—from publicly financed AIDS education have been widely reported in mass media. Educational material has been recurrently censored by those who find any depiction of sexuality offensive and likely to encourage sex. Within the Reagan administration, Secretary of Education Williams piously counseled chastity, while the surgeon general pressed for information on condoms, surmising that Americans—in particular, young Americans—are not going to remain chaste until a cure for AIDS is found. The secretary of communications for the U.S. Catholic Conference of Bishops objected to condom advertisements specifically because "such ads might promote 'safe sex,'" while Joseph Cardinal Bernardin of Chicago reiterated that although the immediate aim of such advertising might be "good — the prevention of disease" it is unacceptable because it "questions the normativeness of heterosexual marriage as the proper context for sexual intimacy, or artificially separates the love-making and life-making dimension of marital intimacy" in the institution which cannot be questioned, heterosexual marriage (Hirsley 1988:A17). Avoiding even implicit questioning of heterosexual marriage (and information about a form of birth control within it) suffices to justify attempts to suppress the exercise of the constitutionally guaranteed right of free speech in a state constitutionally separated from the directives of any church. "Medical necessity" is an accepted rationale for intervening in the lives of stigmatized populations in the United States, but is insufficient for any initiatives which might offend the religious feelings of sex-negative Christian churches by advertising the existence or increasing the availability of prophylactics. This is a social fact. The result of subordinating the concern for effective outreach to those most at risk of HIV transmission to avoiding anything which might offend someone with the moral susceptibilities of Senator Helms's rhetoric is that

> not a single piece of government-sponsored education about AIDS for young people in Canada or in the U.S. has been targeted at a gay audience. . . Government officials, school board members, public health officials, Catholic cardinals insist that AIDS education must be sensitive to "community values." But the values they have in mind are those of no existing community affected by AIDS. When "community values" are invoked, it is only for the purpose of imposing the purported values of those (thus far) unaffected by AIDS on the people (thus far) most affected (Crimp 1988: 270, 265).

Needles

AIDS has also been used to reinforce condemnation of drug users—at least low status users of street drugs. As of mid-1987 28 percent of U.S. AIDS patients were IV drug users. After a restudy of 1982–86 drug-related deaths in New York City, the Department of Health concluded that "AIDS-related deaths involving intravenous drug users accounted for 53 percent of all AIDS-related deaths in New York City since the epidemic began [sic.: was recognized], while deaths involving sexually active homosexual and bisexual men accounted for 38 percent" (*New York Times*, 22 Oct. 1987, p. B1). In New Jersey, where IVDUs account for 53 percent of diagnosed cases, the mean time between diagnosis and death is only 18 days, a statistic which in itself indicates that lack of contact between IVDUs and medical services (and education). Watters, Iura and Iura (1987) found that 90 percent of San Francisco IVDUs continue to share needles. The average needle-user shared needles with thirty-seven different people a year.

In order to combat needle sharing, some public health officials proposed needle exchange programs, such as those underway in Great Britain, Australia, and the Netherlands. As with condoms, making shooting heroin safer is an unpalatable tactic even to liberal politicians. San Francisco Mayor Dianne Feinstein delivered her opinion that "it is a terrible and truly offensive idea which would put the health department in the position of aiding and abetting drug addiction" (*San Francisco Chronicle*, 26 July 1986).

Routine testing

If condoms and clean needles were used, transmission of HIV or whatever agent in the blood causes AIDS could probably be blocked at relatively low costs. Supposed fiscal conservatives claim that avoiding the costs of big government (especially in cases where the costs can be privatized) is one of their major concerns. Avoiding even the appearance of "condoning" private behavior of consenting adults apparently is more important than saving tax dollars or than doing anything effective in AIDS education, however, because money is appropriated for mass HIV testing. In advocating HIV testing as a routine part of marriage application, President Reagan claimed that his reason was to measure the scope of HIV's spread through the population (*New York Times*, 1 June 1987). An interest in accurate numbers is spectacularly out of character for Ronald Reagan, whose administration attempted to dismantle a wide range of longitudinal data sets. Moreover, if the interest were genuine, such a self-selected sample would provide a biased estimate. Routine testing for death certificates would provide far more useful data without affecting life chances, but apparently no one in the federal government is interested in finding evidence of HIV-infection in "reputable" members of the president's own generation. Rather, marital testing is aimed at the young and at distinguishing possible "deviants."[35]

The rationale for military testing is just as specious: the battlefield transfusions which the Department of Defense maintained they were protecting hardly ever occur. Blood volume expanders have superceded the technology of transfusions, as the National Academy of Science (1986: 122) report noted. As Mohr (1988:179–81) suggests, the HIV antibody test is another in a long line of indicators seized upon by the American military to distinguish possible homosexuals (and secret drug users): "Knowing a soldier's antibody status will not help the army to take better care of him. The paternalistic argument is wholly bogus. In no other area is the army suddenly concerned with the better care of its personnel."

The sudden concern for the health of prison inmates — at the same time that nothing is done to curb prison rape or to reclassify condoms from being contraband in prisons — is similarly suspect. Then U. S. Attorney General Edwin Meese recommended to federal and state parole boards that a positive HIV antibody test be considered a reason not to parole prisoners, who gravitate to child care positions (*New York Times* 9 June 1987)! We find it difficult to believe that ex-cons gravitate to child care or that they would be permitted to take jobs in that sector if they sought them. Although it appears to us that this incredible concern was a passing attempt to increase parental anxiety about day care facilities (and, thus, directly part of the administration's promotion of "traditional" families), no questions about it were raised when the news was reported.

In all these instances, the President, Secretary of Defense, and Attorney General of the United States did not even bother to concoct remotely plausible rationales for costly testing. The rationales given are transparently unrelated to the needs for epidemiological information or to protecting military personnel, prisoners, or anyone else who tests positive. It is more difficult to establish what their real motivation is, but it certainly appears likely that their aim is to ferret out and punish "secret deviants." Suitable sacrifices reaffirm the moral order, according to Durkheim and Foucault. In this case, the death of "deserving" cases may deter experimentation with drugs or sexual adventures. An "innocent"/"deserving" distinction is at least implicit in the Reagan administration's approach: IV drug users and male homosexuals in the late 1970s and early 1980s should have known of the risks of a yet-to-be-identified disease; unborn babies and those receiving transfusions could not. The moral status of those born black in Haiti or central Africa is not exactly clear in this theodicy, nor is it clear why "God's punishment" of homosexuality passed over those who engage in female-female sex.

Conclusion

In public health thought (discourse), AIDS was immediately added to the class of exotic diseases transmitted by promiscuous sex. Although promiscuous needle use and heterosexual "promiscuity" now supplement homosexuality within the paradigm of immoral excess, the explanatory model persists among medical researchers at least in accounting for transmission of a virus believed to be the cause of AIDS, and for many non-scientists as the "real cause." Because a syndrome was initially identified among gay men, it was obvious to medical researchers that whatever it was must be sexually transmitted. The preference for a sexual explanation persisted, obstructing consideration of drug use by those already "explained" as "homosexuals." Between mid-1983 and late-1986, the anomaly to this explanation posed by the existence of heterosexual Haitian and African cases was avoided by assuming the Haitians were lying and the Africans were engaging in heterosexual anal intercourse (and were also probably lying). There was never any evidence that Haitians or Haitian-American men are more likely than men of other origins to conceal homosexual behavior when suffering from fatal diseases. There is no evidence that central Africans are more likely to engage in heterosexual anal intercourse than are North Americans. (Questions about how, when, and by whom exclusively heterosexual male African AIDS cases were anally penetrated were also begged by the extension of the anal explanatory model).

In addition to homosexuality, beginning in 1984, another "sexual deviance," prostitution, was medicalized to account for AIDS—with no attention to prostitutes' drug habits, or even to their sexual habits. Again, "being a prostitute" rather than behavior was the focus of attention. Given the apparent difficulty of female-to-male sexual transmission, this broader conception of "promiscuity" does not explain aetiology, but reinforces attempts to condemn and eliminate extra-marital sex. A focus on prostitutes is certainly consistent with the CDC taste (paradigm) for multiple-partner sexual transmission as an explanation of whatever they can't explain without the help of emotional reactions to "immorality." In American epidemiological work in central Africa, other avenues (razors and needles used for tattooing, knives used for circumcision, and the common reuse of needles in Western-style hospitals in Africa) to bloodstreams (especially male ones) are not explored, while questions about visits to prostitutes and the number of sexual partners are a source of seemingly endless fascination.

The commitment to the inadequate sexual transmission theory derives from more fundamental features of American medicine than the homophobia and erotophobia of some clinicians and researchers. As has been widely noted, American doctors prefer to deal with acute diseases amenable to capital-intensive, high-tech remedies involving considerable control over patients. No such remedies are available for AIDS. A disease that kills previously healthy men in their twenties and thirties is both personally and professionally distressing. It is even a threat to the reputation of medicine in American society. We believe that doctors need to explain AIDS away as "their own fault," quite apart from pre-existing hostility to homosexuality, prostitution, and recreational drug use, or of contempt for drug users and prostitutes. The sexual transmission of AIDS has been used by opportunistic politicians (inside and outside public health) to legitimate reinstituting prohibitions of homosexual acts that are exceedingly unlikely to transmit the AIDS virus (e.g., fellatio, see Winkelstein et al. 1987b: 323). Under the guise of public health, homosexuality *en toto* has been remedicalized, and new extensions of social control of sexually active adults are proposed daily to protect a "public health" in which the "public" is only a righteous elect.

Notes

1. The "client" for American medicine includes the state as well as patients and families of patients.

2. An instance of possibly direct importance for federal government epidemiologists was the congressional inquiries about the failure to establish the cause of "legionnaire's fever": see Culliton (1976). Despite the label of a "lifestyle choice" in the name, legionnaires were not considered a menace, and their deaths were not seen as divine punishment for conventioneering in Philadelphia. Perhaps, the briefness of the outbreak spared those who died from being blamed for their illnesses.

3. For compelling analysis of sensationalism of the promiscuity paradigm to fit conventional prejudices within mass media coverage of AIDS, see Albert (1984 et seq.), Crimp (1988), and Gilman (1988:245–72). The focus of the present paper is on the conceptions, selective attention, and actions of public health professionals and organizations.

4. In 1987 New York City Department of Health reexamined 1982–86 drug-related deaths and classified many as AIDS-related, but did not extend the analysis to the late 1970s "junkie pneumonia" (Crimp 1988: 249, n11).

5. The set of labels used before the consensus on "AIDS" was achieved are listed in Murray and Payne (1988). It bears noting that GRID (gay-related immunodeficiency) was not a locution used (at least in print) by epidemiologists. It was used in the gay press, and in a clinical abstract by the discoverer of AIDS (Gottleib 1982). An interesting contrast is the mysterious series of deaths still known as "legionnaire's fever."

6. The subtext of much scientific and most popular AIDS discourse is that gay men went shopping outside conventional morality and acquired a syndrome, like acquiring a leather jacket. Presumably a celibate nun (or a monogamous, heterosexual man) injected with blood containing HIV in the 1970s was no more choosing to acquire a syndrome of infections than was a man exposed to HIV at the same time while engaging in homosexual activity, yet transfusion cases (along with children born with congenital syndromes of immunodeficiency) are often presented as "innocent victims," although there is no difference in the ignorance about the existence and risks of AIDS, and, therefore, no difference in the degree of agenthood in running the risks.

7. To avoid potential misunderstandings, we do not question that viruses, including the putative AIDS-causing virus, HIV, can be transmitted during anal intercourse. Direct transmission to the bloodstream, however, not sexual orientation nor even the number of sexual partners in itself (i.e., independent of the sexual behavior engaged in), is salient. Exposure to HIV or something else co-occurring with HIV (if HIV-infection is an indicator rather than the cause of AIDS) appears to be a necessary but insufficient condition for damage to immune functioning (see Duesberg 1987, 1988; Levy and Ziegler 1983; and "the need for a virus" section below).

8. The general public conflates cause with transmission. Some of the difficulty health and school officials have had in convincing parents that pupils with AIDS going to school with their children do not constitute a threat to their children can be attributed to the dissemination of the hepatitis analogy. This equation did not originate among the masses!

9. See Shilts 1987 on the official claims of adequate funding.

10. Bayley et al. (1985: 360) and Rodriquez et al. (1985:1099) provide the most compelling evidence)

11. "It actively infects only 1 in 10^4 to $>10^5$ T cells. Under these conditions HIV cannot account for the loss of T cells, even if all infected cells die, because during the two days it takes HIV to replicate, the body regenerates about 5% of its T cells, more than enough to compensate for losses due to HIV" (Duesberg 1988: 514).

12. As one anonymous referee noted, "Research on the relationship between drug use and AIDS has continued to be hampered by moralistic focus on 'street' drugs."

13. Hessol et al. (1988) found statistically significant correlations between the progression of HIV infection to AIDS and earlier use of hallucinogens and of tranquilizers, cautioning that the correlation might be because use of these drugs is an indicator of a lifestyle of indiscriminate mixtures of recreational drugs rather than any direct effects of the specific substances.

14. Canadian and French cases linked to Haiti are not included. Detailed secondary analysis of Haitian-linked AIDS cases is contained in Murray and Payne (1989).

15. Frequency of listings in gay guidebooks is highly correlated with U.S.-Caribbean island air travel (Murray 1988b).

16. There are questions on travel to or sex with persons native to Haiti and Zaire within the previous two years in the CDC's current Multi-Area Cohort Study (MACS) questionnaire (except for West Coast cities). No rates of positive response to this question have been published. Data on the most recent two years can hardly be expected to bear on behavior prior to 1981, or indeed on Human Immunodeficient Virus (HIV) infection, given the official estimate of a 7.8 year mean incubation period it (Lui, Darrow and Rutherford 1988).

17. See the critique of the sensationalism and ficitionalizations in Shilts (1987) by Crimp (1988: 238–49). In particular, Crimp shows how the unsubstantiated portrait of Patient Zero is made of the genre conventions of a villain seeking to destroy the innocent and the stereotype of uncontrolled homosexual male promsicuity. It was this story based on conventional American demonology that was serialized in newspapers across America and on "60 Minutes." With this focus, purporting to be "the facts" about how AIDS came to California (or America in some versions), the portrait of federal government unconcern and inaction in the book was ignored. Gaetan Dugan, not Ronald Reagan or the Department of Health Services in his administration could be blamed for the spread of AIDS. Leaving aside questions about the basis for Shilts's knowledge of what Dugan thought about whether

Kaposi's sarcoma was contagious, the time between his sexual contacts and the appearance of opportunistic infections regarded as AIDS was too short to be consistent with the current model of HIV incubation into AIDS (Moss 1988).

18. In contrast Schultz et al. (1984: 296) reported a 59% drop in rates of rectal gonorrhea in Manhattan — from 485 per hundred thousand in 1980 to 201 in 1983.

19. Bayer (1989:43) had access to the communication of the findings of no distinct risk factor to Dr. Silverman from the principal CDC epidemiologist working on AIDS, William Darrow. The existence of this finding was reported in the April 1984 *Coming Up!* Bayer also reports that Silverman and his deputy for communicable diseases, Dean Echenberg, complained about the finding to Darrow's superiors at CDC. It is extremely difficult to imagine data showing sex clubs were a risk factor for AIDS being suppressed in an administration signally insensitive to the gay community and to civil liberties. Not issuing a report exonerating gay institutions is far more in character for the Reagan administration, its Department of Health and Human Services et al.

20. As they had left the state, the case did not go to trial. In earlier years as a homophile activist in the Society for Individual Rights, Littlejohn participated in challenging medical authority and pushing the American Psychiatric Association to remove homosexuality from the list of mental illnesses.

21. It seems that Littlejohn, Matlovich, and Shilts chose the battleline and did not attempt to see if anyone would "pay attention" to educational programs. I have heard allegations that there was another sense of no one paying attention to these men in the bathhouses that undergirded their "revenge" (see Hippler 1989:87).

22. Shilts (1987:436–41), who can be taken as an accurate reporter of the views and machinations of the Milk Club clique, details the "squeeze play" of telling gay leaders that Silverman would close the baths and Silverman that there was community support and its failure when an open meeting showed that Shilts's friends had been misrepresenting a consensus that did not exist.

23. Traditionally, clubs requiring membership have been called "private member clubs" rather than "public places." Bayer (1989) who is ostensibly concerned with the boundaries of private and public does not question the semantic sleight in Feinstein, Silverman et al. relexifying private assembly as "public" because such establishments are licensed by the county. It should be obvious that the county also issues marriage licenses without claiming that this provides a basis for regulating conduct within **that** institution. Building codes, public recording of deeds, etc. involve the state in homes, so that "public concern" has precedent there (as well as in hotels, a locale which the

New York Health Commissioner included within the bounds of his AIDS policy jurisdiction). The analogy of seatbelt laws and motorcycle helmet requirements is less apt in that governments build and maintain roads in addition to licensing drivers (besides which the clear medical evidence about motorcycle helmets has only intermittently led to the state protecting persons from conduct dangerous to their health and costly to the public). I can also report from personal experience that smoking was still permitted in meetings within the Department of Public Health at the time.

24. The relevance of "commercial" in this is unclear (see note 6 above). It might also be observed that the overwhelming majority of acts observed in these places were not and have not been proven dangerous. Of course, the whole safe/unsafe distinction so carefully nurtured by the Department of Public Health in San Francisco prior to 9 April 1984 was abandoned in the blanket proscription of sex in gay clubs.

25. It cannot be assumed that the sex reported by the bath sample occurred exclusively in the baths. Perhaps owing to the professional bias of psychologists for constructing personality patterns, no attempt was made to distinguish how many sex partners bathgoers had sex with in the baths from how many outside. The cherished notion of the promiscuous personality, of course, undercuts the rationale for government interference with the operations of the specific institution of the baths. Since at the time the questionnaire was prepared and distributed the official public health view was that if the baths were closed, gay men would go elsewhere, the explanation for this failure might be historical rather than occupational, i.e., the authors did not anticipate that their results would be used to justify a policy shift.

26. The persistence with which promiscuity was attacked as the problem, continuing despite the gradual shift in epidemiological discourse from number of sexual partners to particular behaviors as the mechanism of transmission (see Darrow, Jaffe and Curran 1983 for the most important statement of this revision) did not bolster confidence in "authoritative" public health pronouncements (see Murray and Payne 1989). McKusick et al. (1983:19–20) betrayed none of their informants' uncertainty about which "safe sex" policy to adopt. They were, thus, able to distinguish those (30 percent) "who have responded appropriately in terms of eliminating contact with the infective agent" (which had not at that point been identified, let alone shown to be in any particular bodily substance) and the "alarming number" (62 percent) "still engaging in high-risk behavior which, according to current [and notably unstable]epidemiological thinking [which was undergoing a paradigm shift at the time] has not removed them from danger of infection." The other eight percent so appalled McKusick et al. that they were not discussed. McKusick et al.'s key to "appropriate adaptation" is clear in their rhetoric of overcoming the "resistance" to commit to a primary relationship: doctors have prescribed monogamy; uncompliant masses have resisted.

27. In the 13 July 1984 *MMWR* (p. 377) slightly different preliminary figures from the San Francisco City Clinic Study were available: 25 percent (of 48) in 1980 to 65 percent (of 215) in 1984. This latter figure was used as the best estimate of HIV-infection among sexually active gay men in deliberations by Silverman and other San Francisco physicians concerned with AIDS (personal communication from a BAPHR member), although it is now regarded as an overestimate due to the biased basis for recruitment into the study (cf. Winkelstein et al. 1987).

28. This figure includes insertive as well as receptive; thirty of eighty-four reported both roles in the same night.

29. At least some justification for such an extrapolation is the earlier heightened visibility of AIDS and AIDS prevention efforts in San Francisco, including the bathhouse closure controversy. Also, the Winkelstein et al. (1987a) data from San Francisco census tracts show a similar (to the Los Angeles bathgoer sample) proportion of the gay population continuing to engage in anal intercourse without a condom.

30. Bayer (1989:61) quotes a 9 October 1985 memorandum from Director of the New York City Office of Epidemiological Surveillance and Statistics Alan Kristal to Health Commissioner David Sencer which says, "The prevalence of infection in the sexually active gay population is already so high that the environment from which one selects sexual partners has little relevance."

31. Silverman (1986:33) also asserted that six months after the bath closure "mail from the gay community was over 60 percent in favor of closing the bathhouses." Just how many letters he was receiving at that point is not specified. It would be surprising if there were large numbers of letters suggesting re-opening the bathhouses. The civil rights precedent was already set, although Silverman has continued to fail to understand a distinction between admiration for the bathhouses and opposition to state interference in constitutionally-guaranteed rights.

32. The same is true for the actions of the Health Commissioner of the State of New York in October 1985. David Axelrod claimed to change the state's policy on the basis of "new evidence" rather than political pressure (New York Times, 25 October 1985, p. B3). One can hardly expect public health officials explicitly to state that they are subordinating their professional judgement to political demands.

33. "[African] patients often express a strong preference for parenteral rather than oral therapy... belie[ving] that parenteral medication is more effective... As with injections, patient expectations and medical overuse of blood transfusion may contribute to the potential spread of HIV" (Quinn et al. 1986: 959).

34. Except when one's own son or daughter or brother or sister is implicated. An analogous widespread fantasy exists in which seduction is necessary to explain homosexuality, which then becomes irresistable, so that heterosexuality cannot compete in a free market.

35. To claims that the intent might be to protect unsuspecting women (who are presumed not to have had sexual intercourse with the men they are applying to marry), Richard Mohr (1988: 180) noted, "The legal institution of marriage is shot through with regulations, legal commitments, binding obligations, and risks affecting major life components about which the partners typically know nothing and about which, indeed, they are socially and legally encouraged to stay in ignorance."

References

(Note: For articles with more than four authors, only the first is listed)

Albert, Edward H. 1984. "AIDS and the press." Society for the Study of Social Problems meetings, San Antonio.

Altema, Reynald and Leslie Bright 1983. "Only Homosexual Haitians, Not all Haitians." *Annals of Internal Medicine* 99: 877–78.

Altman, Dennis 1986. *AIDS in the Mind of America.* Garden City, N.J.: Doubleday.

Altman, Lawrence K. 1983. "Debate Grows on U.S. Listing of Haitians in AIDS Category." *The New York Times* 31 July, pp. 1,18.

Astor, Gerald 1983. *The Disease Detectives.* New York: New American Library.

Barre-Sinoussi, F. et al. 1983 "Isolation of a T Lymphotropic Retrovirus from a Patient at Risk for AIDS." *Science* 220: 868–70.

Barton, S.E. et al. 1985. "HTLV-III Antibody in Prostitutes." *Lancet* 8469:1424.

Bayer, Ronald 1989. *Private Acts, Social Consequences.* New York: Free Press.

Bayley, A.C. et al. 1985. "HTLV-III Serology Distinguishes Atypical and Endemic Kaposi's Sarcoma in Africa." *Lancet* 1: 359–61.

Bell, Alan and Martin Weinberg 1978. *Homosexualities.* New York: Simon & Schuster.

Bérubé, Alan 1984. "The History of Gay Bathhouses." *Coming Up!* 6, 3: 15–19.

Boncy, Madeleine et al. 1983. "AIDS in Haitians." *New England Journal of Medicine* 308: 1419–20.

Bosk, Charles L. 1979. *Forgive and Remember: Managing Medical Failure.* Chicago: University of Chicago Press.

Bourguignon, Erika 1976. *Possession.* San Francisco: Chandler & Sharp.

Brandt, Allen M. 1985. *No Magic Bullets.* New York: Oxford University Press.

——— 1988. "AIDS: From Social History to Social Policy." Pp.146–70 in E. Fee & D. Fox (eds.) *AIDS: The Burden of History.* Berkeley: University of California Press.

Brenky-Fadeux, D. and A. Fribourg-Blanc 1985. "HTLV-III Antibody in Prostitutes. " *Lancet* 8469: 1424.

Bullough, Vern L. 1974. "Homosexuality and the Medical Model." *Journal of Homosexuality* 1:99–110.

——— 1976. *Sexual Variance.* Boston: Wiley.

Carrier, Joseph M. 1975. *Urban Mexican Male Homosexual Encounters.* Ph.D. dissertation, University of California, Irvine.

———. 1976. "Cultural Factors Affecting Urban Mexican Male Homosexual Behavior." *Archives of Sexual Behavior* 5: 103–24.

Centers for Disease Control 1981a "Pneumocystis Pneumonia — Los Angeles." *Morbidity and Mortality Weekly Reports* 30: 250–52.

———1981b. "Kaposi's Sarcoma and Pneumocystis Pneumonia among Homosexual Men - New York City." *Morbidity and Mortatilty Weekly Reports* 30: 305–08.

———1985. "Heterosexual Transmissionof HTLV-III/ LAV." *Morbidity and Mortality Weekly Reports* 34: 561–63.

Clumeck, N. et al. 1984. "AIDS in African Patients." *New England Journal of Medicine* 31.: 492–97.

Cohen, Judith B. et al. 1987. "Prevalence of HIV Antibody among Prostitutes in the San Francisco Bay Area." *San Francisco Epidemiology Bulletin* 3,4: 14–15.

Connor, Steve and Sharon Kingman 1988. *The Search for the Virus.* New York: Penguin.

Conrad, Peter and Joseph W. Schneider 1980. *Medicalization and Deviance.* New York: Mosby.

Crimp, Douglas 1988. *AIDS: Cultural Analysis, Cultural Activism.* Cambridge, MA: MIT Press.

Culliton, Barbara J. 1976. "Legion Fever: Postmortem of an Investigation that Failed." *Science* 194:1025–27.

d'Adesky, Anne-Christine. 1986. "Haiti: the Great AIDS cover-up." *New York Native* 14 April. 15–17.

Davis, Wade. 1986. *The Serpent and the Rainbow.* New York: Simon & Schuster.

Duesberg, Peter H. 1987. "Retroviruses as Carcinogens and Pathogens." *Cancer Research* 47: 199–1220.

——— 1988. "HIV is Not the Cause of AIDS." *Science* 241:514–17.

Fettner, Ann G. 1986. "A Place to Die and a Drink of Water." *New York Native* 157 21 April.: 22–26.

Fischl, Margaret A. and Gordon M. Dickinson 1984. "AIDS among Haitians." *Transactions of the New York Academy of Science* 437: 352–53.

Fitzgerald, Francis 1986 "The Castro." *New Yorker* (28 July).

Fleck, Ludwig 1979 [1935]. *The Genesis of a Scientific Fact.* Chicago: University of Chicago Press.

Foucault, Michel 1980. *Power/Knowledge.* New York: Pantheon.

Fox, Renée C. and Judith P. Swazey 1978. *The Courage to Fail.* Chicago: University of Chicago Press.

Fry, Peter 1987. "Male Homosexuality and Afro-Brazilian Possession Cults." Pp. 55–91 in S. Murray ed., *Male Homosexuality in Central and South America.* New York: Gay Academic Union.

Galliher, John F. and John H. Cross 1983. *Moral Legislation Without Morality.* New Brunswick, NJ: Rutgers University Press.

Gilman, Sander L. 1988. *Disease and Representation.* Ithaca, NY: Cornell University Press.

Good, Byron J. 1977. "'The Heart of What's the Matter': The Semantics of Illness in Iran." *Culture, Medicine & Psychiatry* 1: 25–58.

Goodfield, June 1982. *Science and the Public.* Washington: National Academy of Science.

Gottlieb, Michael S. et al. 1982. "GRID." *Clinical Research* 30:349A.

Herskovits, Melville J. 1937a. *Life in a Haitian Valley*. New York: Knopf.

———. 1937b. "African Gods and Catholic Saints in New World Negro Belief." *American Anthropologist* 39: 635–43.

Hessoll, Nancy A.et al. 1987. "The Natural History of HIV-Infection in a Cohort of Homosexual and Bisexual Men." Paper presented at the International AIDS Congress in Washington, D.C.

——— 1988. "Cofactors for Progression of HIV Infection in a Cohort of Homosexual and Bisexual Men." Paper presented at the International Conference on AIDS in Stockholm.

Hippler, Mike 1989. *Matlovich*. Boston: Alyson.

Hirsley, Michael 1988. "Catholics Oppose TV Condom Ads." *San Francisco Examiner* and Chronicle (9 October): A17.

Humphreys, Laud 1975. *Tearoom Trade*. Chicago: Aldine.

Jones, Brian 1984. "The Doctor and the Gay Pols." *Bay Area Reporter* 14,15: 6.

Kayal, Philip M. 1985. "'Morals,' Medicine and the AIDS Epidemic." *Journal of Religion and Health* 24: 218–38.

Kitsuse, John I. and Malcolm Spector 1973. "Toward a Sociology of Social Problems." *Social Problems* 20:407–19.

Kleinman, Arthur 1980. *Patients and Healers in the Context of Culture*. Berkeley: University of California Press.

Koch, Robert 1890. *Ueber Bakteriologische Forschung*. Berlin: Verlag von August Hirschwald.

Koenig, R.E. et al. 1987. "Prevalence of Antibodies to HIV in Dominicans and Haitians in the Dominican Republic." *Journal of the American Medical Association* 257: 631–34.

Kreiss, Joan K. et al. 1986. "AIDS Virus Infection in Nairobi Prostitutes." *New England Journal of Medicine* 314: 414–18.

Krieger, Terry and Cesar A. Caceres 1985. "70% of AIDS Patients Have Been Drug Abusers." *National Coalition of Gay STD Services Newsletter* 7,2: 53.

Kuhn, Thomas S. 1962. *The Structure of Scientific Revolutions*. Chicago: University of Chicago Press.

——— 1977. *The Essential Tension*. Chicago: University of Chicago Press.

Landes, Ruth 1940. "A Cult Matriarchate and Male Homosexuality." *Journal of Abnormal and Social Psychology* 35: 386–97.

Landesman, Sheldon A. 1983. "The Haitian Connection." Pp. 28–37 in Kevin Cahill ed., *The AIDS Epidemic*. New York: St. Martin's Press..

Lauritsen, John 1985. "CDC's Tables Obscure AIDS/Drug Connection. *Coming Up!* 6,7: 6–18.

Lee, John Alan 1978. *Getting Sex*. Toronto: General.

Leigh, Carol 1988. "Further Violation of Our Rights." Pp. 177–82 in Douglas Crimp ed., *AIDS: Cultural Analaysis, Cultural Activism*. Cambridge, MA: MIT Press.

Lemp, George F. et al. 1990. "Projections of AIDS Morbidity and Mortality in San Francisco." *Journal of the American Medical Association* 263:1497–1501.

Leonidas, Jean-Robert and Nicole Hyppolite 1983. "Haiti and AIDS." *Annals of Internal Medicine* 98:1020–21.

Lessor, Roberta and Katarin Jurich. 1985. "Ideology and Politics in the Control of Contagion: the Social Organization of AIDS Care." Society for the Study of Social Problems meeting, Washington, D.C.

Levine, Martin P. and Richard Troiden 1988. "The Myth of Sexual Compulsivity." *Journal of Sex Reseach* 25: 347–63.

Levy, J. A., and J. L. Ziegler 1983. "AIDS is an Opportunistic Infection and Kaposi's Sarcoma Results from Secondary Stimulation." *Lancet* 2: 78–81.

Lieberson, Jonathan 1986. "The Reality of AIDS." *New York Review of Books* 16 Jan. 43–48.

Lipton, Jack P. amd Alan M. Hershaft 1985. "On the Widespread Acceptance of Dubious Medical Findings." *Journal of Health and Social Behavior* 26: 336–51.

Lui, Kung-Jong, William W. Darrow and George W. Rutherford III 1988. "A Model-based Estimate of Mean Incubation Period for AIDS in Homosexual Men." *Science* 240:1333–35.

McCombie, S.C. 1986. "The Cultural Impact of 'the AIDS test.'" *Social Science and Medicine* 5:455–59.

McKusick, Leon, William Horstman and Arthur Carfagni 1983. *Report On Community Reactions to AIDS Survey*. San Francisco: Department of Public Health.

———1984 *Reactions to the AIDS Epidemic in Four Groups of San Francisco Gay Men*. San Francisco: Department of Public Health.

———1985 "AIDS and Sexual Behavior Reported by Gay Men in San Francisco.." *American Journal of Public Health* 75: 493–96.

McKinlay, John B. and Sonja M. McKinlay 1977. "The Questionable Contribution of Medical Measures to the Decline of Mortalities in the United States in the Twentieth Century." *Milbank Memorial Fund Quarterly* 55:405–28.

Merton, Robert K. 1968. *Social Theory and Social Structures.* New York: Free Press.

Métraux, Alfred. 1959. *Voodoo in Haiti.* New York: Oxford University Press.

Mohr, Richard D. 1987a. "Aids, Gays and State Coercion." *Bioethics* 1:35–50.

———1987b. "Policy, Ritual and Purity: Gays and Mandatory AIDS Testing." *Law Medicine and Health Care* 15: 178–85.

Moss, Andrew R. 1988. "Letter" *New York Review of Books*

Murray, Stephen O. 1979. "The Institutional Elaboration of a Quasi-Ethnic Community." *International Review of Modern Sociology* 9:165–78.

———1980a. "The Invisibility of Scientific Scorn." 198–202 in R. de Mille ed., *The Don Juan Papers.* Santa Barbara: Ross-Erikson.

——— 1980b. "Lexical and Institutional Elaboration: the 'Species Homosexual' in Guatemala." *Anthropological Linguistics* 22: 177–85.

——— 1984. *Social Theory, Homosexual Realities.* Gai Saber Monograph 3.

——— 1987a. *Male Homosexuality in Central and South America.* Gai Saber Monograph 5.

———1987b. "A Loaded Gun: Some Thoughts on American Concentration Camps and the AIDS Epidemic." *New York Native* (27 July): 15–17.

——— 1988a. "The San Francisco Gay community during the 1980s." Paper presented at the annual meetings of the American Anthroplogical Association in Phoenix.

——— 1988b. " The International Transmission of AIDS: A Case Study in the Failure of Organization Skepticism in Science." MS.

Murray, Stephen O. and Kenneth W. Payne. 1985. "The Remedicalization of Homophobia: 'Scientific Evidence' and the San Francisco Bathhouse Closure Decision." Paper presented at the annual meetings of the Society for the Study of Social Problems in Washington , D.C.

——— 1986. "The Political Semantics of AIDS." Paper presented at the annual meetings of the Society for the Study of Social Problems in New York City.

——— 1989. "The Social Classification of AIDS in American Epidemiology." *Medical Anthropology* 10:115–28.

Nachman, Steven R. 1986. "Haitians and AIDS in South Florida." Partially published in *Medical Anthropology Quarterly* 17:32–33.

National Academy of Science 1986. *Confronting AIDS*. Washington: National Academy Press.

Norman, Colin 1986. "Sex and Needles, Not Insects and Pigs, Spread AIDS in Florida Town." *Science* 234: 415–17.

Novick, Alvin 1985. "Quarantine and AIDS." *Connecticut Medicine* 49: 81–83.

Oppenheimer, Gerald M. 1988. "In the Eye of the Storm." 267–300 in E. Fee & D. Fox (eds.) *AIDS: The Burden of History*. Berkeley: University of California Press.

Payne, Kenneth W. and Stephen Risch. 1985. "The Politics of AIDS." *Science for the People* 16,5:17–24.

Perlstadt, Harry and Russell E. Holmes 1987. "The Role of Public Opinion Polling in Health Legislation." *American Journal of Public Health* 77: 612–614.

Pivar, David J. 1973. *Purity Crusades*. Westport, CT: Greenwood.

Quinn, Thomas C., Jonathan M. Mann, James W. Curran, and Peter Piot 1986. "Aids in Africa." *Science* 234: 955–63.

Reiss, Albert J. 1961. "Social Integration of 'Queers' and 'Peers.'" *Social Problems* 9:102–20.

Richwald, Gary A. et al. 1988. "Sexual Activites in Bathhouses in Los Angeles County." *Journal of Sex Research* 25: 169–80.

Rodriquez, L. et al. 1985. "Antibodies to HTLVIII/LAV among Aborginal Amazonian Indians in Venezuela." *Lancet* 2:1098–1100.

Ross, Michael W. 1984. "Psychosocial Factors to Admitting to Homosexuality in Sexually Transmitted Disease Clinics." *Sexually Transmitted Diseases* 12: 83–87.

Roth, Julius 1957. "Ritual and Magic in the Control of Contagion." *American Sociological Review* 22: 310–14.

Schultz, S., S. Friedman, A. Kristal and D. J. Sencer 1984. "Declining Rates of Rectal and Pharyngeal Gonorrhea among Males in New York City." *Morbidity and Mortality Weekly Report* 33:295–97.

Seale, John 1985. "How to Turn a Disease into VD." *New Scientist* 1461: 38–41.

Shilts, Randy 1987. *And the Band Played On.* New York: St. Martin's Press.

Silverman, Mervyn F. 1986. "Addressing Public Health Concerns of the City of San Francisco." Pp. 27–35 in M. Witt (ed.) *AIDS and Patient Mangement.* Owing Hill, MD: Rynd.

Simpson, George E. 1942. "Sexual and Familial Institutions in Northern Haiti." *American Anthropologist* 44: 655–74.

Sontag, Susan 1978. *Illness as a Metaphor.* New York: Farrar, Straus, Giroux.

Stelling, Joan and Rue Bucher. 1973. "Vocabularies of Realism in Professional Socialization." *Social Science and Medicine* 7: 661–75.

Strauss, Anselm, Shizuko Fagerhaugh, Barbard Suezek and Carolyn Wiener 1985. *Social Organization of Medical Work.* Chicago: University of Chicago Press.

Styles, Joseph 1979. "Insider/outsider: Researching the Gay Baths." *Urban Life* 8: 135–52.

Trauner, Joan B. 1978 "The Chinese as Medical Scapegoats in San Francisco, 1870–1905." *California History* 57: 70–87.

Van de Perre et al. 1985. "The Female Prostitute: a High Risk Group for HIV-III Infection in Central Africa." *Lancet* 8469: 524–26.

Vieira, Jeffrey et al. 1983. "AIDS in Haitians." *New England Journal of Medicine* 308: 125–29.

Watters, John K., Dena Midori Iura and Kelly Wakaye Iura 1987. *AIDS prevention and education services to intravenous drug users through the Midcity Consortium to Combat AIDS.* Sacramento: California Department of Alcohol and Drug Programs.

Weinberg, Martin S. and Colin J. Williams 1975. "Gay Baths and the Social Organization of Impersonal Sex." *Social Problems* 23: 124–36.

Weinberg, Thomas S. 1978. "On 'Doing' and 'Being' Gay." *Journal of Homosexuality* 4: 143–56.

Werdegar, David et al. 1987. "Self-reported Changes in Sexual Behaviors among Homosexual and Bisexual Men from the San Francisco City Clinic Cohort." *Morbidity and Mortality Weekly Report* 36: 171–173.

Winkelstein, Warren et al. 1987a. "Reduction in Human Immunodeficiency Transmission among Homosexual/bisexual men, 1982–86." *American Journal of Public Health* 76: 685–89.

——— 1987b. "Sexual Practices and Risk of Infection by the Human Immunodeficiency Virus." *Journal of the American Medical Association* 257: 321–25.

——— 1988. "Continued Decline in HIV Servoconversion Rates among Homosexual/bisexual Men." *American Journal of Public Health* 78:1472–74.

Zola, Irving K. 1972. "Medicine as an Institution of Social Control." *Sociological Review* 20:487–504.

DRUG FORUM, Vol. 6(1), 1977–78

THE SENSUOUS HIPPIE PART II: GAY/STRAIGHT DIFFERENCES IN REGARD TO DRUGS AND SEXUALITY

JOHN A. NEWMEYER, PH. D.
Epidemiologist
Haight-Ashbury Free Medical Clinics

ABSTRACT

This paper derives from an extensive questionnaire study of the sexual practices and drug use of a sample of clients of the Haight-Ashbury Free Medical Clinics in San Francisco, California. A separate paper described how the "junkie" and "nonjunkie" portions of this sample differed [1]; the present paper attempts a similar analysis of the "straight" and "gay" subsamples.

Heterosexual/Homosexual Patterns of Drug/Alcohol Use

An exhaustive survey of the literature unearthed very few studies dealing with heterosexual/homosexual patterns of drug or alcohol use. There were a few case studies of a nonrepresentative sort, and also a few studies which tested with generally negative results – the psychoanalytic notion that alcoholism is linked to repressed homosexuality. Cain in a study of forty alcoholics of varying ages, sexes, social classes, and ethnic backgrounds, concluded that "homosexuality occurs no more frequently among alcoholics than among nonalcoholics [2]." On the other hand, Greenberg (1973) found that the incidence of illicit drug use, mostly marijuana, was higher among his sample of eighty-six homosexual men than among a control group [3]. Greenberg's sample, generally a youthful, college-educated group, was obtained through homophile organizations – which may have given him a "drug-liberal" biased selection of the gay population. Saghir's sample of eighty-nine gay men was also drawn from homophile organizations, but was carefully matched with a sample of thirty-five *unmarried* straight men similar in distribution by age, race, and occupation [4].

He found that the incidence of excessive drinking among the gays was somewhat higher than among the straights, but that actual alcohol dependence was similarly low for both groups. However, a significantly higher proportion of the gays than of the straights admitted to the use of nonprescription drugs, mostly marijuana but also amphetamines, psychedelics, barbiturates, and amyl nitrite. The study of Bluestone et al of thirty-one adolescent homosexuals in a New York City prison concluded that imprisoned homosexuals have higher educational levels, better work histories, and less drug addiction than do other prisoners [5]. Finally, Springer's study of drug-dependent adolescents discerned no increase in homoerotic activity as a result of nonprescription drug use [6]: these drugs seemed actually to decrease sexual appetite and to redirect latent homoeroticism into the desexualized shared ecstatic union of the drug "high." It is clear that no conclusive answers are available to the question of whether or not a gay population uses drugs or alcohol more than a demographically similar straight population.

The present study's sample was obtained by approaching every third client on random days of operation of the Clinics' Medical Section, and on random days of operation of the Clinics' Drug Detoxification Section, during the Spring of 1974. A two-dollar incentive was provided, to minimize the refusal rate on what was after all a fairly extensive (137 item) questionnaire. By this means, some ninety-five completed forms were obtained. One item asked the client to characterize his present "choice of sexual partners" as "heterosexual," "bisexual," or "homosexual"; those making one of the latter two responses were classified, for the purposes of this study, as "gay."

The "gay" group consisted of nineteen males and eleven females. A similar sex ratio obtained in the "straight" group, with forty males and twenty-five females. The two groups were very similar in terms of age, the median for both being just over twenty-five years. Both groups were likewise similar in racial composition, with about three respondents in four being Caucasian. The gays, however, were rather better off in terms of occupation: a significantly higher proportion were employed, and of those employed, the gays had a higher proportion holding down middle-class jobs. (See Table 1.) This difference was noted for both sexes. In regard to years of education, though, only among females was a difference in favor of gays noted. Both the gay males and straight males had about a three-fifths proportion who had had at least some college.

Findings

Nothing much was found that would shed light on the etiology of a gay or a straight sexual style among the present sample. The gay males and straight males described the same median age of learning about masturbation, intercourse, pregnancy, menstruation, orgasm, and homosexuality; the gay and straight females were likewise similar in their age of learning about these issues.

Table 1. Occupation v. Sex-Orientation Group

	Straight Males	*Gay Males*	*Straight Females*	*Gay Females*
White-Collar	10	9	4	5
Blue-Collar	16	5	2	1
Unemployed	16	3	18	5

Our inquiries about the experience of various sexual activities turned up some interesting differences. Among males, there were of course certain activities that one group or the other favored because of their sexual orientation — but aside from these, the gay men were found to be more enthusiastic about (i.e., wished to experience for the first time, or wished to continue past experiences) masturbation, group nudity, group sex, and the use of dildos or other mechanical devices. The straight men were more enthusiastic about attending erotic films, spanking their partner, having sex with a prostitute, and accepting money for engaging in sex. The relative preferences among gay females were for group nudity, group sex, sex with an animal, having sex with a prostitute, committing adultery, transvestism, anal intercourse, spanking, being spanked, cunnilingus, and masturbation. In no respect — even those relating to heterosexual activity — were the straight women more "into" sexuality than their gay counterparts.

The inquiry into current sexual activity showed some remarkable trends. Naturally the gay group had had much more homosexual activity. But both the gay males and females matched their straight counterparts in the extent of heterosexual activity — which means our "gay" groups might better be termed "bisexual" groups. The gay men actually reported a lesser incidence of premature ejaculation during heterosexual intercourse than did the straight men, but the latter group claimed to have enjoyed recent heterosexual activity more. The gay men and particularly the gay women were more into masturbation than the straight men or women: they had started it earlier, enjoyed it more, and had engaged in it more during the past year.

It was fascinating to note that nearly three-quarters of the straight men reported having "accidently hurt their lover," while only one-half of the gay men reported thus. A slightly higher rating of "your own body's sensitivity as compared to others" was given by the gays, but the gay men also slightly exceeded the straight men in their preference for touching their partner rather than being touched.

The gay men's attitudes toward masturbation and (of course) toward homosexuality were significantly more favorable than the straight men's. The gay women exceeded the straight women in their favorability toward masturbation, "discipline"-type sex, women's sexual liberation, and homosexuality.

Thus the gays – and especially the gay women – showed a rather more libertarian attitude toward sexual activity in general.

A slightly higher proportion of the straight men than of the gay men reported having a steady sexual partner at present. However, those gay men who were involved with a steady partner reported a somewhat higher level of satisfaction with their situation. No such differences were noted among the women. Among both sexes, the gays reported somewhat greater satisfaction with their current sex lives in general (see Table 2). The gays of both sexes also appeared to be rather more active sexually, of late (see Table 3).

The group was asked, "How do you feel your knowledge of sex compares with that of your friends?" It was intriguing to note that the gay men significantly exceeded the straight men in claiming "more knowledge than others," while the reverse relationship was found among the gay and straight women.

LIFETIME USE OF DRUGS

The group was asked about their lifetime use of various drugs, their use of drugs during the last two months, and their use of drugs "to make sex better." In terms of claimed lifetime experience, the straight men spoke of more contact than the gay men with psychedelics, amphetamines, cocaine, heroin, and tobacco

Table 2. Enjoyment of Recent Sex v. Sex-Orientation Group

	Straight Males	*Gay Males*	*Straight Females*	*Gay Females*
"Pleasant"	27	12	19	8
"Neither Pleasant nor Unpleasant"	5	3	1	0
"Unpleasant" or "None"	5	0	1	0

Table 3. Frequency of Sexual Intercourse During Past Six Months v. Sex-Orientation Group

	Straight Males	*Gay Males*	*Straight Females*	*Gay Females*
Twice a week or oftener	22	10	17	8
Three to five times/month	6	4	4	1
Twice or less per month	11	4	4	1

The gay men exceeded the straights only in regard to amyl nitrite ("Poppers" act as short-term smooth-muscle dilators, and hence permit a rush of oxygen-rich blood to the brain through dilated blood vessels. The psychic "peak" thus obtained has an active, directed quality that is perhaps more consonant with the male than the female orgasm. This differential quality might in turn account for the observation [1] that gay men were the first to use amyl nitrite widely.) As for recent drug experience, psychedelics, barbiturates, and quaaludes were evidently more in current favor among the gay men, while only tobacco had a greater extent of claimed use among the straight men. The two types of men had a very similar pattern of use of drugs "to make sex better," although the gay men seemed to favor alcohol somewhat more. Among the women, all the differences were in favor of the gays. For nearly every drug, the gay women spoke of a more extensive lifetime use than did the straight women, and their recent use of marijuana, cocaine, alcohol, tobacco, amyl nitrite, and quaaludes was also higher than the straight women's. The gay women apparently were also more prone than the straight women to use psychedelics, cocaine, and amphetamines to enhance their sexual experience, and were more likely to say that their sex lives were better since they started using drugs. The query, "If you could do any drug of your choice or have sex with anyone of your choice, which would you do?" was answered overwhelmingly in favor of sex by the gay men and largely in favor of sex by the straight men and the straight women – but fully half of the gay women opted in favor of drugs, particularly cocaine (see Table 4). Nevertheless, all four groups were about fifty-fifty as regards enjoying sex "more while you are straight" or "more while you are high." And only the straight males claimed to any extent that "drugs increased your attraction to possible sexual partners."

About two-thirds of the gay males claimed that sexual contacts were "quite seldom" related to drug-using situations. This proportion dropped to one-third for the straight males and straight females, and to nearly zero for the gay females. (See Table 5.) A similar trend was noted in reply to the question, "In the evolution of your sexual behavior, have you found drugs helpful when trying something new?" (See Table 6.) The role drugs play in the sexuality of this particular group, therefore, seems to have a peculiar correlation: the more females

Table 4. Choice of "Sex With Anyone of Your Choice" or "Drug of Your Choice" v. Sex-Orientation Group

	Straight Males	*Gay Males*	*Straight Females*	*Gay Females*
Drug	8	1	6	5
Sex	31	15	13	5

Table 5. "How Often Are Sexual Contacts Related to Drug-Using Situations" v. Sex-Orientation Group

	Straight Males	*Gay Males*	*Straight Females*	*Gay Females*
"90% or more of the time"	12	2	2	3
"About 2/3 of the time"	4	1	7	4
"About 1/3 of the time"	10	3	6	2
"Quite seldom"	14	11	8	1

Table 6. "In the Evolution of Your Sexual Behavior, Have You Found Drugs Helpful When Trying Something New?" v. Sex-Orientation Group

	Straight Males	*Gay Males*	*Straight Females*	*Gay Females*
Yes	17	5	7	7
No	21	12	16	4

(from zero to two) involved in a pairing, the greater the likelihood that drugs will be involved!

It was fascinating to find that the majority of the gay females and one-third of the straight females reported having been raped. And fully six of the gay males – plus two of the straight males – claim themselves to have been raped. By contrast, the incidence of rape *reported to the police* in San Francisco is about 500/year, or only about one rape for every 160 females between fifteen and thirty.

These findings emphasize the notion that gay males must be discussed separately from gay females – at least, the gay males of this sample strike one as having active but separate enjoyment of both drugs and sex, while the gay females tended to combine the two types of enjoyment. Both gay groups seem active sexually (including heterosexually), seem happy with their sex lives, and are widely experienced and open to more experience. The early 1970's were a time of great improvement in the social consciousness of gays; perhaps this accounts for these observations among the gays of our sample. Or perhaps the age-group and city of residence of this group explains some of the above-noted findings.

The straight males appear to be somewhat less evolved in their attitudes and practices than do the other three groups. However, this group appears to be from a somewhat lower social-class background than the other groups, and this may account for most of the differences.

In general, conclusive answers regarding gay *v.* straight drug use must await studies which carefully control for all the major demographic variables: marital status, age, occupational status, education, size of city of residence, and ethnicity. Such studies should also separate the predominantly homosexual subgroup from the bisexual subgroup, and should also begin to examine differences in the style of use of certain drugs (amyl nitrite, alcohol, barbiturates) in gay and straight social milieux. Finally, it is probably best to select the sample from the population at large and then determine their sexual orientation, rather than to attempt to select separate gay and straight samples.

REFERENCES

1. G. R. Gay, et al., The Sensuous Hippie: I. Drug/Sex Practice in the Haight-Ashbury, *Drug Forum, 6:*1, pp. 27-47, 1977-78.
2. A. H. Cain, Homosexuality and Alcohol, *Sexology, 30,* pp. 296-298, 1963.
3. J. Greenberg, A Study of Male Homosexuals (Predominantly College Students), *Journal of the American College Health Association, 22:*1, pp. 56-60, October, 1973.
4. M. T. Saghir, et al., Homosexuality: III. Psychiatric Disorders and Disability in the Male Homosexual, *American Journal of Psychiatry, 126:*8, pp. 1079-1086, 1970.
5. H. Bluestone, E. P. O'Malley, and S. Connell, Homosexuals in Prison, *Corrective Psychiatry and Journal of Social Therapy, 12,* pp. 13-24, 1966.
6. A. Springer, Some Aspects of the Problem of Sexual Behavior of Drug-Dependent Adolescents, *Zeitschrift Nervenheilkunde, 31:*2, pp. 139-155, 1973.

Direct reprint requests to:

John A. Newmeyer, Ph.D.
Epidemiologist
Haight-Ashbury Free Medical Clinics
529 Clayton Street
San Francisco, California 94117

SEX DIFFERENCE AND MALE HOMOSEXUALITY IN FRENCH MEDICAL DISCOURSE, 1830–1930*

Robert A. Nye

Near the end of the nineteenth century, psychiatrists first began systematically to identify and describe a spectrum of sexual disorders they called "perversions." Around 1900, however, Frenchmen who imagined themselves the guardians of the public welfare believed themselves justified in singling out the perversion of male homosexuality as a particularly grave danger to the nation. In the words of the politician Ernest Charles, "If there is one vice or sickness especially repugnant to French mentality, to French morality, to French health, it is—to call things by their name—pederasty."[1] A public pronouncement of this kind would have been literally unthinkable only a few decades earlier, but, despite the fact that private homosexual activity was not illegal under the French penal code, a widespread consensus had emerged which held male homosexual behavior to be, at the very least, a symptom of profound individual pathology, and, at worst, a sign of imminent national collapse.

In this paper I hope to reconstruct the reasons male homosexuality reached this high level of public visibility by 1910, concentrating in particular on the role that medical language played in shaping its image. The layman Ernest Charles may have hesitated about whether to call "pederasty" a "vice" or a "sickness," but in characterizing it a threat to the "health" of the fatherland, he demonstrated a dependence on a medical discourse on sexual perversions shared by many of his contemporaries. This discourse was of relatively recent historical vintage. It linked together effeminacy and reproductive sterility in male homosexuals, and masculinity and sterility in lesbians—invoking a kind of elementary *inversion* of the "normal" qualities of each sex. I wish to focus here on the reasons such a linkage was made for males; but, as we shall later see, in the binary classificatory system that regulated sexual identity in that era, changes admitted on one side of the sex/gender spectrum entailed proportional changes on the "opposite" side.[2]

* A version of this paper was presented at the sixty-first annual meeting of the American Association for the History of Medicine, New Orleans, Louisiana, 5 May 1988.

[1] Ernest Charles, *La Grande Revue*, 25 July 1910.

[2] For a discussion of some of the implications of historical studies of sex/gender systems, see Joan W. Scott, "Gender: a useful category of historical analysis," *Amer. Hist. Rev.*, 1986, *91*: 1053–75.

Bull. Hist. Med., 1989, *63*: 32–51

The reciprocal dependence of the medical conceptions of male and female identities permits me to argue that "mannish" lesbians and "effeminate" homosexuals—the dominant images of the fin de siècle—were in part a product of the misogynous outlook of male doctors, who believed themselves obliged to defend ferociously the traditional system of sexual differentiation and all the social consequences that flowed from it.

In order fully to explain why the fin de siècle medical image of the homosexual was constructed the way it was, I will discuss the general biological context that shaped medical speculation about a spectrum of sexual types in the early nineteenth century and try to show where the place occupied after 1880 by "homosexuals" was usually located. I will then indicate how and why sexual preference for one's own sex was "pathologized" near the end of the century by psychiatrists and doctors of legal medicine. I hope to explain this development by discussing changes within French medicine, by analyzing cultural and social anxieties about the nation's geopolitical situation, and by considering the changing relations between the sexes. Finally, I hope to show that the acceptance and perpetuation of the medical image of male homosexuality owes much to early literary apologists for homosexuality, who uncritically adopted the discourse on the subject previously established by doctors.

It is certainly an exaggeration to say that "homosexuality" was *invented* in the fin de siècle. The word itself was of recent origin, to be sure, but there were a number of French words signifying male love—*sodomy* and *pederasty* chief among them—which may be traced to the Middle Ages. These and other words taken from *argot* were used, willy-nilly, in European legal, ecclesiastical, and medical texts to describe such behavior, to deplore it, and to outlaw it.[3] Considering the origin of these terms,[4] it is not surprising that in their earliest appearances in the French medical lexicon a tone of moral outrage took precedence over one of clinical detachment.[5] Later in the century, as urban vice squads made more vigorous efforts to repress "outrages to public decency," medical specialists attached to the police prefecture and to prisons took greater interest in "pederasts" as a type of sexual deviant.[6] It was roughly during the last quarter of the nineteenth century

[3] On "homosexualität," a neologism of the German literary figure K. M. Benkert, see the entry "Homosexualité" in Claude Courouve, *Vocabulaire de l'homosexualité masculine* (Paris: Payot, 1985), pp. 129–38. See the entries on "Pédéraste / Pédérastie," pp. 169–78; and "Sodomie / Sodomite," pp. 191–98. On the *argot* used to characterize homosexuals in the first half of the nineteenth century, see p. 24.

[4] On this point in general, see John Boswell, *Christianity, Social Tolerance, and Homosexuality: Gay People in Western Europe from the Beginning of the Christian Era to the Fourteenth Century* (Chicago, Illinois: University of Chicago Press, 1980). On the evolution of public perceptions of sodomy in seventeenth-century England, see B. R. Burg, *Sodomy and the Perception of Evil: English Sea Rovers in the Seventeenth-Century Caribbean* (New York: New York University Press, 1983), pp. 2–41.

[5] For instance, see the definition of "Pédérastie" by Pierre Reydellet, on the "eternal shame" of these seducers of young boys, in *Dictionnaire des sciences médicales*, 60 vols. (Paris: Panckoucke, 1812–22), 40: 44.

[6] See on this period, Pierre Hahn, *Nos Ancêtres les pervers: la vie des homosexuels sous le second empire* (Paris: Olivier Orban, 1979), pp. 41–50.

that psychiatric nosologies began systematically to incorporate the varieties of sexual deviance.[7] No one could perform this task better than the doctor, who, in the words of Jean-Paul Aron and Roger Kempf, was the "guardian and good Samaritan of the bourgeoisie, above all suspicion, [who could] speak of filth without getting himself dirty."[8] In the words of a turn-of-the-century psychiatrist: "Science purifies what it touches."[9]

The biological concepts that informed the medical outlook on human sexual variations in the nineteenth century may be briefly summarized. The human sexual economy was believed to function according to a quantitative model of energy flow in which "moderate" expenditures of (sexual) energy were most consonant with health and with reproductive fertility. Extreme expenditures of this energy (in masturbation or coitus) were regarded as pathological and as leading to impotence, sterility, or both. Low expenditures were *already* signs of morbidity, whether they were a product of inheritance or the result of previous excesses. The key concept in this model was the capacity to engender. Only "moderate" sexual function was believed to be consistent with healthy fertility; all forms of sexual activity departing from this reproductive ideal were consigned to the realm of the abnormal.[10] Thus, medical science imagined a spectrum of possible rates of sexual function varying from low rates (sexual indifference) to high rates (sexual excess) through a moderate range corresponding to normal sexual function. But scientists also believed they could plot other sexual characteristics on this spectrum, correlating them with rate of sexual function. Genital morphology, secondary sexual characteristics, and the typical "moral" features corresponding to each point on the spectrum were gradually included.

Until the 1880s this physiological spectrum of sexual variation was regarded as compatible with the classical system of anatomical teratology completed in 1837 by Isidore Geoffroy Saint-Hilaire which was widely cited through the century. It was Saint-Hilaire's aim in his four-volume compendium to identify the general laws of anatomical variation in the animal kingdom governing the "anomalies" and "monstrosities" observed in nature.[11] All departures from the "representative" (average) type of the species or

[7] Jacques Léonard discusses this era in depth in *La Médecine entre les pouvoirs et les savoirs: histoire intellectuelle et politique de la médecine française au XIXe siècle* (Paris: Aubier Montaigne, 1981).

[8] Jean-Paul Aron and Roger Kempf, "Triumphs and Tribulations of the Homosexual Discourse," in *Homosexualities and French Literature: Cultural Contexts, Critical Texts*, ed. George Stambolian and Elaine Marks (Ithaca, New York: Cornell University Press, 1979), p. 146.

[9] E. Marandon de Montyel, *Obsessions et vie sexuelle* (Evreux, France, n.d.), p. 291.

[10] See, in general, Georges Canguilhem, *Le Normal et le pathologique*, 3d ed. (Paris: P.U.F., 1975), esp. pp. 19–25, 34–40. On masturbation in particular, see Jean Stengers and Anne Van Neck, *Histoire d'une grande peur: la masturbation* (Brussels: Editions de l'université de Bruxelles, 1984).

[11] Isidore Geoffroy Saint-Hilaire, *Histoire générale et particulière des anomalies de l'organisation chez l'homme et les animaux, des monstruosités, des variétés et vices de conformation, ou traité de tératologie*, 4 vols. (Paris: J. B. Baillière, 1832–37), 1: 99. See also the discussion on monsters in Georges Canguilhem, *La Connaissance de la vie*, 2d ed. (Paris: Vrin, 1985), pp. 171–85.

race were the consequence, he argued, of an excess or deficit of development in the volume of an organ or organs, resulting in anomalous variations of size or number, or the displacement of parts in an organism.[12] In Saint-Hilaire's system the principal evidence for human sexual variation was located in genital morphology, the teratological sign par excellence of deviation from the "representative" sexual norm. By ordering the known genital anomalies of each sex in a rank corresponding to whether they were the product of an "arrested" or "excessive" embryological development, Saint-Hilaire hoped to provide doctors of legal medicine in particular with a descriptive, ontological, and phylogenetic scheme for resolving practical cases of sexual identity.[13]

Saint-Hilaire envisions a spectrum of sexual differentiation isomorphic with the spectrum for physiological function described above. Males are grouped on one side of the spectrum and females on the other. The portion in the middle is composed of "hermaphroditic" anomalies inclining to one half or the other, depending on their genital structure. Saint-Hilaire deals with several particularly knotty cases, but he decisively places them on either the "male" or the "female" portion of the spectrum, because, as he explains, to these "great classes belong not only different but nearly *inverse* functions in the family and in society. In that sense there are no intermediaries; our laws do not admit their existence or foresee their possibility."[14] Bisexuality, which he defined as the capacity to both impregnate and be fecundated, was therefore an actual and formal impossibility.

It is tempting to conclude here that this system of anatomical variation and sexual difference, as Saint-Hilaire's statement suggests, was predicated on the Napoleonic code; it took its marching orders, so to speak, from the civil obligations given doctors of legal medicine to establish the sex of individuals in disputes arising from marriage, paternity, inheritance, military service, or crime. In an article on "hermaphroditism" he published much later in the century, the physician Gabriel Tourdes wrote in nearly identical terms,

> The difference of sex establishes in all societies two categories of persons who dispose of different rights and duties; our laws do not admit the existence or even foresee the possibility of any intermediary condition. Sex determines not only civil status, but also the entire direction of life.[15]

The argument has been made recently, by Thomas Laqueur, Laura Schiebinger, and others, that an "anatomy and physiology of [sexual] incommensurability" was generated as a by-product of the era of the eighteenth-

[12] Saint-Hilaire, *Histoire générale*, 1: 116, 179.
[13] *Ibid.* (1836), 2: 33–44, esp. the chart on p. 36.
[14] *Ibid.* (1836), 3: 573. This and subsequent translations by author.
[15] Gabriel Tourdes, "Hermaphrodisme (Tératologie)" in *Dictionnaire encyclopédique des sciences médicales*, 4th ser. (Paris, 1888), 13: 643.

century bourgeois revolutions to replace the old "metaphysical" hierarchy those revolutions had destroyed.[16] This suggestion seems admirably suited to the French case, where, in the biology of sexual differentiation, it seems especially difficult to separate clearly the political and cultural from the scientific influences.

This anatomical and physiological hypostatization of sex difference, by clearly distinguishing the unique qualities of each sex, contributed to the construction of the "separate spheres" of public, productive (male) life and domestic, reproductive (female) life. In this system women were effectively restricted, by their natures, to the home and child-rearing, while men were guaranteed a monopoly of the great world beyond. But there were some unpleasant implications for males in such a system. Since genital morphology, secondary sexual features, fertility, and "moral" qualities were believed to be in correspondence with one another, the appearance of an atypical, nonmasculine feature on the body or in the behavior of a male served as a sign that his place on the spectrum of sexual variation was sliding toward the lower end of the male range; here, "female" features appeared in higher proportions as the "representative" male type approached the ambiguous, "hermophroditic" zone at the spectrum's center. Thus, impotence, sterility, effeminate behavior or tastes, feminine secondary sexual characters, or a "vice" in genital conformation were symptoms, in this system, of demasculinization. Individuals at the extreme or "hypermasculine" end of the spectrum displayed none of these qualities, but they faced the danger of an overexpenditure of sexual energy which could relocate them in the low end of the spectrum, where feeble sexual economies were the rule.

As the result of a number of developments in France after midcentury to which doctors and psychiatrists were particularly well suited to respond, the spectrum of sexual variation underwent some important changes. As I have argued elsewhere, rising rates of alcoholism, insanity, crime, syphilis, and other organic and social pathologies bred widespread fear among critics of culture and the political elite that *La grande nation* was in a state of irremediable *biological* decline.[17] Most industrializing societies experienced similar changes in vital signs in the era, but in France the situation was complicated by the weakened geopolitical status brought about by the German military victory of 1870.

French doctors adapted the medical concept of degeneration to an explanation of these symptoms of national decline and helped set in motion a number of programs designed to treat them. Of particular concern to

[16] These remarks are Thomas Laqueur's from "Orgasm, Generation, and the Politics of Reproductive Biology," in *The Making of the Modern Body: Sexuality and Society in the Nineteenth Century*, ed. Thomas Laqueur and Catherine Gallagher (Berkeley and Los Angeles: University of California Press, 1987), p. 2. This is also a point generally argued by Scott, "Gender," pp. 1070–75.

[17] I discuss these matters at length in *Crime, Madness, and Politics in Modern France: The Medical Concept of National Decline* (Princeton, New Jersey: Princeton University Press, 1984).

medical and scientific observers was the fact that the French birth rate was significantly lower than the birth rates of the surrounding industrial powers, in particular the newly unified German empire. There was also a disturbing decline in the ratio of male to female live births, from 107:100 in 1840 to 104:100 in 1900. These figures raised concern about depopulation and the "degeneration" of the French "race."[18] Doctors asked openly if there was a weakened masculine "will" to reproduce in France. And, since it was believed that males were desirable, and that male births depended on the sexual vigor and male identity of the father, then it was the duty of France's most masculine citizens to procreate.[19] Individual French couples were not adequately moved by the desire for offspring to sacrifice their own standard of living for the good of the nation, but the abundant rhetoric on repopulation, a vigorous campaign against birth control, and the consideration of eugenical measures designed to improve the quality, if not the quantity, of the population testify to the general cultural anxieties this desire provoked.[20]

These pressures for men to exercise their generative faculties for the good of the nation were building simultaneously with the appearance of a vigorous feminist movement demanding the vote for women and equal access to occupations, and with changes in the sexual behavior of women.[21] Men were being asked not only to dismantle their comfortable monopoly in the public domain, but to give greater sexual satisfaction to the women who were to be their future competitors. Such developments were bound to produce reassessments of traditional sex roles and identities. It is certainly no accident that one finds in fiction from George Sand through 1914 the image of weak men and strong women in great abundance, as though novelists, men and women alike, were testing in their fiction the social and psychological consequences of the new relationship between the sexes. A recent student of this fin de siècle literature, indicating the number of themes involving a husband's helpless resignation in the face of his wife's

[18] I discuss the statistics and the medical and social scientific response to the population issue, *ibid.*, pp. 135–44. On the hygienic and demographic literature, see Joseph Spengler, *France Faces Depopulation* (Durham, North Carolina: Duke University Press, 1938), pp. 135–74. On the search for the social and biological causes, see Nye, *Crime, Madness, and Politics*, pp. 132–70. See also René Worms, *La Sexualité dans les naissances françaises* (Paris: W. Giard et Brière, 1912), pp. 55–60.

[19] On the influence of masculine and feminine qualities on the sex of offspring and the medical literature and lore on this subject, see J. C. Bénard, "Fille ou garçon à volonté: un aspect du discours médical au 19e siècle," *Ethnologie française*, 1981, *11:* 63–76.

[20] See, on these issues, Francis Ronsin, *La Grève des ventres: propagande néo-malthusienne et baisse de la natalité française (XIX–XX siècles)* (Paris: Aubier Montaigne, 1980); William Schneider, "Toward the improvement of the human race: the history of eugenics in France," *J. Modern Hist.*, 1982, *54:* 268–91.

[21] Laure Adler has surveyed the nineteenth-century marriage manuals in *Secrets d'alcove: histoire du couple de 1830 à 1930* (Paris: Hachette, 1983), pp. 67–99. On feminism and the associated medical implications, see Angus McLaren, *Sexuality and Social Order: The Debate over the Fertility of Women Workers in France, 1770–1920* (London: Holmes and Meier, 1983); Karen Offen, "Depopulation, nationalism, and feminism in fin-de-siècle France," *Amer. Hist. Rev.*, 1984, *89:* 648–76. Steven C. Hause and Anne R. Kenney, *Women's Suffrage and Social Politics in the French Third Republic* (Princeton, New Jersey: Princeton University Press, 1984).

adultery or flight, concluded, "With the emancipation of women, something has been refused males which seemed so much constitutive of their identity that they felt themselves totally rejected as men."[22]

Since they were already occupied with the elaboration of a medical explanation of national decline which included a variety of inherited and acquired pathologies, it was perfectly logical for doctors to consider these new developments within this frame of reference. It should not surprise us that they perceived them to be different manifestations of a single pathology, namely, a diminution or redistribution of the vital sexual energy required to guarantee both (traditional) sexual identity and reproductive fertility in men and women. Encouraged in this outlook by the profoundly conservative fears of French society, doctors sought to reaffirm the traditional sexual identities of both sexes and ground them more strongly than ever in "normal" reproductive fertility.

In practice this medical effort to undergird traditional sexual difference meant that doctors identified the types of sexual behavior which departed from the model of heterosexual reproduction and incorporated them into a new psychiatric nosology of abnormal sexual deviance. They thus helped to construct a new medical discourse of perversions which transformed sexual *behavior* into sexual *identities*, or, in Michel Foucault's terms, sought to locate sexual abnormalities "to strew reality with them and incorporate them into the individual."[23]

This was a task essentially for psychiatrists and doctors of legal medicine, who, among medical practitioners, most frequently encountered the varieties of human sexual behavior in their work. These specialists relied heavily on the old tradition of teratological classification, but they were also interested in the most recent biological findings on human fertilization, and on the evolution of sex. These findings more or less agreed with their own socially conservative agenda: sexual reproduction was "superior" to evolutionarily antecedent and more primitive forms of reproduction such as simple fission or hermaphrodism; sexual reproduction depended in the higher animals on a highly distinctive sexual dimorphism, on highly aggressive reproductive behavior in the male, and on coyly passive behavior in the female.[24] It is important to note here that most of the psychiatrists who were

[22] The quotation is from Annelise Mauge, *L'Identité masculine en crise au tournant du siècle, 1871–1914* (Paris: Rivages, 1987), p. 103; see also Isabelle de Courtivron, "Weak Men and Fatal Women: The Sand Image," in Stambolian and Marks, eds., *Homosexualities and French Literature*, pp. 210–27. Carroll Smith-Rosenberg discusses some of the scholarly literature on these themes in literary modernism in "The New Woman as Androgyne: Social Disorder and Gender Crisis, 1870–1936," in her book *Disorderly Conduct: Visions of Gender in Victorian America* (New York: Oxford University Press, 1985), pp. 287–88.

[23] Michel Foucault, *The History of Sexuality*, 4 vols. (New York: Vintage, 1980), 1: 44.

[24] See Maurice Caullery, *Les Problèmes de la sexualité* (Paris: Alcan, 1913), *passim*; L. Tillier, *L'Instinct sexuel chez l'homme et chez les animaux* (Paris: Doin, 1889); André Cresson, *L'Espèce et son serviteur (sexualité, moralité)* (Paris: Alcan, 1913); Alfred Fouillée, "La Psychologie des sexes," *Revue des Deux Mondes*, 1 September 1893, pp. 397–429; *idem*, "Le Tempérament physique et moral d'après la biologie contemporaine," *ibid.*, 15 July 1893, p. 292.

busy dividing up the world into sex-specific behavior and illnesses probably regarded themselves as political progressives engaged in a Republican crusade against monarchy, the church, and superstition. By identifying and treating individuals, mostly women, who were afflicted with "reactionary" religious delusions or who displayed hysterical symptoms of religious zeal, they acted in a politically correct manner but also gave expression to their own misogynous impulses and those of the society around them.[25]

Until the mid-1880s the old anatomical taxonomies of sexual type held sway. The decisive benchmarks for evaluation of male sexual identity were the "typicality" of the genitals, secondary sexual characters, and, most tellingly, functional potency with a normally constituted member of the "opposite" sex. A man who did not possess a full complement of these features felt "wounded in his pride, . . . degraded; he [found] it difficult to dwell on his infirmity; his intellect and moral qualities [were] alter[ed], and his equilibrium [was] broken."[26] As we have seen, in the outlook of mid-nineteenth-century medicine, unmanly sentiments were associated with so-called hermaphrodites, eunuchs, or men afflicted by gynecomasty, hypospadias, cryptorchidism, or some other form of physical abnormality.[27] When male homosexuals entered the orbit of the medical cosmology in the 1880s, they were naturally integrated into this anatomico-physiological framework and located near hermaphrodites somewhere on the lower end of the spectrum of male gender identity, where masculine features merged insensibly into feminine ones and where, of course, their immediate neighbors were "masculine" women.

The energy flow charts and equilibrium models constructed earlier in the century continued in service in the fin de siècle; sexual energy was still a finite resource and its overexpenditure a disaster for the organism. But in the new organicist psychiatry of the era, dominated as it was by the model of degenerative inheritance, rates of vital function which were too high or too low were also a disaster for the species (read "race"). *Perversion* was the term which eventually emerged to characterize the excesses or deficits of sexual expenditure which departed from "normal" reproductive activity, so the spectrum of the normal and the pathological was still composed of infinite variations measured in quantitative terms, despite the invention of a

[25] On the anti-clerical aspects of this development, see Jan Goldstein, "The hysteria diagnosis and the politics of anti-clericalism in late nineteenth-century France," *J. Modern Hist.*, 1982, *54:* 209–39.

[26] Paul Moreau, *Des abérrations du sens génésique* (Paris: A. Helm, 1880), p. 81.

[27] For an analysis of the consequences of these deficiencies in the Old Regime, see Pierre Darmon, *Le Tribunal de l'impuissance: virilité et défaillances conjugales dans l'ancienne France* (Paris: Seuil, 1979), and the preface of Dominique Fernandez to the eighteenth-century *Traité des eunuques* of Charles Ancillon (Paris: Ramsay, 1978). For typical medical reaction to a "hermaphrodite," see the large number of medical commentaries from the late 1860s gathered by Michel Foucault relative to the case of Herculine Barbin, in *Herculine Barbin, dite Alexina B.* (Paris: Gallimard, 1978), pp. 135–56. For late nineteenth-century medical reactions, see Jean Borie, *Le Célibataire français* (Paris: Le Sagittaire, 1976); Pierre Garnier, *La Stérilité humaine et l'hermaphrodisme* (Paris: Georges Carré, 1894).

new nosological semiology of apparently qualitative type.[28] However, it was now admitted that a normal equilibrium was rare enough that, in the words of Eugene Gley, "Every man has, in effect, some weak point in his mind or body, and there is no such thing as an *absolutely* normal condition for the one or the other."[29]

Within the framework of these general developments there was an evolution over the period from medical characterizations stressing the anatomical features of homosexuals to those placing more weight on their psychology. In 1857 the physician Ambroise Tardieu claimed in his *Étude médico-légale sur les attentats aux moeurs* that the pederasts picked up by the Paris vice squad possessed penises shaped like those of dogs, and their passive partners the soft and rounded contours of women.[30] Because the "active" and "passive" modes corresponded to received ideas about sexual attraction, Tardieu and some of the first commentators on pederasty insisted that the "active" pederasts were wholly masculine in nature.[31] By 1880, however, the view that the "males" in the typical pederastic couple were anatomically distinctive was decisively challenged;[32] the masculine features of the active partner disappeared with his doglike penis, since it was now held that merely engaging in such behavior "made the most solid types effeminate and gave rise to cowardice."[33] These are the first indications of the growing tendency to equate homosexuality with effeminacy and "unmasculine" behavior.

Until the 1880s French doctors seem to have preferred the term *pederasty* to refer to homosexual acts, despite the fact that such usage involved a considerable narrowing of meaning from earlier centuries.[34] This term continued in use, particularly in medico-legal circles, for a while longer, and

[28] Georges Lantéri-Laura, *Lecture des perversions: histoire de leur appropriation médicale* (Paris: Masson, 1978). I must disagree here with Lantéri-Laura (especially his pp. 26–29), who wishes to see sexual perversions as qualitative, not quantitative, disorders. I think he is taking the signs of degenerate semiotics too seriously as signifying particular syndromes with autonomous states, though psychiatrists warned against doing this. See Jean-Martin Charcot and Valentin Magnan, "Inversion du sens génitale," *Archives de neurologie*, November 1882, *4:* 320.

[29] Eugene Gley, "Les Abérrations de l'instinct sexuel," *Revue Philosophique*, 1884, *17:* 92.

[30] Ambroise Tardieu, *Étude médico-légale sur les attentats aux moeurs* (Paris, 1857). On Tardieu, see also Jean-Paul Aron and Roger Kempf, *Le Bourgeoisie, le sexe et l'honneur* (Paris: Editions Complexe, 1985), pp. 45–87; and Hahn, *Nos Ancêtres les pervers*, pp. 65–70. In this era there was literally no word for the passive partners of what the doctors called pederasts.

[31] M. Masbrenier, "Pédérastie et assassinat," *Annales d'hygiène publique et de médecine légale*, 3d ser., 1879, *1:* 254–56. In Germany around the same time the forensic physician Johann Ludwig Casper was publishing similar views on pederasty. See *Klinische Novellen zur gerichtlichen Medicin: Nach eignen Erfahrungen* (Berlin: A. Hirschwald, 1863).

[32] Paul Brouardel, "Étude critique sur la valeur des signes attribués à la pédérastie," *Annales d'hygiène publique et de médecine légale*, 3d ser., 1880, *4:* 182–89.

[33] F. Carlier, *Les Deux Prostitutions (1860–70)* (Paris: Dentu, 1887), p. 276.

[34] Claude Courouve demonstrates that until the end of the eighteenth century *pederasty* did not refer strictly to sexual relations, but was used in a number of more general senses, including the "amour des garçons." *Vocabulaire de l'homosexualité*, pp. 170–72. The term *sodomy* all but disappeared from the medical vocabulary because the act was decriminalized during the Revolution and did not figure in the Napoleonic code.

seemed able to incorporate convincingly the newest psychiatric findings.[35] However, following Carl Westphal's important article on the "contrary sexual instinct" in 1870, psychiatrists gradually developed new terminology, which enabled them to introduce the phenomenon into the domain of mental illness.[36]

The first French text in this development was the 1882 paper by two of the most influential psychiatrists of the era, Jean-Martin Charcot and Valentin Magnan, on the "inversion of the genital sense." Here, Charcot and Magnan treated inversion as a weakening or "perversion" of the affective faculties which produced a "strange order of ideas" giving rise to a genital appetite for the same sex.[37] But inversion was not, in their account, an illness sui generis; rather, it was one of a host of other fetishistic attachments, such as obsession with nightcaps, aprons, or shoe nails, which, in the case of inversion, had fixed on a person of the same sex. Apart from the occasional reference to unusual genital conformations, Charcot and Magnan had taken a decisive step away from the earlier generation's faith in anatomical signs. They did not break with a constitutional analysis, however, because this degenerative disorder could be inherited from an ascendant, or could be provoked by masturbation or "vicious excess," which by "weakening" the "natural" instincts opened the door to obsessive ideas.[38] They not only preserved the link between inversion and the quantitative model of sexual excesses and deficits but extended this link to the whole culture by suggesting that sexual inversion was one of the "degrading consequences of a weakening of morals in a profoundly vitiated society."[39]

The primary themes developed by Charcot and Magnan were preserved and elaborated in the major French sexological texts through the 1930s. The appearance of homosexual love and a number of other forms of nonreproductive sexuality was treated as a tragedy for individuals and as a moral tale of grave consequence for France. This critique assumed its characteristic form in Alfred Binet's important article "Fetishism in Love" (1887). Binet, a student of Charcot's, modernized Etienne Esquirol's old category of erotomania for the new organicist medicine. All love, he argued, was to some extent fetishistic, for how else could we account for the odd pairings one observed between ugly and beautiful individuals? But in some predisposed beings, a kind of "hypertrophy" in the "normal level" of genital excitement occurs, and, often by accident, the full attention of the erotic

[35] Alexander Lacassagne refers frequently to "inversion" and "psychic hermaphrodism" as typical qualities of pederasts in his article "Pédérastie," *Dictionnaire encyclopédique des sciences médicales*, 2d ser. (Paris, 1886), 22: 239–59.

[36] Carl Westphal, "Die conträre Sexualempfindung: Symptom eines neuropathischen (psychopathischen) Zustandes," *Archiv für Psychiatrie*, 1870, *2:* 73–108.

[37] Jean-Martin Charcot and Valentin Magnan, "Inversion du sens génitale," *Archives de neurologie*, January 1882, *3:* 53–54.

[38] *Ibid.*, pp. 54–57; Charcot and Magnan, "Inversion du sens génitale" (November 1882), pp. 297–98.

[39] Charcot and Magnan, "Inversion du sens génitale" (January 1882), p. 54.

impulses is focused on a single feature or object. This "exaggerated" and "pathological" behavior was a true "perversion" of the sexual instinct.[40] The bewildering variety of forms assumed by fetishistic attachments ought not to confuse us, because it is the "perversion itself which is the characteristic fact."[41] The very appearance of these multiple obsessions is the consequence of the unique need

> so frequent in our epoch, to augment the causes of excitation and pleasure. Both history and physiology teach us that these are the marks of enfeeblement and decadence. The individual does not look for strong excitations with such avidity but when his power of reaction is already in a weakened state.[42]

Eventually this "love against nature" produces "an impotence of psychic origins," so that the fetishist is unable to reproduce, which is "entirely logical, because most often these sick individuals are degenerates and the ordinary consequence of degenerescence is sterility."[43]

This analysis was used by psychiatrists to account for any instance where love assumed exaggerated forms: necrophilia, bestiality, masochism, sadism, and exhibitionism, among others.[44] Though the sheer variety of so many objects of sexual desire was a troubling symptom of general cultural disorder, the "hypertrophy of normal love"[45] in fetishistic attachments was particularly worrisome because, as Charles Féré, another student of Charcot's, put it, "The sexual preoccupations [of individuals] are often in inverse ratio to their sexual powers. Nations that perish through sterility are remarkable for licentiousness."[46]

What Féré and other French sexologists of the era were describing was the disruption of a healthy balance between "natural" and "cerebral" passions. The strongest natural drive in the "normal" organism was to engage in reproductive sexual relations with a member of the "opposite" sex. Normally, this drive relentlessly overrode or ignored obstacles separating it from its innate aim, but when the drive was sufficiently depleted, through its own excessive activity or through a congenital weakness, the mind assumed, by default, the power to deflect the organism in abnormal directions.[47] The

[40] Alfred Binet, "Le Fétichisme dans l'amour, étude de psychologie morbide," *Revue Philosophique*, 1887, *24:* 143–44. His words are that fetishism is "pathologique, c'est à dire exagérée" (p. 143).

[41] *Ibid.*, p. 165.

[42] *Ibid.*, p. 166.

[43] *Ibid.*

[44] See Emile Laurent, *L'Amour morbide: étude de psychologie pathologique*, 3d ed. (Paris, 1895), pp. 154–230; also Benjamin Ball, *La Folie érotique* (Paris: J. B. Baillière, 1888), pp. 82–84, 116–24, 130–39, 140–48; see also Paul-Emile Garnier, *Les Fétichistes, pervertis, et invertis sexuels: observations médico-légale* (Paris: J. B. Baillière, 1896), *passim.*

[45] Laurent, *L'Amour morbide*, p. ii.

[46] Charles Féré, *The Evolution and Dissolution of the Sexual Instinct*, 2d ed. rev. (Paris: Charles Carrington, 1904), p. 31.

[47] Variations of this argument are frequent in the medical literature. See Ludovic Dugas, "L'Inversion sexuelle," *Archives de l'anthropologie criminelle*, 1895, *10:* 327; Georges Saint-Paul (pseud. Dr. Laupts), *Perversion et perversités sexuelles: une enquête médicale sur l'inversion* (Paris: Georges Carré, 1896), pp. 202–5;

supreme irony of this development is that psychiatrists believed it affected men more readily than women. In the evolutionary perspective of the era, men were more advanced than women, who represented a case of "arrested" embryological development.[48] The male's superior intellect and capacity to reason, a strength in the struggle for survival, was a liability in love. In the words of Julien Chevalier, women are more instinctive, and so "resemble one another in love, while men, more conscious, more cerebral, love in a particular and personal fashion. This is, in the end one of the reasons for the instinct's fragility insofar as complexity is synonymous with instability."[49]

Judging by the space devoted to it in medical discourse on male sexuality, inversion was regarded as one of the most common and certainly one of the most dangerous of the aforementioned perversions of the sexual instinct. Whether it was considered to be innate or acquired, inversion was most commonly treated as a fetish: "homosexual fetishism," in Pierre Garnier's words,[50] or, in the view of Georges Saint-Paul, an exaggeration of the normal sentiment of male friendship in morbid guise.[51]

However, the most interesting aspect of the medical perspective on inversion at the end of the nineteenth century is its characterization of homosexual desire as a pallid version of "normal" love, not a simple inversion of heterosexual love grafted onto instincts of normal power. A homosexual was born a homosexual not because he possessed an *innate* attraction for his own sex, but because his weakened vital force and tepid genital instincts left him in a state of relative sexual indifference, and therefore prey, as we have seen, to "cerebral passions" which might produce "monstrous attachments." We hear in this an echo of the old teratological formula for hermaphrodites and eunuchs, whose sexual instincts were believed to be exceedingly weak.

As we have also seen, the sine qua non of masculine sexual identity was the capacity for "normal" reproductive fertility. Doctors therefore denied to inverts, and for that matter to all fetishists whose orgasms were dependent

---

Moreau, *Des abérrations du sens génésique*, p. 172; E. Marandon de Montyel, *Obsessions et vie sexuelle*, pp. 250–91; Laurent, *L'Amour morbide*, p. 11; Garnier, *Les Fétichistes*, pp. 18–19.

[48] On the influence of this evolutionary perspective in conceptually organizing gender roles, see Victor J. Seidler, "Reason, Desire, and Male Sexuality," in *The Cultural Construction of Sexuality*, ed. Pat Caplan (London: Tavistock, 1987), pp. 82–112.

[49] Julien Chevalier, *L'Inversion sexuelle: une maladie de la personnalité* (Lyons: Storck, 1893), pp. 414–15. Féré makes a similar point more explicitly in arguing that the appearance of sexual pathologies is a sign of a "dissolution" (reversal) of a generally progressive biological evolution: *Evolution and Dissolution of the Sexual Instinct*, pp. 41–44.

[50] Garnier, *Les Fétichistes*, p. 22. The use of the words *homosexuality* and *homosexual* became popular only in the 1890s; these words never challenged the primacy of *inversion* and *invert* before 1914. Of German provenance (homosexualität), the term was used alongside *inversion* frequently in the medical literature and seems to have been favored over the better-established term by sexual reformers well disposed to the cause of the acceptance of homosexuality (Magnus Hirschfeld, André Raffalovitch). See "Homosexualité / Homosexual" in Courouve, *Vocabulaire de l'homosexualité*, pp. 129–38.

[51] Saint-Paul, *Perversion*, pp. 20–31.

on abnormal sexual stratagems or objects, the capacity for true potency. Their interest in sex was considerably under the average;[52] their orgasms, when they experienced them at all, were troubled by hyperesthesia or "irritable weakness."[53] Because of the unusual demands it made on their sexual economies, coitus with a woman caused inverts to suffer a profound exhaustion that often endured for several weeks.[54] Finally, in the most extreme cases, or as a consequence of a progressive degeneration, the invert assumed a wholly passive or oral attitude in sexual relations, experienced little pleasure, enjoyed no orgasm.[55] Thus, homosexual love was practically a contradiction in terms; when it could be sustained at all, it was often "platonic" or consisted of mutual caresses leading nowhere in particular.[56]

As noted above, the anatomical spectrum of sexual identity had posited a direct relationship between "normal" potency, genital conformation, and secondary and behavioral sexual characteristics. Inverts, with their weak genital drives, were thus presumed in advance to be effeminate in appearance, in manner, and in taste, so the appearance of any of these features was set down as clinical evidence for the condition. Many doctors acknowledged that episodes of homosexual behavior in youthful sex-segregated situations, if temporary, did not automatically provoke effeminization in its participants.[57] But any appearance of feminine qualities in adult males was a universally recognized sign of a congenital or acquired sexual disorder, of which inversion was the most common type.

Though doctors frequently praised the "feminine" qualities of steadfastness, sensibility, and tenderness in women, they presented these same features in men in the most negative way imaginable, revealing the savage misogyny that undergirded the conservative medical perspective on sex and gender. Effeminate men were held to be "timid,"[58] "wicked and pusillanimous,"[59] or to be "lacking a grandeur of mind and spirit [and therefore] incapable of vast enterprises or of spontaneous expressions of courage and

[52] Henri Legludic, *Notes et observations de médecine légale: attentats aux moeurs* (Paris: Masson, 1896), pp. 224–25; Louis Reuss, "Des abérrations du sens génésique chez l'homme," *Annales d'hygiène publique et de médecine légale*, 3d ser., 1886, *16*: 311; Garnier, *Les Fétichistes*, pp. 144–45; Chevalier, *Inversion sexuelle*, p. 343.

[53] Louis Thoinot, *Attentats aux moeurs et perversions du sens génital* (Paris: Doin, 1898), p. 308; Féré, *Evolution and Dissolution of the Sexual Instinct*, p. 191.

[54] Thoinot, *Attentats aux moeurs*, p. 312.

[55] Antoine Luyt, *Les Fellatores* (Paris, 1885), p. 43; Paul Brouardel wrote of passive pederasts in 1880 that to the extent they lacked the normal "ardor" of the male, "they undergo rather than provoke the genital activity in which they participate" ("Étude critique," p. 189). In *L'Inversion sexuelle*, Chevalier writes that "active" pederasts become, by degrees, "passive" ones, and descend finally to "oral onanism, the last stage of depravity and the termination of all genital potency" (p. 173).

[56] Chevalier, *L'Inversion sexuelle*, p. 377. Smith-Rosenberg has noted similar material in the medical literature on lesbianism: "New Woman as Androgyne," p. 275.

[57] Chevalier, *L'Inversion sexuelle*, pp. 203–21; Saint-Paul, *Perversion*, pp. 30, 78–79; Dugas, "L'Inversion," pp. 328–29.

[58] Dugas, "L'Inversion," p. 330.

[59] Emile Laurent, *Les Bissexués, gynecomastes et hermaphrodites* (Paris: Georges Carré, 1894), p. 103.

devotion."[60] Louis Thoinot deplored their vanity, their tendency to gossip and commit "indiscretions,"[61] and Julien Chevalier found them "capricious, envious, and vindictive" and given to lying, men for whom "writing an anonymous letter is the most exact expression of their courage."[62] Since such beings were an "homme incomplet, femme manqué," in a formula of Emile Laurent's,[63] a true invert was "capricious, vain, cowardly, envious, vindictive, susceptible, uniting all the flaws of a woman without balancing them off by any of the qualities of a man; thus he will be equally detested by both sexes."[64]

In Georges Saint-Paul's account, homosexuals were either "born inverts" (incurable and "vicious") or "feminoform," a condition, which, depending on the degree of hereditary predisposition, was potentially reversible.[65] In his scheme the degree of pathology corresponded to the degree of feminized behavior, so that, by definition, the "male" character in a typical homosexual union was the "accidental" or "occasional" type. Doctors, in their efforts to present the differences between the sexes as harmonious and complementary, were ordinarily constrained in their analysis of females to discuss their feminine (nonmasculine) nature in a positive manner, not as a simple "negative" of "positive" masculinity. However, they were under no such constraints in discussing these feminine features in men, where the mask of solicitude for the "weaker" sex they customarily assumed could be temporarily and revealingly set aside. Carroll Smith-Rosenberg has persuasively documented the misogynous impulses that informed the medical description of "mannish lesbians" in this same period; doctors were busily adding a set of masculine physical and behavioral characteristics to the "barrenness" that typically marked the nontraditional woman.[66]

As noted above, the whole of this medical analysis of homosexuality was embedded in a critique of modern culture and society stressing the vast range of novel stimuli promoting the spread of "cerebral" passions at the expense of natural ones. Garnier blamed bourgeois materialism and the thirst for riches,[67] Lacassagne the "intellectual emancipation" of the age;[68] Emile Laurent believed that excessive leisure, food, and drink were at fault.[69] Julien Chevalier echoed Jean-Jacques's denunciation of *luxure* and

[60] Pierre Garnier, *Impuissance physique et morale chez l'homme et la femme*, 3d ed. (Paris: Garnier Frères, 1882), p. 124.

[61] Thoinot, *Attentats aux moeurs*, p. 309.

[62] Chevalier, *L'Inversion sexuelle*, p. 194.

[63] Laurent, *Les Bissexués*, p. 18.

[64] Reuss, "Des abérrations," p. 131.

[65] Saint-Paul, *Perversion*, pp. 14–20.

[66] Smith-Rosenberg, "New Woman as Androgyne," pp. 259–65. For the standard medical outlook on female sterility in French medicine, see Yvonne Knibiehler and Catherine Fouquet, *La Femme et les médecins: analyse historique* (Paris: Hachette, 1983).

[67] Garnier, *Impuissance*, pp. 18–19.

[68] Alexander Lacassagne, preface to Chevalier, *L'Inversion sexuelle*, p. v.

[69] Laurent, *L'Amour morbide*, p. 319.

sensual excess, which bred a kind of "exhausted and jaded precocity" in which "one excess calls forth another" until normal heterosexual attractions lose their appeal.[70]

In their search for historical parallels to the putative contemporary growth of homosexuality, medical commentators were drawn to the example of ancient Greece whose "turpitudes," one argued, were obvious to those who did not view them through the "brilliant colors of a prism."[71] Less hasty consideration of "amitié antique" might partially exonerate Greek homosexuality on the grounds of cultural relativism,[72] but there could be no question of deploying this argument in defense of the "normality" of homosexuality in the twentieth century:

> While the Greek, who was a homosexual by education and culture, could harmonize his cult of masculine beauty with his sexual potency simply by allowing a considerable latitude in the choice of erotic object, our homosexual, who is endowed with a sexual constitution in *discordance* with the social milieu, suffers most frequently from a weakening of his procreative sexual power; which justifies in turn his classification among the neuropaths and abnormals.[73]

The power of this medico-biological discourse of homosexuality was so great that medical concepts influenced the first reasoned defenses of the phenomenon in France. Literary figures who sought to present a generally more favorable account of homosexuality than could be found in the medical literature were forced to do so on a linguistic and conceptual terrain already marked out by medicine, a fact that invariably vitiated their efforts in behalf of greater tolerance. André Raffalovitch, an energetic propagandist for homosexual rights, sought to establish the existence of a type of homosexuality in which the man had lost none of his manly qualities and often concealed his true nature behind the facade of married life. Raffalovitch accordingly heaped abuse on "effeminate" inverts, arguing that their moral worth was in inverse relation to their degree of effeminacy.[74]

Emile Zola, *Dreyfusard* and noble crusader for unpopular causes, pleaded the cause of inverts in his preface to Georges Saint-Paul's book on sexual perversions. He observed that one does not condemn a hunchback for having been born that way, so "why scorn a man for acting like a woman when he has been born half woman?" But Zola follows this half-hearted plea for understanding with a piece of undigested familialist propaganda:

[70] Chevalier, *L'Inversion sexuelle*, pp. 170–71.

[71] Ball, *La Folie érotique*, p. 142; also Charcot and Magnan, "Inversion du sens génitale" (January 1882), p. 54.

[72] Ludovic Dugas, *L'Amitié antique* (Paris: Alcan, 1922).

[73] Angelo Hesnard, *Traité de sexologie normale et pathologique* (Paris: Payot, 1933), p. 641.

[74] André Raffalovitch, "Quelques observations sur l'inversion," *Archives d'anthropologie criminelle*, 1894, *9*: 216. In England, Havelock Ellis was the most vocal critic of the notion that homosexuals were invariably effeminate. See Jeffrey Weeks, "Havelock Ellis and the Politics of Sex Reform," in *Socialism and the New Life: The Personal and Sexual Politics of Edward Carpenter and Havelock Ellis*, ed. Sheila Rowbotham and Jeffrey Weeks (London: Pluto Press, 1977), pp. 151–55. Also Jeffrey Weeks, *Coming Out: Homosexual Politics in Britain from the Nineteenth Century to the Present* (London: Quartet Books, 1977), pp. 68–84.

> And in the end everything which touches on sex touches social life itself. An invert is a disorganizer of the family, of the nation, of humanity. Man and woman exist to make children, and they will kill life itself on the day they decide to make no more of them.[75]

André Gide, himself a homosexual, attempted to refute such arguments in *Corydon,* a justly famous defense of homosexuality which was begun in 1907 and privately printed in 1911. Gide had Corydon complain, "The only serious books I know on this subject are certain medical works which reek of the clinic from the very first pages."[76] But explicitly acknowledging the force of such texts, Gide took special pains to distinguish what he called "normal homosexuals" from inverts, whom he admitted were effeminate and perhaps even "degenerates."[77] Corydon drew upon the "heroes" of ancient Greece to demonstrate that a society could tolerate homosexuality and still preserve martial values, concluding, "I can think of no opinion more false, and yet more widely held, than that which considers homosexual conduct and pederasty as the pathetic lot of effeminate races."[78] Nor, replied Corydon to a charge of his interrogator, was there some necessary connection between homosexuality and depopulation. Forgetting an earlier statement that "respect for women usually accompanies uranism,"[79] he said that depopulation was a result of "the shameless stimulation of our popular imagery, theaters, music halls, and a host of publications [which] serves only to lure woman away from her duties; to make her into a perpetual mistress, who no longer consents to maternity."[80]

Gide's ideal of homosexuality was subsumed under the ancient term *pederasty,* which had once meant an intimate tutelage of a young boy by an adult male, in contrast to its modern, medicalized, usage. In a note he added to the 1922 edition of *Corydon,* he contrasted this manly relationship to the cases of "inversion, of effeminacy, of sodomy" which Proust had, alas, discussed at such length in his novel.[81] One might ask, however, whether a defense of such a narrow concept of homosexuality, which,

[75] Emile Zola, preface to Saint-Paul, *Perversion,* pp. 3–4.

[76] André Gide, *Corydon,* trans. Richard Howard (New York: Farrar, Straus & Giroux, 1983), p. 17.

[77] *Ibid.,* p. 119.

[78] *Ibid.,* p. 115.

[79] *Ibid.,* p. 116.

[80] *Ibid.,* p. 118.

[81] *Ibid.,* p. xx n. The story of Gide's struggle with his own homosexual impulses has been well told by Gide himself in his *Si le grain ne meurt* and his *Journals.* Jean Delay also discusses the biographical details at some length, underscoring Gide's professed repugnance for "sodomy" (adult male anal intercourse) and "effeminacy." Of particular interest is Gide's acceptance of the advice given him by Paul Brouardel, a professor of the Paris Medical School, whom he consulted about his first homosexual affairs and who told him that his condition was temporary and would be replaced by "natural instinct" after his marriage. For Brouardel, and presumably for Gide, the most hopeful sign was that he was fully "viril," that is, potent with women. See Jean Delay, *La Jeunesse d'André Gide,* 5th ed., 2 vols. (Paris: Gallimard, 1957), 2: 517–20. See also Gerald H. Storzer, "The Homosexual Paradigm in Balzac, Gide, and Genet," in Stambolian and Marks, eds., *Homosexualities and French Literature,* pp. 186–210; also Wallace Fowlie, "Sexuality in Gide's Self-Portrait," *ibid.,* pp. 243–61.

moreover, seems to share the prejudices of the standard medical thinking on the subject, constitutes much of a defense at all.

Marcel Proust's effort to extract what was worthy in the variety of homosexualities from that which was not is much more complicated, but no less troubling, than Gide's. Of course Proust did not attempt to write a defense of homosexuality in his *À la recherche du temps perdu,* but to study objectively its nature and variations, as his numerous botanical and other scientific metaphors are meant to suggest. Many scholars have demonstrated Proust's familiarity with the medical and biological theories of the prewar era, particularly his knowledge of mental pathologies, and literary critics have shown how these theories served the literary aims of the writer in his great novel.[82]

The most extraordinary of these critiques, J. E. Rivers's *Proust and the Art of Love,* convincingly argues that Proust's apparently detached account of life in Sodom and Gomorrah was heavily influenced, and ultimately enriched, by his internalization of the social prejudices against the homosexual impulses in himself. The unflattering accounts of "inverts" in his novel were the result, Rivers argues, of a homosexual self-hatred that moved Proust to deny his own nature and yet express his own unhappiness in portraits that were alternately scornful and pitying.[83]

The "social prejudices" that Proust feared were, it happens, the same as the medical ones we have been considering here. We know that the youthful Proust chose his male friends from among those who were "physically well made, sportive, at once aristocratic and liberal."[84] We also know that Proust fought a duel in 1897 with Jean Lorrain over the insinuation of a homosexual relationship, and nearly provoked another a decade later when a young friend did not strenuously enough deny to a third party the suggestion that Proust was homosexual.[85] In yet another incident, when Proust was 49, Proust scolded Paul Souday for attributing to him a "feminine" sensibility in terms that leave little doubt about the precise nature of his fears:

> At a time when *Sodome et Gomorrhe* is about to appear—a time when, since I will be talking about Sodom, no one will have the courage to come to my defense—you are blazing the trail (without malice I am sure) for those who *are* malicious by treating me as being "feminine." From "feminine" to "effeminate" is one short step. Those who served me as seconds in my duel will tell you whether I have the softness of effeminates.[86]

[82] Among the most recent of these are Serge Béhar, *L'Univers médical de Proust* (Paris: Gallimard, 1970); Bernard Straus, *Maladies of Marcel Proust: Doctors and Disease in His Life and Work* (New York: Holmes and Meier, 1980).

[83] J. E. Rivers, *Proust and the Art of Love: The Aesthetics of Sexuality in the Life, Times, and Art of Marcel Proust* (New York: Columbia University Press, 1980), p. 73.

[84] Béhar, *L'Univers médical de Proust,* p. 32.

[85] Rivers, *Proust and the Art of Love,* pp. 33–37.

[86] *Ibid.,* p. 32.

In the brillant opening passages of *Sodome et Gomorrbe* Proust reveals to his readers that, in an unguarded moment, a certain gentleness and spirituality could be seen in the face of the imperious Baron de Charlus, "who prided himself so upon his virility, to whom all other men seemed odiously effeminate, what he made one suddenly think of, so far had he momentarily assumed her features, expression, smile, was a woman."[87] Charlus is suddenly transformed in the narrator's eyes into a "new person" whose whole being became more "intelligible" in light of this discovery. The narrator then speculates that Charlus belongs to "that race of beings, less paradoxical than they appear, whose ideal is manly simply because their temperament is feminine and who in their life resemble in appearance only the rest of men";[88] Charlus is a male invert with an "incurable malady" of a degenerative kind, the chief symptom of which, as Proust reveals in later volumes, is a diminished capacity to conceal his progressive effeminization.[89]

Proust admits of a kind of love between inverts, but only where the gap between the more masculine and feminine of them resembles the "normal" dimorphic attraction of men and women, as is the case with Charlus and Jupien. The invert's normal fate, "for every creature follows the line of his own pleasure," is to "seek [love] in a sex complementary to his own."[90] The tragedy of homosexuality in Proust's novel is that, in practice, homosexuals "fall in love with precisely that type of man who has nothing feminine about him, who is not an invert and consequently cannot love them in return."[91] The close kinship of the "hermophroditic" invert and women ensures their "sterile" relations, and leads Proust to admit that the kind of self-fertilization that typifies hermaphrodites leads inevitably to "degeneracy and sterility,"[92] but he speculates that in the "moral sense" one invert may fertilize another with his "music, or his fragrance or his flame."[93]

Though Proust occasionally endows the inverts in his novel with masculine features, as in Saint-Loup's personal bravery and energetic patriotism, he more frequently reflects the unforgiving views expressed in the medical perspective of "inverts" as sterile, repellently effeminate, unstable, and afflicted with a congenital disorder whereby their abnormal sexuality is hypostatized into a "mode of selfhood" and a "category of identity."[94]

The widespread fear of effeminization and homosexuality that was

[87] Marcel Proust, *Cities of the Plain* (French title *Sodome et Gomorrbe*), trans. C. K. Scott Moncrief (New York: Vintage, 1970), p. 5.

[88] *Ibid.*, p. 13.

[89] Rivers, *Proust and the Art of Love*, pp. 188–89.

[90] Proust, *Cities of the Plain*, p. 17.

[91] *Ibid.*, p. 13.

[92] *Ibid.*, p. 4.

[93] *Ibid.*, p. 22.

[94] Rivers, *Proust and the Art of Love*, p. 198. On Saint-Loup, Rivers writes: "One could read *Sodom I* and decide that the national security of any nation depends on the exclusion of homosexually oriented men—those hermaphroditic sexual mutations—from the armed services. Or one could read the story of Saint-Loup's heroism and come to an entirely different conclusion" (p. 203).

common elsewhere in Western Europe in the decades before the war was certainly stimulated by growing military tensions, a number of prominent homosexual scandals, and the multiple strains put on traditional sex roles by the progressive emancipation of women. These pressures produced in Germany and England, in particular, the same anti-homosexual animus that prevailed in France, and resulted in similar defensive denials by homosexuals and their defenders that homosexuality was incompatible with manliness or constituted a threat to the national security.[95]

Carroll Smith-Rosenberg has recently argued that in its dual capacity to empower and restrain, a dominant discourse such as the medical assessment of homosexuality may create new models that individuals so labeled might employ for their own emancipation, thus confounding the discourse's original meaning. She shows convincingly how the medical image of the androgynous lesbian was used by women to construct a new "ideal" for female behavior. This androgynous ideal, because it broke with traditional notions of passive and domesticated femininity, served as an inspiration and model for feminist writers in the 1920s and 1930s who were seeking not only new horizons of love but an entirely new vision of a being who had broken the mold of woman as wife and mother.[96]

But if women, especially in the Anglo-Saxon nations, could make a positive virtue of the dominant medical discourse on "lesbian" androgyny, male homosexuals and their defenders could not do the same with the image of effeminacy, at least not without gravely threatening the relatively more narrow and tenuous foundation on which male identity was believed to rest. This was nowhere more true than in France, where the unusual concerns about depopulation and infertility encouraged the development of a medical prophylaxis that stressed the connections between normal sexuality, traditional family life, and national survival. These linkages also made doctors the natural experts in these matters, and provided a widespread currency, as we have seen, for the medical discourse they generated on male sexuality in particular. In the words of Georges Saint-Paul:

> Truly normal love is very rare, I must confess, at least in that state of perfect normality in which not only the vital ends of generation and the purity of race, but also the social aims of patriotic grandeur, the conservation of the family and the purity of morals are all bound together.[97]

The threat to "French mentality, to French morality, to French health" which Ernest Charles had claimed to discover in "pederasty" testifies elo-

[95] On the homosexual scandals in Germany, see Isabel V. Hull, *The Entourage of Kaiser Wilhelm II, 1888–1918* (Cambridge: Cambridge University Press, 1982), pp. 109–45; James D. Steakley, "Iconography of a scandal: political cartoons of the Eulenberg Affair," *Stud. Visual Communication*, 1983, *9*: 20–51. George Mosse has recently discussed these issues in England and Germany in *Nationalism and Sexuality: Respectability and Abnormal Sexuality in Modern Europe* (New York: Howard Fertig, 1985), pp. 1–47.

[96] Smith-Rosenberg, "New Woman as Androgyne," pp. 287–96.

[97] Saint-Paul, *Perversion*, p. 232.

quently to the power of a biological and medical discourse of male homosexuality in the fin de siècle. There is no escaping the existence of what Jean Borie has called the pervasive "ordre familial," which doctors elaborated throughout the century and which even found its way into the literary formulas of those who sought to combat it.[98] The adherents of this "order" viewed sexual behavior through the lens of legitimate reproductive fertility; men who could not attain to this ideal, or feared falling short of it, risked forfeiting that solid status residing in being a father and husband, a man with heirs and his manhood beyond question. At stake for men, and no doubt for women, too, was a self-identity for which their sexuality had become the sign. As Pierre Hahn has written in his study of the invention of homosexuality, "By the end of the century, no man could call himself sane or normal if he could not affirm his sexual identity from head to toe."[99]

[98] Borie, *Le Célibataire français*, pp. 9–14, 24, 52, 66.
[99] Hahn, *Nos Ancêtres les pervers*, p. 82.

Discrimination and AIDS

1. Introduction

Most normative moral theories embrace something like the following:

> (A) It is morally wrong to discriminate against a moral being (or class of moral beings) unless that being (or class of beings) possesses a morally relevant differentiating property.

where

> A differentiating property is a property possessed by an individual (or class of individuals) and not possessed by the other members of the relevant population.

(A) appears to be a corollary of some principle of universalisability: Moral beings which possess the same morally relevant properties should be treated in a morally equivalent manner. But in this paper we shall not be concerned with the origin of (A), or even its justification. Nor are we concerned with extending (A) to cover positive discrimination in addition to the common negative discrimination to which (A) is relevant.

In this paper the focus of our concern is the morality of discriminatory treatment of persons with the HTLV III (or AIDS) virus, or, more specifically, with the circumstances in which

Copyright 1987 by *Social Theory and Practice*, Vol. 13, No. 2 (Summer 1987)

discriminatory treatment of such persons is justified. But as an important preliminary we need to sort out what constitutes a morally relevant differentiating property. This we do in Section 2. In Section 3 we shall look at the question of whether being infected with the HTLV III virus *is* such a morally relevant differentiating property, or whether some other AIDS related property constitutes such a morally relevant difference. In Section 4 we shall look at some cases which illustrate the kinds of moral obligations those infected with the HTLV III virus (or likely to be so infected) have if they are to avoid discrimination, while in Section 5 we look at some cases where discrimination does seem to be morally justified.

2. Morally Relevant Differentiating Properties

How do we justify the claim that a differentiating property *P* is morally relevant in the manner required in (A)? Here is a rough suggestion:

> (B) If to treat the members of a moral population which have a differentiating property *P* in the same manner as the members of the population which do not have *P* would have morally undesirable consequences for the population as a whole, then *P* is a morally relevant differentiating property.

(B) is consequentialist in nature, but is neutral as to what features of the consequences are relevant. Utilitarians will obviously be interested in those consequences which are pleasurable or painful, but other moral theories may consider additional features of the consequences.

We take it as essential that discrimination involves consideration of consequences, even within the context of a moral theory which is not wholly or generally consequentialist. For surely, when we consider discriminating because of *P*, we must be concerned with the *effects* that allowing those with *P* unrestricted equal membership of the population will have upon the population as a whole. And if we are interested in such effects, surely we are considering consequences.

Of course it is *possible* to take into account things other than the consequences, but we find it difficult to think this really happens. It may be urged that we should be concerned with (say) the justice of some piece of discrimination. But then we believe that it is a consideration of justice that led us to our general principle (A). Obviously justice considerations will be outweighed in some cases, and it is these cases where discrimination is justified. These are the cases where the consequences of non-discrimination are bad enough. So considerations of justice lead us again to concentrate on consequences, and similarly with considerations of freedom, privacy, respect for persons, and so on. We realise that some will say that our notions of justice and the like are too restricted and formal and that richer notions with more genuine content will resolve the question of discrimination without an independent consideration of consequences. But it is our view that these richer notions have really subsumed the consequentialist considerations.

Some may still maintain that matters other than consequences should be considered. But then it seems that we would not find enough general agreement on this "extra" for it to provide any significant influence on the content of a social policy.

It should not be unexpected that the consequences with which we are here concerned are those that can reasonably be predicted, and to which some appropriate level of probability can be attached. Furthermore *all* such consequences must be considered: short term and long term, and also the consequences of the discriminatory practice itself (especially if the discrimination is to be unfair or unjust). Also the nature of the discriminatory practice proposed will be of the utmost importance when considering the morality of the nature of the proposal.

(B) cannot stand alone as determining morally relevant differentiating properties. There are further restrictions on *P*. Here are at least some of these additional requirements we must take together with (B).

(i) The consequences must be bad *enough*. For example, slightly unpleasant consequences may not do, but life threatening ones may. Of course it is more complicated than this. Also relevant is how widespread the consequenes will be. Mildly bad consequences for all members of the population may well be enough, while mildly bad consequences for a small sub-population may not be.

(ii) (B) must be read probabilistically. It is not required that the population must actually experience the consequences, or that it be certain that it would unless the discrimination is enforced. What is required is that it can be predicted with an appropriate level of probability that the consequences would occur unless discrimination is effected. There are two elements here: one is that there be sufficient level of probability, and the other that this probability have sufficient weight.

The sufficient weight requirement means that the probability is based on both a suitable and sufficient body of evidence to make it rational to act on the probability estimate.[1] The sufficient level of probability requirement is that the chance of the bad consequences occurring, given no discrimination, is significant. Of course there is the difficult question of what level of probability constitutes a significant probability. Obviously this will not be determined independently of the nature of the consequences. What is clear is that a mere *possibility* of bad consequences is not sufficient.

If we take life threatening consequences for all the population, we would tolerate only a very small probability before discriminating (unless the discrimination itself carries with it a higher probability of equally bad consequences), but for mildly unpleasant consequences for a sub-population the probability tolerable would obviously be higher.

(iii) *P* must be maximally specific. Suppose *P* is a differentiating property, and for those with property *P* there is a significantly high probability that they will produce undesirable consequences for the population as a whole. But now suppose those who have property *Q* in addition to *P* have an even higher probability of producing those same bad consequences, while those who have not got *Q* but have *P* (that is they have the compound property *P* and not *Q*) have a probability which is below the threshold significance level. It seems that we should discriminate with respect to the differentiating property *P* and *Q*, but not with respect to the differentiating property *P*.

(iv) There are certain epistemic and pragmatic requirements on *P*. It must be discernible (in a practical and realistic manner) whether or not *P* obtains. If ascertaining whether or not *P* obtains itself produces bad consequences, then it might not be appropriate to discriminate with respect to *P*. That will depend on the nature of those consequences, and the level of the probability that those consequences will be actualised. What level of certainty is required will depend upon the consequences for the population as a whole, the probability that those consequences will be actualised, and also upon the consequences for those with property *P* of the proposed discrimination.

(v) There may be moral restraints on which properties may be appropriately used as the basis for morally justifiable discrimination, but this depends on the normative moral theory from which one is operating more than do the other requirements. Suppose a life threatening disease can be inflicted on both sexes, but only transmitted by one sex. It could be argued on grounds of justice or fairness that only discrimination on the basis of having the disease should be allowed, and discrimination on the basis of having the disease and being of a particular sex is unacceptable. A more extreme example is where one component of a maximally specific differentiating property could only be present if the individual fails to act in an immoral manner, for instance, perhaps you could only avoid the property by harming another person. And what if the property is picked out using definite descriptions of a set of identified individuals which in fact make up a high risk group? And what if the consequences of discrimination change markedly if one uses one differentiating property rather than another (as, for example, use of the property of being of a particular race)?

Again, suppose the differentiating property picks out a minority group already identified in the population and already subject to unfavourable treatment. At least there is a question of whether we should (morally) use such a property for discrimination even if it is agreed that it might be "good for the population as a whole" in simple consequentialist terms. More argument may be required.

Consequentialists will feel this moral requirement *is* adequately met by taking the *total* consequences into account. But those not of a consequentialist persuasion may well believe that there are additional moral restraints pertaining to the acceptance of a differentiating property as a morally relevant differentiating property.

We have argued that property *P* satisfying (B) does not in itself establish that we are justified in discriminating against those with property *P*. Satisfaction of the list (i) - (v) of additional requirements is necessary for the specification of a morally relevant differentiating property. We believe that some such list of requirements ultimately will adequately refine (B) and indirectly our principle (A). Undoubtedly (B) will need to take still more on board, but we think we have now done enough for our purposes here.

So from now on we will use (A) on the understanding that a morally relevant differentiating property must satisfy (B) together with requirements (i) to (v) above, plus any relatives that we should need to add. We will call such a differentiating property a *proper* morally relevant differentiating property. This is obviously a fairly complex matter, but at this point it is sufficiently clear for us to proceed.

Undoubtedly some will object to the whole tenor of this discussion of discrimination. The objection we anticipate is the charge that our entire argument is essentially consequentialist despite its billing as being normative theory neutral, and thus some will reject our contention that for matters of discrimination at least, consequences are determinate of morality. They will say we are too reductionist on matters of justice, and so forth, and such reductionism is not acceptable to the non-consequentialist. While we maintain our view that our argument is largely normative theory neutral, we offer a sketch of an alternative route to what we take to be, at least in all important respects, the same position.[2] Most people agree that "harm to others" gives *prima facie* grounds for the state to interfere with the actions of the individual, although the reasons offered for such a view can vary enormously. Now this gives *only prima facie* grounds. Whether actual interference is justified will depend, finally, on other matters. So when asking whether the state should interfere with those with property *P* because they may harm others in virtue of having *P*, we have to consider such questions as: how bad is the harm; how likely is it that the harm will come about; is *P* the kind of property which will make it feasible for the state to be able to interfere, and is it morally acceptable to interfere with individuals because they have *P*? And these are exactly the same questions we posed when asking if *P* is properly morally relevant. So although what follows is couched in terms of discrimination, the essential features could be made in terms of morally acceptable interference with the individual by the state.

3. AIDS and Discrimination

We are concerned with the question of discrimination against those who have been infected with the HTLV III (or AIDS) virus. Let us briefly review the medical picture of this virus, and of those who have been infected with it.

The most serious cases of infection are those where the individuals have AIDS proper. Such individuals paradigmatically have severe, life-threatening, opportunistic infections,[3] such as certain kinds of pneumonia and cancer, due to deficiencies in their immune systems. This is frequently referred to as AIDS category A or (just) AIDS. AIDS category B includes individuals with Lymphadenopathy Syndrome (LAS) and those with other symptoms which constitute what is referred to as the AIDS Related Complex or ARC. These individuals are not in immediate likelihood of losing their lives, but are in very poor health and great discomfort. Finally, AIDS category C includes those individuals who have a confirmed antibody positive test result for the HTLV III virus, or would have if tested, but have no symptoms (that is, they are quite healthy). Persons of all categories are potentially contagious.

The AIDS virus has now been found in all bodily fluids: blood, urine, semen, saliva, and even tear drops. This is at first sight alarming. But there is, as yet, no evidence of the virus being transmitted via saliva or tear drops in casual contacts.

What the evidence does point to is that AIDS is transmitted through (a) sexual contact involving exchanges of bodily fluids and (b) through contact with contaminated blood/blood products/hypodermics. As such, the HTLV III virus is importantly different from the various flu viruses which are frequently transmitted via aerosols of infected saliva. Also important is the fact that a virus (any virus) can infect a person only by first entering the cells of his or her body, because a virus is entirely dependent upon the enzymes in living cells for its own reproduction. In the case of the HTLV III virus, entry into the bloodstream seems to be necessary.

The prognosis for individuals infected with the HTLV III virus is far from rosy. As the disease has been monitored only since 1981 definitive pronouncements are still not possible. However using mathematical models it has been predicted that the mean incubation period of the disease is six to eight years, and the range from one to fifteen.

Using the data acquired during the last three years it has been esitmated that within three years of infection, 5 percent to 15 percent of people will develop AIDS, and another 25 percent to

35 percent will develop LAS. These figures may well increase with time.[4]

Because AIDS is (a) serious and undesirable, (b) non-curable, and (c) contagious, it has very serious consequences for the community. It is most prevalent in male homosexuals and intravenous drugs users, but is by no means restricted to these groups. Prostitutes, those who have had involvement with a bisexual (even via an intermediate step), and those who are dependent on blood products are also at risk.

Highly reliable tests to screen for the HTLV III virus have been developed. Those currently used within Australia are the ELISA and the Western Blot. The procedure employed is to first use an ELISA. If the result is positive a second ELISA is used. If the result is still positive the blood is then subjected to the Western Blot which is both a more complex and more expensive procedure for looking at the same reaction, but is also more reliable.

Since no antibody test is perfect there will be some individuals whose results are positive, while they do not actually have any HTLV III virus within their blood. Such results are referred to as false positives. A false positive is not much fun for the individual who has tested positive. However, with respect to securing the purity of the blood supply and generally identifying high risk groups, these false positives are unproblematic. It is rather the false negatives--individuals who test antibody negative but who have been infected with the HTLV III virus--that are the problem.

The incidence of false negatives using the ELISA is believed to be quite low. However, it may be as high as three percent.[5] The most probable cause of a false negative is the failure of the development of antibodies to the HTLV III virus. The development of such antibodies may take up to nine weeks. This gives us another category of AIDS--call it Category D--and such persons are contagious. If a category D individual donates blood or has interaction conducive to contagion between the time of infection with the HTLV III virus and the development of antibodies he (or she) will be putting others at serious risk, and this will be undetectable by testing as he (or she) will test negative.

Is having AIDS (category A, B, C or D) a proper morally relevant differentiating property? More simply, since being HTLV III antibody positive is reliably detectable and means that one may pass the virus on, is being HTLV III antibody positive a proper morally relevant differentiating property?

Prima facie, it is. Close personal interaction can spread AIDS and clearly having AIDS or ARC has highly undesirable (life threatening) consequences. Also the probabilities are of a sufficient level, in the appropriate circumstances, of the undesirable consequences being brought about. But while we believe that being antibody positive is clearly a differentiating property of moral relevance, we do not think it is a property that measures up as a proper morally relevant differentiating property. It fails some of those *extra* requirements that mark off the properly morally relevant.

There are indeed three ways in which it fails to meet the requirements. It fails to meet the epistemic and pragmatic requirement in two different ways, and it fails to be maximally specific.

Consider then its failure to meet the epistemic and pragmatic requirement:

(1) It is difficult to identify the group that is antibody positive and, because of category D, even more difficult to identify the group that has been infected by the HTLV III virus. There are of course the tests mentioned above. But realistically, the tests can only be used at the request of a member of a high risk group. It is not practical to require regular universal testing, and those who are merely HTLV III antibody positive may have no symptoms and therefore be unaware that they are antibody positive. And Category D could not be identified even if there was regular universal testing. It is not even clear that the related property of being at high risk of being infected is any better. While promiscuous male homosexuals and intravenous drug users may know they are at high risk, the wives of bisex-

ual men and other such persons are also at high risk and yet may have no idea that they are at risk.

(2) To require that people be tested may itself have very bad consequences for some individuals. It is not easy to live with the news that you are antibody positive when the prognosis is so bad, and this consequence is fairly likely for those who test positively. Some have even argued that it may outweigh the supposedly good consequences of the testing program, and hence some advisory services advise individuals against being tested. This is not surprising given the connection between AIDS and homosexuality, and the discrimination which homosexuals already suffer within our society. And it is not clear that the *entire* high risk group could be adequately identified in practical terms for a testing program.

Consider now the failure of the property of being infected by the HTLV III virus, or the property of being HTLV III antibody positive, to meet the requirement of maximal specificity. The epistemic and practical considerations mentioned above may lead us to consider the property of believing that one is at risk of being antibody positive or being infected, rather than being antibody positive or being infected by the HTLV III virus. But now consider the more specific property of believing that one is at high risk of being HTLV III infected and being morally responsible. It seems that this group has a much lower probability of causing undesirable consequences for the population, in fact a probability lower than the threshold significance level (though, of course, there is always the chance of an accident). Being HTLV III antibody positive or even believing that one is at risk of being HTLV III infected is not a sufficiently specific differentiating property.

These kinds of considerations, together with further epistemic considerations push us in the following direction. We should only discriminate in those cases where it is reasonable to believe that there is a high risk that a person is infected by the HTLV III virus and will not act responsibly.

This may seem very weak. For we are suggesting that discrimination should not be automatic for those in a high risk group, or even for those who are antibody positive, but only where it is probable both that a person has been infected and will not behave responsibly. But we have found that "stronger" properties do not measure up as properly morally relevant.

We should note here that one very desirable feature of this differentiating property is that most of those at high risk will have reason to believe that they are. If they act responsibly (and thus avoid discriminatory treatment), this will reduce the chance of creating other people at risk who are unaware that they are at risk--for example, the wives of bisexual men and those sexually involved with intravenous drug users.

We shall, in what follows, concentrate on this differentiating property. In Section 4 we will discuss what constitutes morally responsible behaviour for a person who believes he (or she) may be infected with the HTLV III virus, and in Section 5 we shall look at cases where discrimination is justified on the grounds that there is good reason to believe that persons cannot, or will not, behave responsibly.

4. Morally Responsible Behaviour For Those Who Are Infected With The HTLV III Virus

Let us look at three cases to elucidate what constitutes morally responsible behaviour for those who believe they are at high risk of having been infected with the HTLV III virus.

(a) HTLV III Infected Persons In The Workplace. While it is true that the probability that an individual will pass on the HTLV III virus in an office environment is very low, it is clearly possible for him to do so. It is possible, though not at all probable, that he could maliciously set about to infect another at his workplace by contaminating food, or by some other action (such cases have been reported). It is even possible that he could do this non-maliciously if his behaviour was excep-

tionally unusual. If he did, he would be behaving in a morally irresponsible manner. To behave morally responsibly in this kind of work environment is very easy--an individual would have to go to some lengths to be able to behave irresponsibly. Sharing office, coffee room, and bathroom facilities in a normal fashion involves only an infinitesimal risk.

An individual who works in a blood bank, on the other hand, would be in a very different position. Since blood is one medium in which the HTLV III virus thrives, an individual could, even while behaving cautiously, infect blood or blood products--maybe by a small cut or a needlestick. A morally responsible individual who knows or believes himself to be HTLV III virus infected therefore should either inform the blood bank of this fact or find another job.

When it comes to the question of policies with respect to employment it is our view that the Australian Public Service decision not to discriminate against antibody positive individuals is correct. It is morally correct because it is reasonable to believe that individuals who are antibody positive will behave in a responsible manner (at least in a minimally responsible manner), and the probability of the virus being passed on in any other manner in an office situation is infinitesimal. Admittedly individuals (even individuals belonging to selectively similar groups) do behave in a variety of ways. It is possible that there is a malicious contaminator. But this behaviour is sufficiently improbable that it would be unjust to discriminate against the whole class of individuals in question given the fact that the vast majority of individuals can be expected to behave responsibly, and given the other kinds of risk which our society tolerates. Of course if, for whatever reason, we believe that some infected individual is not responsible, that individual should be subject to some appropriate form of discrimination.

(b) The Bisexual Husband. Suppose Pat and Chris have been married for many years. Pat is a traditional housewife with conservative values. She believes that she is living within a monogamous relationship and her husband has encouraged this

belief. But Chris, who is bisexual, also has casual homosexual relationships.

Chris becomes aware of the fact that he may be HTLV III infected. What is he to do? Confession to his wife could result in the collapse of their relationship. If he says nothing and continues to have sexual relations with her she may be further exposed to the risk of infection.

At this point there seem to be at least two ethically acceptable courses of action open to him. On the one hand he could tell her he is at risk and that she may be too. On the other he could have the antibody test, find an excuse not to have sex for six months, and then have a second antibody test.

Suppose Chris chooses the latter alternative. If both results are clear he will know Pat is not infected (or at least not by him). He then has a second choice. Either he can resume sexual relations with Pat, and not resume his other sexual relations, or he can tell her about his other sexual relations, explain the risks and let her make her own decision. Now suppose that Chris is antibody positive. In this case he should tell Pat his antibody status and let her decide what to do about their relationship. For to continue sexual relations is to further expose Pat to risk. If Pat is a woman of child-bearing age she may become pregnant and a large percentage of babies born to antibody positive women go on to develop AIDS. Finally, if Pat does not know she is at risk she may donate blood (remember tests are not completely effective) and so place yet more individuals at risk.

We should make it quite clear at this point that we are not saying that there exists any absolute obligation for a person, like Chris, at risk of being infected with HTLV III virus to be tested. Nor is there any absolute obligation to inform the spouse that she may also be at risk. There are alternative ways in which one may initially handle the situation. But the bottom line (morally speaking) is that it is irresponsible to continue to expose to risk a non-consenting spouse. And it is also irresponsible to fail to provide information that may prevent the spouse being the cause of another individual's suffering or death.

(c) The One-Night Stand. A more difficult case is that of the one-night stand. Is there here an obligation to reveal one's antibody status to one's prospective partner? Of obvious relevance here is what one intends to do, or what it is reasonable to believe will happen. Also of the utmost relevance are what dangers adhere to the activities in question, and the probability that such dangers will be actualised.

It is here extremely plausible to argue that the information in question is vital if the individual is to be able to make an informed decision. It is one thing to consent to have sex where there is a belief that there is no incipient danger to health and life that will flow from that action. It is quite another thing to consent believing such a danger is present. If the matter of HTLV III is not explicitly raised what exactly is one consenting to? Is one consenting to HTLV III-free sex? Is one consenting to taking a risk that the other individual is infected with the HTLV III virus?

The notion of consent includes a legal factor and its interpretation is a legally complex issue. But there is certainly a social/moral issue here too. In a community where the dangers of HTLV III have been widely publicised and discussed, if an individual is not coerced into non-safe sex is it reasonable to charge his (or her) antibody positive partner with socially irresponsible behaviour? Suppose the individual asks; is the respondent obliged to give a straight answer? Suppose the individual does not ask; is the other party obliged to volunteer the information?

At this point we will construct an analogous situation. Suppose I own a grocery store and stock just one, very popular, brand of baby food--Brand X. Suppose also that recently there have been a few "strange" infant deaths and it is suspected that some cans of Brand X baby food with the 007 serial number are responsible. But (for whatever reason) no government action has yet been taken to prohibit the sale of Brand X baby food with the 007 serial number. Perhaps it is because the probability is very low. However there has been a lot of publicity implicating it.

Suppose I am approached by a customer who is well informed about the infant deaths but she still wishes to buy some Brand X from me. I have some in stock but it is all of the 007 serial number. Do I have an obligation to tell her that it has the suspect serial number? More specifically, do I have an obligation to answer her truthfully if she asks me explicitly, and do I have an obligation to volunteer the information if she does not ask?

It is our view that moral responsibility dictates an affirmative answer to all these questions, even if the probability of a particular can being contaminated is low (even very low). And insofar as the risks are of a similar magnitude, and the consequences of similar severity, one's answers to these questions, and those raised by the one-night stand case, should be consistent.

When the consequence of a course of action is very serious and the risk that this consequence will be actualised non-negligible, then the conclusion one is forced toward is one in which the relevant information is supplied whether (or not) a request for such information is tendered. This then is a requirement for morally responsible behaviour in such a situation. We note that is also the basis of the legal response to AIDS in the Australian state of New South Wales.

In summary, we have taken the view that it would of course be generally desirable not to discriminate (socially or legally) against those who are HTLV III infected or against those who have a high probability of being so infected. But this view rests on the presumption that such persons will accept certain responsibilities and obligations in their interactions with others. And of course if there is failure to be responsible, or if it is reasonable to believe that some persons will not be responsible, then there will be a strong case for discriminatory treatment. We shall consider some of these cases in the next section.

We have earlier discussed the difficulty in deciding whether a person is HTLV III virus infected, or at high risk of being so infected. It might be thought these epistemic concerns are small change compared to those required in making the judgment of a person's propensity to act responsibly. We can offer no insight into how this is to be done. Rather we rely on the undeniable truth that it is a judgement that we commonly make in a whole range of personal and public situations, and the epistemic status of such judgements is not thereby taken to be automatically impugned.

5. Cases Where Discrimination May Be Justified

To behave in a morally responsible manner is to behave in a way that minimises the probability that (morally) bad consequences will be brought about. We have no intention of embarking upon the difficult and lengthy task of attempting to set up necessary and sufficient conditions for an individual to be morally responsible. The cases in which we are here interested are ones where some piece of behaviour carries with it a significant probability of bringing about a bad consequence. What is obvious here is that a necessary condition of an individual being able to behave responsibly is that he or she has the capacity to act freely, that is to choose, and that there is not compulsion, mental abnormality or mental incapacity, that renders this impossible.

We have argued that discrimination is justified in cases where it is reasonable to believe that an individual (or group of individuals) is at high risk of having been infected with the HTLV III virus *and* will not act responsibly. We shall here consider three such cases to see why discriminatory treatment is justified in the circumstances depicted. We leave aside the extra, difficult question of the exact nature of the discriminatory treatment which is needed. To some extent this is determined by what is needed to avoid the harmful consequences in question. But more is needed to determine the morally best discriminatory treatment, and the morally best legislation to underpin such treatment.

(a) The Psychotic AIDS Sufferer. Certain kinds of psychosis render an agent not responsible for his actions, or at least not responsible while he is undergoing a psychotic episode.

One example of a psychosis which would render an agent likely to engage in actions that may lead to the infection of other individuals with the HTLV III virus, and simultaneously render him not responsible for those actions, is Manic Depression. While in the manic phase an individual, typically, is subject to overpowering libidinal urges. He also is deluded with respect to his own powers and abilities and becomes prone to gross recklessness. (Manic depressives, typically, find it difficult to sustain personal relations because during a manic phase they are prone to do things like spend all the family savings or give away the family car.) These days many manic depressives are successfully managed with drugs. Some, however, do not respond to this treatment, and others cannot be relied upon to take their medications. Both these latter groups therefore would seem to be proper objects of a general discriminatory treatment, since they cannot be relied upon not to engage in activities which impose non-negligible risks upon others.

In a situation where we have reason to believe a psychotic has been infected by the HTLV III virus, and the probable behavior of the psychotic places others at high risk of very bad consequences, restriction of his freedom of interaction is justified.

A special case is that of the malicious psychotic infected with the HTLV III virus, who knows he is infected and who uses this in his malicious activities. The case for discrimination remains, but the kind of discrimination that is appropriate will clearly be different.[6]

(b) Intravenous Drug Users. Intravenous drug users may place at risk themselves, other IV drug users with whom they share their fits, and their sexual partners. But there seems to be no reason to suppose that they will be markedly less sexually responsible than other members of the community, except per-

haps if they turn to prostitution to support their habit. Here then we will be concerned only with transmission via syringes.

In the case of sexual transmission of the HTLV III virus we typically are concerned with sane, adult individuals. But in the case of intravenous drug users, it is not so clear that they do have real control over their actions (and most specifically actions that could lead to infection with the HTLV III virus). An intravenous drug user who is addicted to his (or her) drug may, in its absence, be *compelled* to behave in reckless ways. Both petty and non-petty crime occurs so that drug users can supply their habits. This in itself is some evidence that drugs make individuals more risk-loving,[7] though there is, of course, also the sheer desperation of dependency. The fact that there is some risk of being infected by the HTLV III virus when one injects an intravenous drug will in many cases be given little weight by an individual whose body is in a state of craving for the drug.

Intravenous drug users who are addicted cannot be seen in the same category as the typical sexual adventurer. For the judgement of the IV drug user will often be seriously imparied because of drug addiciton. Using a Millian framework we may therefore place him (or her) with children and lunatics when assessing the appropriateness of paternalistic legislation aimed at protecting the IV drug users from contracting the HTLV III virus. Using the argument of the preceding sections, it also justifies discrimination against him (or her) to protect others whom he (or she) would otherwise be likely to infect.

This of course leaves without an answer the practical question of what it would be possible to do. Criminalising the sharing of hypodermics would be utterly pointless for the reasons already given. If the risk of contracting the HTLV III virus is impotent with respect of curtailing the practice of sharing needles, then we might expect that so would be the threat of a criminal action. (And IV drug users already face the threat of a criminal action in virtue of the fact that they are users!) Nonetheless it is clear that to restrict such a person, if an adequate mode of restriction could be specified, would be justified.

(c) HTLV III Antibody Positive Children. The recent case of Eve Van Grafhorst raises the question of what is to be done with children who have been infected with the HTLV III virus.[8] For instance, should they or should they not be able to attend regular school? In the case of circumstances surrounding infected children, we can concentrate on children who are proven HTLV III antibody positive.

The HTLV III antibody positive child will, like any other child, have much to gain from both the educational and social aspects of the school situation. Each of the other children the infected child comes in contact with will, on the other hand, be at some (at this time still unquantified and perhaps very small) risk of contracting the virus.

Obviously the problem is greater with respect to younger children, who in the normal run of things will suffer from minor cuts and abrasions, may bite each other, and do not always consistently follow the highest standards of hygiene. We believe, on reliable medical assessment, that the probability of infection of a child by contact with an infected child, in an unsupervised situation, is significant, though quite low.

Children, like all of us, are constantly at risk of injury from many sources. These risks may not be high but they do exist. We all risk injury and death, and impose risks of injury and death upon others each time one of us takes out the car. Activities like riding horses or playing football involve certain risks. Adults who engage in these activities voluntarily undertake these risks. Parents who allow their children to engage in these activities allow those children to be exposed to those risks.

We do not brand such parents irresponsible. It is the general view within our society that if a sporting activity is properly supervised and adequate care taken, the advantages--both physical and psychological--which accrue to those children participating in them outweigh the minor risks they simultaneously undertake. Similarly with the risks associated with being a passenger in a car.

There are of course other activities that parents or schools will not allow children to engage in because they are considered too dangerous (or at least too dangerous in certain circumstances). For example, classes using pools are usually not allowed unrestricted use of the high diving board. And children, generally, are not permitted to sky dive.

For parents of children mixing with an HTLV III antibody positive child the situation is one where whatever the risk the children are exposed to, there is, unlike swimming or football, no obvious countervailing gain to the exposed children. So why should parents let their childern be exposed? The only advantage, it would seem, is to the infected child.

We noted earlier that the right to non-discriminatory treatment carried with it the responsibility not to put others at risk. What is so hard about cases involving children is that we cannot always hold children to be so responsible. The reasons are obvious: they may not possess all the relevant information, and even if they did we do not believe they would be responsible just because they are *children*. So, it may be argued, the right to non-discriminatory treatment is lost.

There are two retorts here. First, children can to some degree--perhaps to the degree they approximate responsible adults--be held responsible for their actions. To this extent at least, antibody positive children should be treated like other children. But while this will be relevant with older children, it will not be relevant to the very young.

Second, since it is usual to transfer the responsibilities of children to their parents or supervisory adults, why not do the same here? But it seems that while we can agree that there generally exists a transferral of responsibility to parents or supervisors, it is not clear that they can adequately discharge *this* responsibility if the children are treated in a totally non-discriminatory fashion.

How can a parent act responsibly and the child simultaneously be treated in a non-discriminatory way at school?

Teachers are not usually informed of the HTLV III antibody status of children, and even if they were they might be unwilling to take on the special responsibility. Children are usually unaware of their status or at least of its implications. Schooling usually involves a large number of physical interactions, some of which may carry with them the risk of passing on the virus. Finally, the parents of the other children may not be in possession of all the relevant information, and even if they were they could do nothing, or little, about it.

The one thing that does seem clear is that a parent cannot act responsibly for a child if the parent is unsure about the child's HTLV III antibody status. So it is the responsibility of the parent(s) of any child who has a background that could make the child at risk to clarify the situation. It also seems clear that some degree of discriminatory treatment for such children will be required at least at some stage.

Clearly such discriminatory practices, however they are presented and whatever attempts are made to make them appear more palatable, will have serious consequences for the child and the family of the child. And of course we find such consequences particularly distressing because they seem so unfair and unjust. It *could* well be that the near certainty of these bad consequences will outweigh the highly improbable very bad consequences that go with non-discrimination. Our view is that that decision should finally be determined by the relevant empirical information on the effects of discrimination on the child, and reliable medical estimates of the probability of infection of other children by an antibody positive child (at a particular time, in particular circumstances). As yet there is great vagueness and uncertainty about these empirical matters. What complicates this balancing is that even without discrimination the prognosis for the HTLV III infected child is extremely bad (worse even than for infected adults), so that the choice of the infected child is between a high probability of dreadful consequences, and a marginally higher probability of marginally worse consequences. But our view is that, at least in some circumstances, the balance will probably fall in favour of some discrimination.

There will be hardliners who maintain no risk is acceptable, and that antibody positive children (and perhaps all people infected with the HTLV III virus) should be subject to strict discrimination. But then the question must be raised: why be so intolerant of *this* risk and simultaneously accept other risks of the same magnitude. Put another way, why discriminate against one particular kind of risk? While determining an acceptable level of risk is a difficult matter, it certainly is related to the consequences that are being risked, and the consequences for a number of kinds of risk may be the same or very similar. Also, while it is hard to be precise as to what level of risk is acceptable, some level will be clearly too high, especially for risks with very bad consequences.

Every year a number of children drown in private swimming pools despite stringent safety requirements. One way to prevent these deaths would be to prohibit backyard pools. This is not done, though the existence of these pools constitutes a risk to small children. So some risks to life, and more specifically in this case, risks to the lives of children, are taken to be acceptable risks.

If the risk of a seven year old passing on the HTLV III virus turns out to be of the same order of magnitude as that of a seven-year-old drowning in a pool then it would be unacceptable to exclude the HTLV III antibody positive child from school. The argument that some parents may not be prepared to accept these risks is beside the point. After all the fact that a parent does not accept the risk imposed by other people having pools gives him no leverage. So why should the former nonacceptance? The irrational attitudes of parents provide no moral justification for discrimination.[9]

It should be noted here that the risk that a child will drown in a private pool can be lessened if parents are more vigilant and pool owners fence their pools. Responsible pool owners and responsible parents should act to lessen the risk of *any* child drowning in a pool. Similarly the parents of antibody positive children and government legislators may be able to implement procedures that lower the risk of one school child passing the HTLV III virus on to another: for example, having someone at the school taking some kind of special supervisory role for such a child.

6. Conclusion

AIDS has confronted our community with a new life threatening risk. It is clear that strict discriminatory practices would help allay those risks. But such practices would not completely remove the risk, and in fact would produce further undesirable consequences for the community. If, instead, those who are at risk of being HTLV III infected are encouraged to behave in a socially responsible manner, and given the information and support they need to make such responsible behaviour acceptable, achievable, and practical, we can minimize, though not completely eliminate, the need for discrimination. It will also, in turn, lower the risk of infection to a level even lower then that which might be expected from more dranconian forms of discrimination, since it will lower the probability of a person *unknowingly* being infected.[10]

Notes

1. See B. Davidson and R. Pargetter, "Weight," *Philosophical Studies* 49 (1986): 219-30.
2. We thank John Campbell whose comments led us to add this sketch of an alternative route.
3. An opportunistic infection is one where the infection occurs while the patient is undergoing some treatment where that treatment predisposes the patient toward the acquiring of the infection.
4. I. Gust, "AIDS," *Bioethics* 5 (1985): 10 *et passim.*
5. The "new" AIDS virus HIV II could be expected to augment this figure.

6. Maliciousness poses a general problem which is certainly not limited to those mental illnesses. There may be grounds for discriminating against HTLV III infected persons where malicious intent can be established.
7. If the risk-loving claim were established this would pose particular problems. Free syringes might then do little to help. Doubt would also be cast on the claim that IV drug users are no more sexually irresponsible than the population at large.
8. Eve Van Grafhorst was an HTLV III antibody child whose mother wished for her to be able to attend pre-school in the state of New South Wales, Australia. Initially she was allowed to attend, but after a parental protest she was excluded.
9. The likely irrationality of the parents of other children poses additional problems for those framing policies concerning HTLV III infected children.
10. We wish to thank John Campbell and Robert Young for their responses to earlier versions of this paper. We also acknowledge the useful comments made on the paper in discussion when it was read at the 1986 conference of the Australasian Association of Philosophy.

Robert Pargetter and Elizabeth W. Prior
Department of Philosophy
La Trobe University

Understanding the Homosexual Patient

The ultimate mistake in management is to see patients in terms of their homosexuality alone as this may be a minor aspect of their personality. The diversity among homosexual men and women is as great as that among heterosexuals

*MICHAEL W. ROSS**
Adelaide

It is important to emphasise the fact that there is probably no typical 'homosexual' patient any more than there is a typical 'heterosexual' patient. On the other hand, there are a number of aspects of homosexual life-styles which differ from many aspects of heterosexual life-styles. These are discussed in an attempt to clarify the appropriate medical and professional approach to homosexual individuals who may be patients.

It is equally important to note that until the last few years, sexual medicine courses were not available in medical schools with the result that medical practitioners have little, if any, knowledge about homosexuality over and above that held by the educated layperson. For this reason, it is important firstly to define homosexuality and to place it into a medical context.

The Homosexual-Heterosexual Continuum

Contrary to popular opinion, 'homosexuals' and 'heterosexuals' do not comprise 2 separate classes of people. Kinsey et al. noted that individuals fit into a continuum which has exclusive heterosexuality at one end and exclusive homosexuality at the other (fig. 1) [1]. If one considers that 1 in 3 male patients is likely to have had a homosexual experience leading to orgasm between the ages of 16 and 55 years, and that almost 1 in 5 will have had as much homosexual experience as heterosexual for at least a 3-year period in the same age range, then it is clear that the world cannot be divided into homosexuals and heterosexuals. However, because our society does stigmatise homosexual relations, we tend to divide individuals arbitrarily into 'homosexuals' and 'heterosexuals' and assume that these are absolute classes. In this article we define 'homosexual' as predominantly homosexual at a particular point in time.

* Dr MICHAEL ROSS is Senior Demonstrator in Psychiatry at the Flinders University Medical School, Adelaide, South Australia, and coordinator of the Gender Clinic at the Flinders Medical Centre. His research interests are in the areas of transsexualism, male homosexuality, and the psychosocial aspects of sexually transmitted diseases.

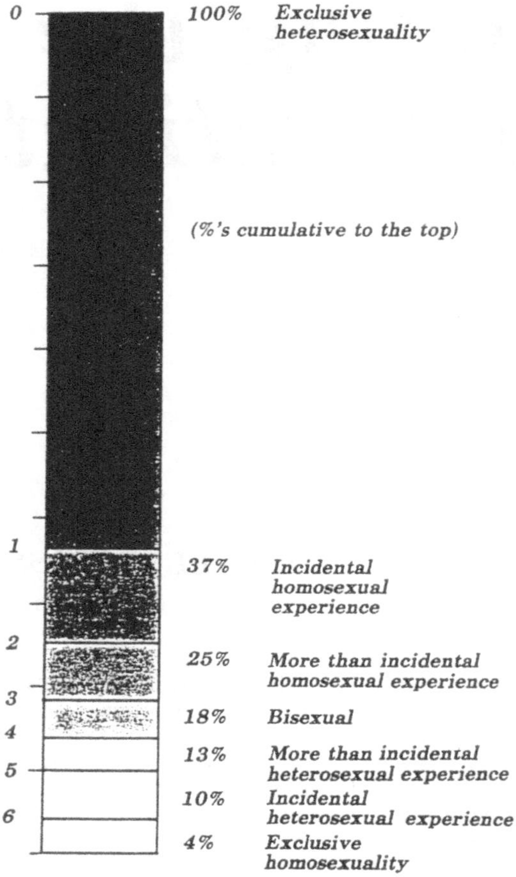

FIG. 1. Kinsey scale and associated proportions of male population.

Homosexual preference may be primary, i.e. having sex is more important than who it is with, or secondary, i.e. the emotional attraction is to the same sex as well. Thus individuals may be behaviourally homosexual but not emotionally or vice versa. It is important to differentiate practice from preference. As an example, McConaghty et al. found in a sample of medical students that over 40% were aware of homosexual feelings, although presumably a much smaller percentage would have acted on these feelings [2]. Within so-called 'homosexual' male samples, Saghir and Robins found that over 48% had had sexual relations with a woman [3] which, as well as illustrating the lack of discrete groups, points to the fact that male homosexuality is not a distaste for female sexual partners but a preference for male ones.

Patients may tell the physician that they are homosexual for a variety of reasons

Disclosure and Medical Attitudes

Those patients who indicate to their medical practitioner that they are homosexual will do so for a variety of reasons, either because they wish to discuss the area with regard to sexual counselling [4] or because they believe that this information will aid medical management. However, not all overtly homosexual patients will share the fact of their sexual preference. Dardick and Grady found that less than 50% of openly homosexual men in the US had told their primary health-care provider that they were gay [5]. One must assume that for those who are covertly homosexual the figure is even lower. In Australia, I found that over 20% of gay men presenting with sexually transmitted diseases did not tell the attending practitioner that their infection was homosexually acquired [6]. Unfortunately, one of the reasons for this is that three-quarters of a sample of 1000 doctors acknowledged that knowing a male patient was homosexual would adversely affect their medical management [7]. As recently as 1980, 84% of American physicians surveyed agreed that homosexual patients hesitate to seek medical care because of physician disapproval [8].

In the light of these findings, it is important to realise that if a male patient volunteers information about his homosexuality the decision has probably not been taken lightly, and that an understanding and accepting response is important. It is also important not to assume that all patients are heterosexual unless one is advised to the contrary. Indeed, between 10 and 20% of gay men are or have been heterosexually married [9], and

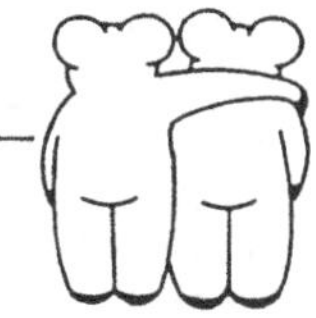

some 54% of homosexual encounters in public conveniences are by married men who define themselves as heterosexual [10].

Areas of Difference in Homosexual Health Care

When a male patient has revealed his sexual orientation, this is usually in the interests of honesty and obtaining more complete health care. There is a tendency to see a homosexual preference as pertaining only to sexual matters, which is a particularly narrow definition. While this information may mean swabbing of additional sites for sexually transmitted diseases if the patient is sexually active (anorectal as well as the usual urethral and oropharyngeal sites), it also has farther reaching implications.

Stigma associated with homosexuality may present as psychological stress or psychosomatic illness

Since a homosexual preference is still stigmatised to a greater or lesser extent in Australasian society, the patient will carry burdens associated with either coping with negative reaction if he is overtly homosexual or, if he is not openly homosexual, coping with the anxieties of keeping sexual orientation hidden and fear of disclosure. The cost of this will be extremely variable. However, there are considerable implications in terms of psychosomatic illness including unexplained headaches, hypertension, gastrointestinal disorders ranging from ulceration to irritable bowel syndrome, and asthma which has a functional component. Psychological stress may also present in a variety of less somatic forms, such as sleep disturbance or generalised anxiety. In most cases the stress is manageable through an accepting clinical interaction or referral to stress management programmes and relaxation training.

On the other hand, the great majority of homosexual men will experience little or no problems with their sexual orientation. It is important to note that homosexuality has not been considered a mental disorder since it was removed from the Descriptive and Statistical Manual (DSM-3) of the American Psychiatric Association in 1973. Nor is there any evidence that, as a group, homosexuals are any different to heterosexuals in their psychological stability and mental functioning. Apart from difficulties with the same range of problems which trouble heterosexual individuals, the homosexual patient may be remarkable in psychological terms only where stigma management presents as an issue.

Stages of Acceptance of Homosexuality

Patients will present in different stages of acceptance of their homosexuality. The best model for describing the path to acceptance of one's sexual orientation has been described by Cass [11]. She has posited 6 stages in the development of a homosexual identity in the individual:

1. *Identity confusion*
2. *Identity comparison*
3. *Identity tolerance*
4. *Identity acceptance*
5. *Identity pride*
6. *Identity synthesis.*

Identity confusion describes the stage where individuals feel that they are different from others and that their feelings or behaviours may be labelled as homosexual. The second stage, identity comparison, is for the individual the first tentative commitment to a homosexual identity and the realisation of being homosexual to a degree.

With identity tolerance in the individual comes the recognition that he or she is probably homosexual and a degree of commitment to this identity arises. By stage four, the identity acceptance stage, the individual accepts the label of homosexual, at least in gay company, and begins to socialise within a gay subculture. The stage of identity pride is marked by wide disclosure and open activism and describes the situation where everything the individual does is defined primarily by his or her homosexuality. At this stage, the central identity of the person is as a homosexual.

The sixth stage of the Cass model is perhaps the one which has stimulated most debate. In the individual, the 'them versus us' view of homosexuals and heterosexuals fades, and is replaced by a situation where the person's homosexual identity is seen as being one of a series of identities, but not one which defines all aspects of the person's life-style. The individual may thus see being homosexual as an incidental matter like political belief or occupation, and not something that he or she is all the time.

Patients' sexuality must be dealt with depending on their own level of acceptance

It is important that we deal with patients' sexuality depending on the level of acceptance they are at and do not try to push them too fast through these stages. We should let them achieve these stages, with encouragement, at their own pace.

Homosexual Relationships

The popular view of the homosexual as promiscuous is not an accurate one for the great majority of gay individuals. A recent survey of gay men in the US found that the median number of lifetime sexual partners of sexually continuously active individuals was less than 50 [12]. It is important to bear this in mind when reading of atypical samples (e.g. many AIDS victims) in which numbers of sexual partners may number in the hundreds or thousands.

A significant proportion of gay men and women will be in homosexual relationships. These relationships have been classified into 4 general categories in a study of Californian homosexual men by Bell and Weinberg [13]. They divided their sample into:

1. *Close-coupleds*
2. *Open-coupleds*
3. *Functionals*
4. *Dysfunctionals.*

The 'close-coupleds' were closely bound together and monogamous, in the sense that the 2 individuals tended to look to one another for sexual and interpersonal satisfactions. They had the lowest level of sexual or psychological problems.

The 'open-coupleds' were living with a special sexual partner, but tended to seek sexual and interpersonal satisfactions with people outside their partnership although this tended to worry them. Psychologically and sexually, they had no more or no less problems than other groups.

The 'functionals' were the equivalent of the swinging singles, and appeared to organise their life around their sexual experiences. They tended to have wide social circles and few sexual and psychological problems.

In contrast, the 'dysfunctionals' were troubled people whose life offered them little gratification and who displayed significantly greater psychological and sexual problems than any other group. This group most closely accorded with the old stereotype of the tormented homosexual.

While this sketch of homosexual relational patterns is brief, it does indicate the great diversity of interpersonal styles which exist within a homosexual life-style.

Sexual Practices and Sexually Transmitted Diseases

To most people, it is sexual practices and gender of partner which sets homosexuals apart from heterosexuals. In practice, however, the same range of sexual activities are practised by both heterosexuals and homosexuals, with the exception of the absence of penovaginal intercourse in homosexuals. It is not generally realised that anal receptive intercourse is practised regularly by 1 in 12 women [14]. While some homosexual men do have a preference for a particular role in anal intercourse or fellatio, the most common situation is for multiple sexual activities to occur in any sexual interaction. Contrary to popular opinion, anal intercourse only occurs in about one-third of male homosexual encounters. Fellatio and mutual masturbation are more common in terms of frequency [15]. In homosexual women, activities will most commonly involve oral or manual stimulation.

From a medical point of view, anal intercourse if carried out with inadequate lubrication or any great degree of vigour may lead to lesions of the rectal epithelium which in places may be only one cell thick, in contrast to the cornified vaginal epithelium. This may act as a portal for pathogens, and thus lead to greater risk than with penovaginal intercourse. The range of sexually transmitted diseases associated with homosexual men includes syphilis, gonorrhoea, non-gonococcal urethritis, hepatitis (A, B, and non-A, non-B), herpes, and the so-called 'gay bowel syndrome' including amoebiasis, giardiasis, shigellosis, Chlamydia infections, anal warts and proctitis [16].

Sexual attitudes affect life-style

While hepatitis and enteric infections are associated with analingus, a practice apparently much more common in the US than in Australasia, it is important to note that the spectrum of sexually transmitted diseases is markedly broader in sexually active homosexual men than was traditionally assumed. To these sexually transmitted diseases must now be added AIDS.

While the great majority of homosexual men will not be at any greater risk of sexually related infections, it is important to expand our previously narrow view of the range of sexually transmitted diseases and to test for additional pathogens in homosexually active men where symptoms occur. As an example, some 37% of Australasian homosexually active men may be surface antibody positive for hepatitis B [17].

Attitudes to Sexuality and Risk Factors in Homosexual Men

From a medical point of view, there are 3 major risk factors for sexually transmitted diseases in homosexual men:

1. *Partner numbers*
2. *Particular sexual practices, e.g. the risks of infection from mutual masturbation are negligible*
3. *Anonymity of partners, which makes contact-tracing difficult.*

In a recent study of the psychological and social factors which influence sexually transmitted disease risks, I found that particular dimensions of sexual attitudes best predicted how the individual managed a homosexual life-style [15]. These dimensions included attitudes to relationships, degree of control of sexual excitement and libido, degree of being visually stimulated by members of the same gender, social comfôrt, acceptance of one's homosexuality, and degree of permissiveness or prudishness. Homosexual individuals may vary across all of these dimensions. It would be a mistake to assume that the simple fact of a homosexual preference can predict anything about how the individual exists as a homosexual. Again, it must also be emphasised that the range of attitudes in homosexual men and women is as wide as the range of attitudes in heterosexual men and women. However, those attitudinal dimensions referred to above do appear to be the important ones in determining what sort of sexual life-style is led.

Homosexual Women

Homosexual women are at much less risk than heterosexual women of contracting sexually transmitted diseases [18] and also enjoy on average much better mental health than heterosexual women [19]. They may still present with the usual range of medical problems as other women, although these are unlikely to be directly related to their sexual preference. Most if not all of the comments made with regard to male homosexuals will also apply to dealing with female homosexual patients, although some of the difficulties faced by homosexual women may include issues such as childrearing. There may also be difficulties with the management of social stigma.

Conclusion

In conclusion, while it is important to have a medical and psychological understanding of the range of problems which homosexual men and women may have, it is also critical that we see these health problems as being neither solely sexually related nor stereotypically homosexual. In understanding and managing homosexual patients, the central issue is to appreciate that homosexual individuals cover the same wide spectrum of humanity as heterosexual persons, and that the division of people into 'heterosexual' and 'homosexual' groups is arbitrary although less psychologically threatening. The ultimate management mistake is to see patients in terms of their homosexuality alone and to ignore the fact that their sexual orientation may be a minor aspect of their identity and personality. The diversity of individuals who may be homosexual precludes generalisation about them from the fact of their sexual orientation alone.

References

1. Kinsey, A.C. et al.: Sexual Behavior in the Human Male (W.B. Saunders, Philadelphia 1948).
2. McConaghy, N. et al.: The incidence of bisexual feelings and opposite sex behavior in medical students. Journal of Nervous and Mental Disease 167: 685 (1979).
3. Saghir, M.T. and Robins, E.: Male and Female Homosexuality: A comprehensive investigation (Williams and Wilkins, Baltimore 1973).
4. Ross, M.W.: Counselling the homosexual patient. Patient Management New Zealand 12: 131 (May 1983).
5. Dardick, L. and Grady, D.: Openness between gay persons and health professionals. Annals of Internal Medicine 93: 115 (1980).
6. Ross, M.W.: Attitudes of male homosexuals to venereal disease clinics. Medical Journal of Australia 2: 670 (1981).
7. Pauly, I.B. and Goldstein, S.: Physicians' attitudes in treating homosexuals. Medical Aspects of Human Sexuality 4: 26 (1970).
8. Sandholzer, T.A.: Physician attitudes and other factors affecting the incidence of sexually transmitted diseases in homosexual men. Journal of Homosexuality 5: 325 (1980).
9. Ross, M.W.: The Married Homosexual Man: A Psychological Study (Routledge and Kegan Paul, London 1983).
10. Humphreys, R.A.L.: Tearoom Trade: A Study of Impersonal Sex in Public Places (Duckworth, London 1970).
11. Cass, V.C.: Homosexual identity formation: A theoretical model. Journal of Homosexuality 4: 219 (1979).
12. Darrow, W. et al.: The gay report on sexually transmitted diseases. American Journal of Public Health 71: 104 (1981).
13. Bell, A.P. and Weinberg, M.S.: Homosexualities: A Study of Diversity among Men and Women (Macmillan, Melbourne 1978).
14. Bolling, D.R.: Prevalence, goals and complications of heterosexual anal intercourse in a gynaecologic population. Journal of Reproductive Medicine 19: 120 (1977).
15. Ross, M.W.: Psychovenereology: Personality and Lifestyle Factors in Sexually Transmitted Diseases in Homosexual Men (Praeger, New York 1985).
16. Ostrow, D.G. and Altman, N.L.: Sexually transmitted diseases and homosexuality. Sexually Transmitted Diseases 10: 208 (1983).
17. Burrell, C.J. et al.: Hepatitis B reservoirs and attack rates in an Australian community: A basis for vaccination and crossinfection policies. Medical Journal of Australia 2: 492 (1983).
18. Robertson, P. and Schacter, J.: Failure to identify venereal disease in a lesbian population. Sexually Transmitted Diseases 8: 75 (1981).
19. Freedman, M.: Homosexuality and Psychological Functioning (Brooks-Cole, Belmont 1971).

Transfiguring Sexual Identity: AIDS & the Contemporary Construction of Homosexuality

STEVEN SEIDMAN

AIDS appeared during a period of significant change in our sexual conventions. A series of movements in the 60s and 70s pointed in the direction of expanded erotic choice and tolerance for diversity. The women's movement struggled for women's erotic autonomy. Feminists demanded that women be able to define and control their own sexuality, and that included choosing a lesbian alternative. Less visible were the struggles by sexually disenfranchised groups like the elderly or the disabled to be accepted as full sexual beings. The counterculture made a more open and expressive eroticism a prominent part of its social rebellion. Furthermore, changes in our sexual norms that reflected long-term trends became evident. For example, the norm that sex is legitimate only as an act of love or a sign of relational fidelity was challenged. Sex discourses and representations (e.g. pornography, sex manuals, radical sex ideologies) appeared that constructed sex as an autonomous sphere of pleasure and self-expression with its own intrinsic value and justification. A libertarian sex ethic accepted sex for its pleasurable qualities in any context of mutual consent and respect. This has expanded the types of relationships in which sex is permitted. Indeed, the exclusivity of marriage as the proper site for sex has given way to a more flexible convention that tolerates sex in varied relational settings. In short, while it would be misleading to assert that a revolution occurred, there did transpire important changes in our sexual norms and behavior during this period.

Indicative of this more liberal sexual culture was the increased tolerance for homosexuality. By the mid-70s gay subcultures were visible in virtually every major urban center.[1] These provided gay people with institutional protection, a source of social support and a mass base for a politics of civil rights reform and gay liberation. Within these gay spaces a cultural apparatus emerged that included gay-oriented publications (books, magazines, newspapers), theatre groups, movies, and so on. Of particular importance is that this new gay intelligentsia articulated affirmative images of homosexuality. Constructions of 'the homosexual' as a morally perverse, deviant or pathological figure were assailed. Homosexuality was reconceived to refer to a morally neutral need or behavior that is not indicative of a distinctive personality type. New models viewed the homosexual as a person with merely an alternative sexual or affectional preference or as a member of an oppressed minority. In fact, some gays endorsed the notion of homosexuals as different but reconceived this in affirmative ways. Finally, gay people made important gains in political empowerment and social inclusion. For example, by the mid-70s more than half the states in the U.S. repeated their sodomy laws; dozens of cities passed anti-discrimination ordinances; the civil service commission eliminated its ban on hiring homosexuals and so on.

The trend towards sexual liberalization and, in particular, the tolerance of homosexuals, encountered a lot of resistance and hostility. In the late 70s this tolerance narrowed considerably as antigay themes became integral to a revived conservative politics. The explanation for this lay perhaps in social developments that paralleled sexual liberalization. Specifically, the conjunction of a series of events including an economic recession, political legitimation problems stemming from Watergate, military setbacks in Vietnam and Iran, and social disturbances arising from the various civil rights, protest and liberation movements, produced a pervasive sense of social crisis and decline. Although social and political responses to this situation were varied, it is not coincidental that a series of purity crusades swept across the country.[2] This was one way people responded to feelings of social danger and sought to gain control over social events. Different groups or phenomena, from pornography to paedophiles, were targeted. However, gay people in particular were singled out. This was not entirely fortuitous. The trend towards the acceptance or at least tolerance of homosexuality challenged the exclusive legitimacy of a heterosexual and marital norm. Moreover, the visibility and political assertiveness of homosexuals, coupled to their symbolic association with social dissolution in a context perceived by many Americans as one of family breakdown and national decline, made them easy prey for scapegoating.

The anxiety and hostility many Americans felt towards recent developments were displaced onto homosexuality. Homosexuals were portrayed as a public menace, as a threat to the family, and as imperiling the national security by promoting self-centered, hedonistic and pacifist values. An antigay backlash crystallized that was initially centered around local and state campaigns to repeal gay rights ordinances. Gradually, it expanded to include national legislation, the resurgence of anti-homosexual discourses, and escalating discrimination and violence toward homosexuals.[3] Its aim was to deny legitimacy to homosexuality; to dismantle gay subcultural institutions; to return homosexuals to a condition of invisibility and marginality; and to reassert a discourse of the dangers of homosexuality.

By the early 1980s the conservative offensive against gay people appeared to be losing some momentum. The Family Protection Act, initially introduced in 1979 and resubmitted in 1981, failed to gain congressional approval. The Briggs initiative, a major piece of antigay legislation, was defeated. Gay rights ordinances were successfully defended or newly enacted. Unfortunately, the marginalization of the antigay campaign suggested by these defeats did not come to pass. The appearance of AIDS and the recognition of its epidemic proportions by 1983 reinvigorated a waning antigay politics. Antigay themes assumed a new prominence in New Right politics as AIDS was seized upon to promote a conservative social agenda. The political ramifications of AIDS have been widely commented upon.[4] I want to press a different point: AIDS has given rise to a far-reaching, perhaps unprecedented, public discussion of homosexuality. Claims about the nature of homosexuality, the identity and culture of homosexuals, and their proper place in the U.S. are being openly debated. AIDS is being used to advocate changes in homosexual identity and behavior. These constructions of homosexuality are likely to be fateful for some time to come.

Specifically, I argue that AIDS has provided a pretext to reinsert homosexuality within a symbolic drama of pollution and purity. Conservatives have used AIDS to rehabilitate the notion of 'the homosexual' as a polluted figure. AIDS is read as revealing the essence of a promiscuous homosexual desire and proof of its dangerous and subversive nature. The reverse side of this demonization of homosexuality is the purity of heterosexuality and the valorization of a monogamous, marital sexual ethic. To be sure, the discourse of homosexuality occasioned by AIDS is not uniform. Liberal segments of the heterosexual media have, in the main, repudiated a politics aimed at the repression of homosexuality. Instead, they have enlisted AIDS in their campaign to construct an image of the "respectable homosexual" and to legitimate a sexual ethic of monogamy and romance. Similar themes are conspicuous in the gay media. In fact, many gays have used AIDS to articulate their own redemptive drama. In imagery that oscillates between the apocalyptic and the millenial, AIDS is seen as marking the failure of a way of life; as signaling, like Stonewall, another critical turning point in the coming of age of homosexuals; and, finally, as the beginnings of a new maturity and social responsibility among homosexuals.

AIDS & Heterosexual Constructions of Homosexuality

In the heterosexual media the identification of AIDS as a gay disease was made early and has proved sustaining despite overwhelming evidence to the contrary. Initially, the appearance of Kaposi's Sarcoma and other rare cancers among young homosexual men led researchers to designate the term GRID (Gay Related Immune Deficiency) for this new syndrome. Taking its cure from medical researchers, the mass media referred to this disease as the "homosexual cancer," the "gay epidemic."[5] These terms suggest an intrinsic tie between homosexuality and AIDS. The causal link was identified as homosexual behavior.

The two most prominent epidemiological theories directly joined AIDS to homosexual acts. The so-called "Overload theory" held that "the gay lifestyle" (the combination of drug use, poor health habits and a history of sexually transmitted diseases resulting from sexual promiscuity) is responsible for the collapse of the immune system. The currently more accepted theory asserts the existence of a virus which combined with other factors breaks down the body's resistance to disease. The introduction of semen into the body during sex releases the virus into the blood stream. The typical scenario that is postulated holds that repeated anal intercourse tears the delicate tissue of the anus. This allows the semen and therefore the virus of the infected person to pass into the blood circulation of the unsuspecting other. Both theories underscore the association between sexual behavior and AIDS among homosexuals. They highlight sexual "promiscuity" as the intermediary or connecting link. The Overload theory posits a more direct, ironic, and insidious dynamic: the immediate sensual pleasures of "promiscuous" sex sets in motion a hidden telos of disease and death. The very act of sexual union—with its cultural resonances of love and the production of life—is turned into an act of death as bodily defenses collapse. Although the viral hypothesis does not view AIDS as the very signature of homosexual behavior, it asserts an indirect tie between promiscuity and AIDS among homosexual men. It is, after all, only under conditions of non-monogamy that sex can threaten viral infection. Both the Overload and the viral theory, then, represent medical frameworks that center on the causality between sexual promiscuity, disease, and death.

In fact, promiscuity became the focal point in the heterosexual media. It has shown a seemingly endless fascination with the quantitative aspects of homosexual behavior. An early and widely reported study by a Center for Disease Control task force in 1981 provided the initial medical justification for this preoccupation.[6] Assuming a connection between gay sexual patterns and the large numbers of male homosexual AIDS cases, CDC researchers compared the sexual patterns of AIDS cases with a male homosexual control group. They reported that the AIDS group had approximately twice as many sex partners as the control group. Although the precise nature of the connection between the number of sex partners and AIDS was unclear, researchers opinioned a causal tie. Serious doubts have been raised about this study.[7] A central flaw is that this study did not define what constitutes a sex act. When does an act between two men count as a sexual act? Does the number of sexual partners suggest a common reference for heterosexuals and homosexual men? If gay men count behavior in which there is no exchange of semen as sex acts (e.g., mutual masturbation, body rubbing, kissing) then the number of sex partners *per se* is irrelevant to AIDS. If the key factor is the introduction of semen into one's blood stream, then the relevant data concerns the number of sex partners with whom there occurred sex acts of this type. Unfortunately the CDC study did not analyze gay sexual patterns in terms of types of sex acts. In fact, the comparisons between the AIDS cases and the control group along the key dimension of exposure to semen revealed no statistically significant differences. Whatever the causal link between homosexual behavior and AIDS the initial CDC study provided few credible clues.

Despite the obvious flaws of the study, the heterosexual media played up the angle of gay promiscuity. The mass media repeatedly concentrated on the number of sex partners homosexual men have per night, week, month, year, and lifetime. These reports did not interpret these figures in the context of gay subcultural life nor in relation to the broader changes in the sexual patterns of Americans. In a sense, the heterosexual media was simply following the pronouncements of the medical establishment. Yet, it is unfortunately not that simple. The medical scenarios, especially through 1983, were highly tentative, conjectural and often contradictory. The mass media didn't merely report the facts but constructed the very reality of AIDS by drawing selectively on medical data and framing this information in a non-medical interpretive schema. By featuring the number of sex partners as the key causal link without further qualification or contextualization, the heterosexual media was, in fact, offering its own particular image of homosexuality.

In the heterosexual media response to AIDS, promiscuity became the defining property of gay sexuality. Headlines and feature stories in all the major national media dramatized a gay lifestyle, a fastlane life of indiscriminate casual sex. A piece in *The San Francisco Examiner* found in AIDS confirmation of the conventional wisdom that gays are "a population whose lifestyle is based on a freewheeling approach to sex."[8] John Fuller in *Science Digest* observed that AIDS is simply further evidence of what science has told us about homosexual men. "Sociologists and psychologists had long noted that the constant search for new sexual partners is a persistent pattern among many gay males."[9] Some commentators underlined the paradoxical aspects of homosexuality. "Ironically, the freedom, the promiscuity . . . that many gays declared an integral part of their culture have come to haunt them."[10] I want to here underscore a key point regarding this discourse: the promiscuity of homosexual men is not considered incidental or a historically specific behavioral property of homosexuality. Rather, it is viewed as essential to homosexuality. In other words, this discourse resurrects an older notion of the male homosexual as a type of person with unique physical, emotional and behavioral traits. His essence is that of a hyper-sexual human type. Homosexual men sexualize themselves and others; they reduce persons to eroticized bodies; they frame sex as mere physical release or pleasure-seeking. Promiscuity manifests the lustful, amoral nature of the homosexual. Homosexual desire symbolizes pure sexual lust or unrestrained desire subject only to the quantitative limitations of physical exhaustion. It is this compulsive, hyperactive, insatiable desire that compels homosexuals to eroticize the forbidden and to transgress all moral boundaries, rendering them dangerous. Homosexuality is constructed as the very antithesis of the heterosexual marital ideal where sex is joined to romance, love and relational permanence and fidelity.

The AIDS discourse on homosexuality is a moral one. The juxtaposition of homosexuality and heterosexual romantic love carries a moral distinction between dangers the dangers of homosexual promiscuity and the purity of heterosexual love and monogamy. From this vantage point, AIDS reveals not only the truth of homosexuality but is its just punishment. Some commentators have seen in AIDS proof of the unnaturalness or perversity of homosexuality. "The poor homosexuals—they have declared war upon nature, and now nature is exacting an awful retribution," writes President Reagan's former Aid Patrick Buchanan.[11] Reverend Charles Stanley, head of the 14.3 million member Southern Baptist Convention remarked: "It [homosexuality] is a sinful lifestyle, according to the scripture, and I believe that AIDS is God indicating his displeasure and his attitude towards that form of lifestyle."[12] Finally, arriving at the same moral judgment but framed within a medical-scientific discourse, Dr. James Fletcher writes in the *Southern Medical Journal*: "If we act as empirical scientists can we not see the implications of the data [AIDS and STD's among homosexual men] before us? Might not these 'complications' be 'consequences' [of homosexuality]? Were it so a logical conclusion is that AIDS is a self-inflicted disorder . . . Indeed from an empirical medical perspective alone current scientific observation seems to require the conclusion that homosexuality is a pathologic condition."[13]

In the above moral rhetorics, AIDS represents a just punishment for homosexuals since they have violated a basic law of God, Nature and Society. There is, however, another more subtle logic of moral judgement presented in the AIDS phenomenon. AIDS is seen as the homosexual's death wish turned upon himself. In modern mythology, homosexuality indicates an unconscious will to subvert and destroy society. Images of subversion surround the homosexual. The ubiquitous association of homosexuals with the corruption of children—the very symbol of purity and social order—is indicative of their link to death. It is, I believe, precisely because in our symbolic universe homosexuality is constructed as a social danger evoking resonances of decline and chaos, that AIDS is seen not only as the truth of homosexuality but as its just punishment. AIDS signals the wish for the annihilation of 'the other' being turned inward, back against the homosexual himself. It's because homosexuality symbolizes a threat to life and society that even in the face of the mass suffering and death among homosexuals the public reaction has often been complacent, indifferent, and vengeful. For threatening social existence and "killing the innocent," homosexual men have received their just desert in AIDS. This, at least, appears to be a perhaps unconscious moral sentiment conveyed in the heterosexual response to AIDS.

AIDS has contributed to reviving a notion of the homosexual as a dangerous and polluted figure. Moreover, the revitalization of a discredited image of homosexuality structured the public response to AIDS. As the principle victim of AIDS but also identified as its chief perpetrator, homosexual men were doubly victimized: by the disease and by society's response to it. Blamed for their own affiliation, accused of spreading disease and death to innocent people, criticized as a drain upon scarce national resources, homosexual AIDS victims felt socially scorned and shunned.[14] Stories circulated of hospital staff, police, and criminal justice personnel refusing physical contact with AIDS victims, of AIDS victims left unattended in hospitals leaving friends and family responsible for their care. Feature stories told of AIDS victims being fired from their jobs, evicted from their homes, ejected from public places. Numerous reports narrate how homosexual AIDS victims had to manage, often alone, a social death in anticipation of their physical one.

AIDS served as an ideal pretext for upgrading the surveillance and oppression of homosexuals. By the end of 1985 demands were being made for stepped up state regulation of homosexual AIDS cases through administering an "AIDS" test as a condition of employment, military service, health and life insurance, blood donation, and so on. Quarantining AIDS cases was seriously discussed and in some states statutes were amended to give the government the power to implement a quarantine.[15] Suggestions were heard to empower the state to rehabilitate sexually promiscuous homosexual men through drugs or confinement. Beyond the repressive measures sought in response to AIDS, backlash forces held that the AIDS crisis rendered homosexuals a public health threat. By claiming that AIDS has produced a national health crisis, backlash forces tried to enlist the state to dismantle gay subcultural institutions. Efforts to close gay bars and baths were part of a broader strategy of withdrawing public tolerance for homosexuals. There were renewed efforts to press for the remedicalization and recriminalization of homosexual behavior. For example the Dallas Doctors Against AIDS issued the following declaration. "Such a sexual public health concern must cause the citizenry of this country to do everything in their power to smash the homosexual movement in this country to make sure these kinds of acts are criminalized."[16] Movements in support of gay rights ordinances were frustrated and efforts to reinstitute or endorse antisodomy laws were given a fresh impetus. At a more immediate level, gay men felt the intensification of oppression through an increase of reported acts of discrimination, harassment and physical assault.[17]

The response to AIDS in the heterosexual media was not uniform. For liberals, AIDS was seen less as disclosing the universal truth of homosexual desire than as revealing the failure of the sexual revolution. Instead of criticizing a hypostatized homosexual desire, liberals identified the urban male gay subculture and its libertarian sexual ideology as the key causal link between promiscuity and AIDS among homosexual men. At times, it must be said, the line between liberal "historicism" and conservative "universalism" or the line between tolerance and repression collapses. After criticizing conservative attempts to enlist AIDS in their politics of repression, Charles Krauthammer, writing in *The New Republic*, alludes to a possible natural link between homosexual behavior and this disease. "In reality no one knows whether AIDS is accidently a homosexual disease or intrinsically so."[18] Moreover, without a historical analysis of the development of the gay subculture, the liberal perspective simply shifts the hypostatization of the promiscuous homosexual from an abstract homosexual desire to an equally ahistorically conceived gay subculture. Liberals have, however, consistently opposed backlash efforts to use AIDS to reinstitute a harsh regime of homosexual oppression. They have criticized the AIDS hysteria and attempts to exploit it to further fuel an antigay backlash.

Although the liberal media has sought to avoid the politicizing of AIDS, liberals have seized on AIDS, no less than conservatives, to propagate their own sexual morality. They have used AIDS to reaffirm the morality of monogamy and romantic love. In fact, the liberal media has sought to rehabilitate a pre-gay liberation ideal of the "respectable homosexual": discreet, coupled, monogamous, and cohabitating.

The *New York Times*, for example, has virtually campaigned to create and legitimate this ideal of the respectable homosexual.[19] Its coverage of AIDS has regularly included interviews with prominent figures in the gay community or relevant "experts" who uniformly criticize the immature and irresponsible promiscuous lifestyle accepted in the gay subculture of the 1970s. Articles appeared that reported changes in the behavior of homosexuals. Key indicators of the fastlane gay lifestyle, e.g., numbers of sex partners, STD's, bathhouse attendance were scrutinized to detect indications of a retreat from promiscuity. Reports of a new emphasis upon dating, courting, and nonsexual attendance were scrutinized to detect indications of a retreat from socializing were given prominence. The *Times* did more than report these developments; it clearly endorsed them. In fact, by virtue of its prestige and its enlisting of experts and community leaders, the *Times* became a major social force in promoting these changes. It ran pieces on homosexual couples who were obviously intended to serve as role models to a crisis-ridden and anomic gay community. One such piece entitled, "Homosexual Couple finds a Quiet Pride," focuses on two professional men who have lived together for some forty years. They are, in appearance, indistinguishable from conventional heterosexuals. In other words, there is no trace of a more unconventional gay subcultural style to their self-presentation. There is an implied discreetness to their homosexuality and their demeanor exudes an almost exaggerated sense of staid respectability. They are described as preoccupied with typical heterosexual concerns such as career, family, domestic affairs, hobbies and anniversaries. The "success" or longevity of their relationship is summed up by the remark, "You have to work at it." Quite clearly, the *Times* is offering them or its construction of them as a model of what is an acceptable homosexual style. With moral codes and identity-models in flux, and with homosexuality itself assailed by backlash forces, this image of a discreet, monogamous, coupled and conventional homosexual life is endorsed as an alternative to more unconventional gay socioerotic models. In fact, the principle thesis of the article is that a "heterosexual model" is now being adopted by homosexuals. "In recent years, some homosexual couples have begun to adopt many of the traditions of heterosexual marriage. Besides having wedding and anniversary parties, couples are exchanging vows . . . in religious services known as 'gay unions.' They are drawing up contracts, wills . . . to provide legal, protections for themselves and their partners. They are adopting children . . .".[20] Setting aside for the moment the credibility of this argument, the message seems indisputable: AIDS is a positive catalyst encouraging homosexual men to adopt heterosexual relational patterns. Because of AIDS homosexual men are rediscovering the charm, civility, security and safety of romance and monogamy. Liberals, no less than conservatives, have exploited AIDS for their own moral purposes. Whereas the latter enlist AIDS as part of their backlash politics, the former use AIDS to relate a moral tale of the virtues of romantic love and monogamy.

AIDS & The Crisis of Homosexuality in the Gay Community

There is a common theme running through the liberal heterosexual and gay AIDS discourse. Segments of the gay community have used AIDS to criticize gay subculture for propagating an ethic of sexual promiscuity. At times the gay media appears to endorse the heterosexual caricature of the profligate homosexual. In fact, AIDS has occasioned within the gay community a turn to a medical language of normality and pathology in an effort to induce behavioral changes among homosexual men. Finally, there is a rather insidious aspect to the gay response whereby AIDS takes on a redemptive significance. AIDS manifests the failure of an ideology and a way of life. It has, moreover, initiated a period of self-criticism and reform of the gay community. A rebirth of sorts is being enacted and AIDS is the principal catalyst. In other words, the suffering brought on by AIDS is made meaningful by rendering it a period of personal and collective rebirth.

Gay men were among the earliest defenders of the Overload theory. This might seem odd since the basic message of this theory is that homosexuals have brought AIDS upon themselves through their own promiscuous behavior. Yet, gay proponents of the Overload theory have been perhaps its most enthusiastic supporters. In a much discussed early piece in the gay press, "We Know Who We Are," Michael Callen, Richard Berkowitz, and Richard Dworkin surmise "that their is no mutant virus and there will be no vaccine. We must accept that we have overloaded our immune system's with common viruses and other sexually transmitted infections. Our [promiscuous] lifestyle has created the present epidemic of AIDS among gay men."[21] An anonymous gay physician was even more succinct in interpreting the message of AIDS: "depravity kills!" The full moral weight of this self-incriminatory rhetoric is partially displaced by targeting the gay subculture as the source of the "gay lifestyle" and therefore of AIDS. Callen assails the norms and conventions of a sex-obsessed urban gay subculture. "Throughout ten years of promiscuity, I have tried to be a good gay and wear my STD's as red badges of courage in a war against a sex-negative society."[22] Callen's severely critical attitudes towards the gay subculture is not exceptional. For example, writing in *The Village Voice*, Stephen Harvey comments: "For years, gay men have been prey to a brand of propaganda perpetrated among themselves which, in its subtle way, has been scarcely less insidious than the harangues aimed at the community from without . . . Co-ghettoists have implied . . . that there was something stunted and incomplete in the lives of any gay men who couldn't get into those obligatory Saturday nights of mass euphoria in the dark . . . To cast doubt on any aspect of the way we habitually behave has been decided out of hand as reactionary . . . In this town at least . . . what gay solidarity means is the high times you have with regulars of the bars, disco, bathhouse of your choice."[23] For many gay men, AIDS symbolized the failure of a gay subculture and lifestyle.

Although the sexual norms and social conventions of the gay subculture are targeted as the main causal tie between promiscuity and AIDS, the individual is not absolved from guilt. Quite the contrary, a salient dimension of the gay reponse to AIDS is that it implicates the individual in his own victimization. Thus, Callen appeals to those promiscuous gays "who know who they are to acknowledge and change their lifestyle. We have remained silent because we have been unable or unwilling to accept responsibility for the role that our own excessiveness has played in our present public health crisis. But, deep down, we know who we are and we know why we're sick."[24] David Goodstein, the recently deceased owner and editor of *The Advocate*, insists that AIDS is the responsibility of individual gay men. "As gay men, AIDS is our responsibility. By responsibility I mean that we are the cause of who we are, what we have and what we do."[25] The moral weight of individual responsibility and guilt is a constant message in the wave of articles on homosexual men whose stories are narrated as an individual odyssey from promiscuity to AIDS to death.

Sexual promiscuity stands at the center of the gay media response to AIDS. It is seen as a product of a historically unique gay subculture. It is, moreover, seen as having a direct causal relation to the current epidemic and to the antigay backlash. For homosexual men with a traditional cultural background, for older homosexuals who came of age in a milieu emphasizing heterosexual models, for those men uncomfortable with their sexuality, or for gay liberationists whose ideals are perceived to have faded behind a wave of self-indulgence, AIDS has functioned as an appropriate symbol of the failure of current gay life. AIDS provides an ideal opportunity for gays to vocalize their discontents. I am suggesting, to be perfectly clear, that for heterosexuals and homosexuals, AIDS has served as a pretext to speak critically about homosexuality and to advocate reforms of the gay subculture. Perhaps gay men felt that the suffering and intensified oppression they have experienced in the AIDS crises could be somewhat neutralized or even made self-confirming by reconceiving AIDS as a moral drama. AIDS comes to signify the beginnings of a great reformation in gay life.

The notion that AIDS has ushered in a time of trial and marks a turning point for gays is neatly captured in the apocalyptic imagery of Larry Kramer's eloquent and moving piece "1112 and Counting." Kramer frames the AIDS phenomenon as a test of collective survival. "Our continued existence as gay men . . . is at stake . . . In the history of homosexuality we have never been so close to death and extinction before."[26] Survival hinges on a shift from the current hedonistic preoccupations of gay men to a new social consciousness and a responsible erotic ethic. Where Kramer is somewhat pessimistic, other gay men speak in an oddly defiant and upbeat tone of AIDS initiating a new era of maturity and respectability. Toby Marotta observes that "most gays share my view—that [AIDS] is the most profound, maturing incident for the gay community in its history."[27] David Goodstein couples a critical view of pre-AIDS gay life to the prospects for renewal and reform initiated by AIDS. "During the last half of the 1970's, it wasn't chic in gay male circles to place a high value on life-companions or close friendships. Now [i.e., with AIDS] we have another chance for progress: to acknowledge the value of intimate relationships."[28] Stephen Harvey is even more direct in acknowledging the redemptive possibilities of AIDS. "It's a perverse and maybe [!] tragic irony that it took the AIDS outbreak . . . to at last . . . integrate [our] sexual natures with the rest of what [we] are."[29] A central feature of this emerging gay maturity is the appropriation of the behavioral models and rituals of heterosexual interpersonal patterns.

Arthur Bell comments: "Indiscriminate sex with phantom partners in backrooms is beginning to diminish. The grudge and filth bars are losing their appeal. Fistfucking is fading. Barbarity is on the way out. Romance [is] . . . on the way in."[30] Stories abound in the gay press of homosexual men rediscovering the quiet joys and healthy lifestyle of romantic love and monogamy. Typically, such narratives set off a pre-AIDS period which is now described as one of immaturity and indulgence. AIDS marks the great turning point where after a protracted period of soul-searching one is reborn: the profligate, self-destructive ways of the past are given up for the new morality of monogamy and romance. Typical is the piece by Arnie Kantrowitz. "Till death do us part." He begins by recalling the liberating experience of sexual promiscuity. "My experiment in sexual anarchy was a rare delight, a lesson in license, an opportunity to see both flesh and spirit glaringly naked. I will never apologize to anyone for my promiscuity."[31] Yet, that is exactly what he does as he narrates his odyssey of personal growth. From the standpoint of a post-AIDS sexual morality his early sensual delights now appear to him as compulsive and narcissistic. The endless cycle of excitement, release, and exhaustion left him jaded and empty. "I decided to trade self-indulgence for self-respect." Having personally witnessed the guilt-ridden, self-destructive ways of his pre-AIDS days, he "decided to get healthy."[32] Exercise and proper diet replaced drug abuse and sleepless nights. With health and self-respect intact, there could be only one proper dramatic finale. "Finally, I rediscovered the difference between lust and love and began an affair."[33] The transfiguration of AIDS into a moral and mythic drama of reformation and renewal has allowed some gays to be so emotionally distanced from the enormity of suffering it has brought that the current period is defined as one of optimism. One gay writer observes in what is a common motif that "the energy formerly reserved for the sexual hunt [can now be] channeled into the community in other ways [such as] . . . the growth of gay community centers, sports clubs, choruses, and a host of other groups." He concludes by remarking that "all of which I believe makes 1983 a time for optimism and joy."[34]

The intermingling of medical and moral perceptions in the response to AIDS has been criticized by some gay men. In an early essay, "AIDS: The Politicization of an Epidemic," Dennis Altman objects to using AIDS as an occasion for social and moral commentary. Arguing for a historical and incidental connection between homosexuality and AIDS, he advocates the "de-homosexualization of AIDS." "I would like to see the discussion of AIDS shift to one that sees it as a test of . . . medicine and health care, rather than a metaphysical judgement of lifestyles."[35] Yet, in *AIDS and The Mind of America* Altman is unable to resist the very moralizing that he earlier condemned. AIDS surfaces in its apocalyptic guise as representing a "vengeful nature."[36] In an apparently major reversal of his earlier position, Altman interprets AIDS as indicating the errors of a libertarian sexual ethic that he himself helped to legitimate. "It is very difficult in view of . . . AIDS to escape the feeling that those of us who argued for liberating sex . . . were wrong."[37] For Altman, too, AIDS marks the end of an era. There can be no return to the sexual adventurous style of the seventies but neither will gay men embrace conventional heterosexual models. The prospects, indeed, look bleak to this former apostle of sexual libertarianism. "Will AIDS . . . lead thousands to once again deny their homosexuality?"[38]

In a departure from the typical response to AIDS, Michael Bronski assails gay people for capitulating to the "AIDS hysteria."[39] AIDS has unleashed, says Bronski, a moral assault upon gays. Bronski criticizes gay men for accepting the interpretation of AIDS by the heterosexual media which judges homosexual life to be a failure. This makes gay men responsible for their own victimization. It has, moreover, led homosexuals to cede some control over their lives to heterosexual institutions which have traditionally oppressed them. In their readiness to subordinate themselves to the ideological authority of the heterosexual media, Bronski discerns a surfacing of latent guilt among gay men. The AIDS phenomenon is evidence of an insecure and guilt-ridden gay community turning against itself. Bronski criticizes, in other words, the response of gay men or at least some of its key media figures to AIDS, not a gay lifestyle or subculture.

Tim Vollmer articulates perhaps the most compelling alternative response to AIDS in the gay community.[40] Vollmer does not dispute the claim that a unique gay subculture materialized in the 70s and that at its center was an adventurous and pluralistic sexuality. However, he defends gay sexual culture for providing positive images of homosexuality and for its sheer erotic brilliance. Vollmer does not, of course, deny the seriousness of AIDS. Indeed, it threatens to unravel gay communal life. Sex had been a primary basis of gay identity and community. Now it's the bearer of disease, death and social disintegration. In this perilous situation, Vollmer advises gay men to resist heterosexual stereotypical images of the profligate homosexual. Gay people must not relinquish control over their lives to heterosexual authorities. Neither a wholesale rejection of gay life as morally bankrupt nor a mindless emulation of heterosexual models is recommended. Rather, gay men need to innovate new models of identity and interpersonal relationships that build upon existing gay subcultures.

Although Vollmer does not entirely avoid redemptive rhetoric (for example, he dramatizes the current period as a historic turning point and a test of the very survival of gay life), the thrust of his argument does elude apocalyptic or millenial symbolism. He avoids stereotypes and the reductionist descriptive and moral language of much of the AIDS discussion. In this regard, Vollmer defends a pluralistic sexual ethic that accepts flexible and diverse erotic arrangements so long as safe-sex guidelines are followed.

AIDS & Homosexuality: The Limits of a Discourse

The public heterosexual and gay response to AIDS share a common moral theme: the dangers of promiscuity which are asserted to be a defining feature of homosexuality today. The former frequently derives promiscuity from the very essence of homosexual desire. The latter traces promiscuity to the contemporary gay subculture. However, even in this more historicist approach there is an absence of a socio-historical analysis. By positing merely an abstract relationship between the gay subculture and promiscuity, the suspicion remains that a universal homosexual desire is at work. There is no developmental analysis of the social factors that have formed gay life in its present configuration.

Locating homosexuality in a historical and structural framework alters our perspective. We would have to acknowledge continuities between heterosexual and homosexual behavior. The recent epidemic of genital herpes, for example, points to a society–wide trend towards expanded erotic individualism and pluralism. Increased non-monogamy is one manifestation of this development. Adopting a sociological point of view would hasten the de-homosexualization of AIDS as its appearance would be seen as more historically contingent. Similarly, it would compel us to shift at least some responsibility for AIDS from specific individuals or groups to more general properties of our social structure and culture. Criticism would have to be redirected from, say, individual homosexuals or a gay subculture to social conditions like capitalism, mass culture or a expressive-therapeutic ideology which have molded homosexual desire and behavior. In particular, a historical and structural viewpoint would compel critics of the gay subculture to countenance the crucial role of homosexual oppression. A critique of homosexual behavior must be coupled to a critique of a society whose hostility to homosexuality helped to produce conditions conducive to creating endemic health and social problems for homosexuals. From this vantage point, it is not very plausible to advocate that gays adopt heterosexual models without simultaneously abolishing all those institutions, legal and cultural barriers to gay men choosing them.

Notwithstanding widely publicized announcements of changing sexual patterns among male homosexuals, the available research is much less equivocal. To be sure, studies report a decline in certain indicators of non-monogamous sex, e.g., bathhouse attendance or STD's. However, this may simply mean that non-monogamous sex is occurring in different locations and is confined to safe-sex acts. Indeed, the appearance of sex clubs confined to safe-sex and the rise of new forms of eroticism centered on visual stimuli, sex talk or role-playing suggest that there may be little change in this regard. Even if we assume that homosexual men today have fewer partners, this does not amount to a change in sexual patterns. The latter is not defined solely by whether one is monogamous or promiscuous. Such a definition omits the qualitative aspects of sex, e.g., its meaning and emotional content or its moral and interpersonal aspects. Moreover, this one-sided view of sex implies an equally simplistic sexual ethic implying that monogamy by itself can serve as the normative standard for evaluating sexual behavior. The conceptual and moral muddle of this discourse is strikingly revealed in the loose and ambiguous way the concept of promiscuity is used.

In both the heterosexual and gay media, promiscuity is taken as the decisive link between homosexual men and AIDS. It is, moreover, considered the essence of a universal or more historically specific homosexual desire. Yet, one looks in vain for a definition or a serious analysis of its meaning. Its sense, however, is conveyed by references to having many sex partners. This, however, is misleading. Promiscuity cannot be defined by the sheer number of one's sex partners. For example, a serial monogamous pattern which involves a sequence of changing partners is not promiscuous behavior. Similarly, promiscuity is not synonymous with non-monogamy. We would not consider, say, an extramarital affair as promiscuous behavior. In general, we must distinguish promiscuity from polygamy or "sexual pluralism." The latter involves multiple sex partners but there may also be established relationships of intimacy and responsibility with each partner. Promiscuity involves a sexually active person whose sex partners change frequently and with each there is an absence of personal intimacy and extended responsibilities. Furthermore, the line between serial monogamy, polygamy and promiscuity cannot always be drawn in a hard and fast way. A serial monogamous pattern involving a sequence of short-lived, emotionally distant relationships has a promiscuous aspect. A polygamous pattern involving one primary long-term relationship and sex with anonymous others suggests a more salient promiscuous element.

At stake is more than a matter of conceptual clarification. The categories used to describe homosexuality carry moral and practical implications. Homosexual behavior cannot be characterized as promiscuous in some generic or essential way. The available studies of current behavior highlight a diversity of homosexual patterns ranging from a monogamous, marital model to promiscuity.[41] Any attempt to frame homosexual desire as some abstract, universal and homogeneous entity whose essence is promiscuity will not find much empirical support in behavioral research. Researchers agree that a more typical pattern for gay men—at least in the 70s—has been to combine an on-going love relationship with secondary affairs centered on sex.[42] The pattern of these secondary involvements range from having a few erotically-centered relationships involving extended responsibilities to having high numbers of changing, anonymous sex partners. To the extent that the latter is more common than the line between polygamy and promiscuity is blurred. In fact, according to some observers, this more promiscuous style characterized a segment of the urban gay population in the 1970s.[43] Indeed, surveys of sexual behavior show that during this period gay men had, on the average, a much higher number of sex partners—many of whom were anonymous—than heterosexuals and lesbians.[44] It is reasonable to assume *some* connection between this behavior and AIDS among homosexual men. The error is to assume a genetic causal tie between homosexuality, promiscuity, and disease or to take AIDS as evidence of the pathological nature of homosexuality.

There is a series of wrong moves here. Promiscuity is *not* the cause of AIDS but a risk-factor. To be even more precise, it is a risk-factor *if* one engages in high-risk sex and *if* one does so in circumstances where the HTLV-III virus is widely circulated. Homosexuals do *not* have to be promiscuous or non-monogamous to acquire AIDS. It is *not* legitimate to take AIDS as indicative of a particular type of sexual pattern or lifestyle. Furthermore, given its appearance among heterosexuals, who in some nations are primarily afflicted, it is wrong to interpret AIDS as a homosexual disease. There is no evidence that AIDS is congenital or that it is produced by homosexual behavior or that it favors homosexual men. The only statement that can be endorsed unequivocally is that *specific homosexual acts* are today high-risk. This fact does not, however, require that homosexual men adopt any particular lifestyle or sexual ethic. It mandates only safe-sex practices but how these are incorporated into a life style or pattern of intimate relationships is open to diverse possibilities.

Conclusion

Foucault has shown how the original intent and political purpose of a discourse on sexuality can be reversed. For example, the scientific-medical discourse of "the homosexual" as a perverse or pathological human type promoted new forms of social control. Yet, taking the issue of homosexuality out of a religious context and placing it in a scientific one, has allowed an appeal to empirical evidence to challenge stereotypes and, ultimately, to contest the medical model itself. Moreover, this medical discourse contributed to creating a common homosexual consciousness and culture that eventuated in a politic aimed at legitimating homosexuality.

If there is a hopeful sign in the AIDS crisis, it is in the potential unintended consequences of making homosexuality a public issue. AIDS has forced public officials to gather and publicize knowledge about homosexuality. The acquisition of detailed empirical knowledge of homosexuality is deemed essential for public health reasons. The medical profession and the lay public must rely upon social researchers and knowledgeable observers of the homosexual scene for information which is considered vital to controlling AIDS. Much of this research will undoubtedly be done by gay people. It is bound to disclose facts and yield insights and perspectives about homosexuality that will discredit stereotypes. Moreover, there is a need to disseminate credible information about homosexuality in order to facilitate behavior that reduces people's risks of contracting AIDS. The enormous expansion of public talk about homosexuality (in newspapers, radio and television programs, in books, plays, advertisements and ordinary conversations), may contribute to making homosexuality more socially acceptable, especially as stereotypes lose credibility. It is likely that AIDS will prompt renewed efforts at sex education. In so far as AIDS education is part of this effort, the discussion of homosexuality will become more routine. At the very least, these developments would provide a context in which to challenge stereotypes and defend homosexuality.

It is, then, possible that AIDS may have a long-term beneficial effect. AIDS requires credible empirical knowledge of homosexuality. This will stimulate and legitimate research on homosexuals, much of which will challenge stereotypes. Finally, this knowledge will be disseminated throughout society and will be taken seriously because of its link to a health crisis. This could provide a favorable setting for legitimating homosexuality and gaining the social inclusion of homosexuals. In the end, this will not result from merely a process of mass enlightenment. Rather, it will require gay people, in particular, to mobilize in order to play a greater role in shaping public discussions. Homosexuals must have a political presence if they expect to shape public policy decisions emerging from the AIDS crisis.

NOTES

1. Cf. Dennis Altman, *The Homosexualization of America* (Boston: Beacon Press, 1983) and John D'Emilio, *Sexual Politics, Sexual Communities* (Chicago: University of Chicago Press, 1983).

2. See Gayle Rubin, "Thinking Sex," *Pleasure and Danger*. Edited by Carole Vance (Boston: Routledge & Kegan Paul, 1984); Pat Califia, "The Great Kiddie Porn Scare of '77 and Its Aftermath," *Advocate*, October 16, 1980.

3. See Altman, *The Homosexualization of America*, Ch. 4; Larry Bush and Richard Goldstein, "The Anti-Gay Backlash," *The Village Voice*, April 8-11, 1981; Scott Tucker, "The Counterrevolution," *Gay Community News*, February 21, 1981.

4. Cf. Dennis Altman, *Aids and the Mind of America* (New York: Doubleday, 1985) and Cindy Patton, *Sex and Germs* (Boston: South End Press, 1985); Richard Goldstein, "The Uses of Aids," *The Village Voice*, Nov. 5, 1985.

5. For examples of the public identification of AIDS as a homosexual disease, see "Gay Plague has Instituted Fear of the Unknown," *The Philadelphia Inquirer*, June 20, 1982; "New Homosexual Disorder Worries Health Officials," *New York Times*, May 11, 1982; "Killer Gay Disease Spreads to Kids," *New York Post*, Dec. 11, 1982; "Homosexual Plague Strikes New Victim," *Newsweek*, August 23, 1982.

6. CDC task force study, *Annals of Internal Medicine*, V. 99, 8/83.

7. See John Martin and Carole Vance, "Behavioral and Psychological Factors in AIDS." *American Psychologist*, Nov. 1984.

8. "A Hard Look/New Worry About Gay Disease," *San Francisco Examiner*, Oct. 24, 1982, p. 14.

9. John Fuller, "AIDS: Legacy of the '60s?" *Science Digest*, Dec. 1983, p. 85.

10. Vincent Coppola, "The Change in Gay Life-style," *Newsweek*, April 18, 1983, p. 80.

11. Patrick Buchanan, "AIDS Disease: It's Nature Striking Back," *New York Post*, May 24, 1983, p. 31. Cf. William Buckley, "On Handling Gays," *National Review*, March 18, 1983, p. 345.

12. *Times Union* (Albany, New York), Jan. 18, 1986.

13. Quoted in James E'Eramo, "The New Medical Journal Homophobia," *The New York Native*, May 21, 1984, p. 9.

14. For example, Mark Starr and David Gonzalez, "The Panic over AIDS," *Newsweek*, May 4, 1983; John Lee, "The Real Epidemic: Fear and Despair," *Time*, July 4, 1983; Gail Appleson, "Litigation Imminent in AIDS Issues," *National Law Journal*, July 25, 1983; Michael Daley, "AIDS Anxiety," *New York*, June 20, 1983.

15. Richard Goldstein, "The Other AIDS Story: Quarantine." *The Village Voice*, May 1, 1984.

16. Quoted in Patton, *Sex and Germs*, pp. 3-4. Also David Morris, "Texas Drops Sodomy Appeal." *Gay Community News*, March 26, 1983.

17. William Greer, "Violence Against Homosexuals Rising, Groups Seeking Wider Protection Say," *New York Times*, Nov. 23, 1986.

18. Charles Krauthammer, "The Politics of a Plague," *The New Republic*, August 1, 1983, p. 21.

19. Richard Lyons, "Sex in America: Conservative Attitudes Prevail," *New York Times*, Oct. 4, 1983; "Homosexuals Find a Need to Reassess," *New York Times*, May 29, 1983; "Homosexuals Confronting a Time of Change," *New York Times*, June 16, 1983; "AIDS Education Takes on an Urgency Within the Homosexual Community," *New York Times*, Sept. 22, 1985.

20. Georgia Dullea, "Homosexual Couples Find a Quiet Pride," *New York Times*, Dec. 10, 1984.

21. Michael Callen and Richard Berkowitz with Richard Dworkin, "We Know Who We Are," *The New York Native*, Nov. 8, 1982.

22. Michael Callen, letter, *The Body Politic*, April 1983, p. 93.

23. Stephen Harvey, "Defenseless: Learning to Live with AIDS," *The Village Voice*, Dec. 21, 1982, p. 21.

24. Callen, "We Know Who We Are."

25. David Goodstein, "Editorial," *The Advocate*, August 6, 1985.

26. Larry Kramer, "1,112 and Counting," *The New York Native*, March 14, 1983.

27. Quoted in Tom Morganthau, "Gay America in Transition," *Newsweek*, August 8, 1983, p. 33.

28. Goodstein, Editorial, *The Advocate*, August 6, 1985, p.

29. Harvey, "Defenseless," p. 21.

30. Arthur Bell, "Where Gays are Going," *The Village Voice*. June 29, 1982, p.

31. Arnie Kantrowitz, "Till death us do part," *The Advocate*, 1983 p. 26. Cf. Margot Joan Frommer, "Coping," *The Washington Blade*, Jan. 21, 1983.

32. Ibid.

33. Ibid.

34. Steve Martz, "A Quick Look Back and Some Thoughts On The Year Ahead," *The Washington Blade*, Jan. 7, 1983, p. 23.

35. Dennis Altman, "AIDS: The Politicization of an Epidemic," *Socialist Review*, Vol. 14, No. 78 (November-December, 1984).

36. Altman, *AIDS and the Mind of America*, p. 168.

37. Ibid., p. 172.

38. Ibid., p. 170.

39. Michael Bronski, "Our Guilt and Fear," *Gay Community News*, Oct. 7, 1982.

40. Tim Vollmer, "Another Stonewall," *The New York Native*, Oct. 28-Nov. 3, 1985.

41. For example, Alan Bell and Martin Weinberg, *Homosexualities* (New York: Simon and Schuster, 1970).

42. See, for example, Letitia Anne Peplau and Steven Gordon, "The Intimate Relationships of Lesbians and Gay Men," in *Gender Roles and Sexual Behavior*, edited by Elizabeth Allgeier and Naomi McCormick (Palo Alto, CA: Mayfield, 1983); Joseph Harry and William Duvall, *The Social Organization of Gay Males* (New York: Praeger, 1978); C.A. Tripp, *The Homosexual Matrix* (New York: McGraw-Hill, 1975); Edmund White, *States of Desire* (New York: E.P. Dutton, 1980).

43. Cf. Dennis Altman, "AIDS: The Politicization of an Epidemic."

44. See Bell and Weinberg, *Homosexualities*; Karla Jay and Allen Young, *The Gay Report* (New York: Summit Books, 1977); Phillip Blumstein and Pepper Schwartz, *American Couples* (New York: Morrow, 1983).

Comment

DENNIS ALTMAN

Steven Seidman may be surprised to find that I basically agree with much of his thesis, in particular the warning against allowing AIDS to be used as an excuse for repudiating the discourse on sexuality that grew out of the gay liberation movement. If he is surprised that we agree, it is because he has taken six pages from my *AIDS in the Mind of America*, where I speculated on the various consequences AIDS might have for the construction of gay sexuality, and interpreted this as simply "moralizing." Yes, I used the term "vengeful nature." Anyone who read what I wrote carefully would realize, however, that I was trying to explain the fears and feelings AIDS has engendered in gay men, not to argue that these feelings are rationally justified. Thus, I raised the possibility that AIDS would lead men to reject a homosexual identity, as AIDS seemed to reverse the gains made by the gay movement in the preceding decade, a possibility that seems to me consistent with the social constructionist view of sexual identity both Seidman and I hold.[1]

Two years later I am much more doubtful that this will happen, and indeed my hunch is that AIDS has considerably strengthened a sense of gay identity and community. I can't blame Seidman for being unaware of my current views; they are summed up in two papers which are about to be published.[2] What is significant, however, is that Seidman seems quite unaware of the need to locate comments on AIDS very specifically in the context of when they were written. Much of the debate around gay sexual behavior he quotes comes from a period—only three years ago—when we knew much less than we do now about the ways in which the HIV virus is transmitted. The pamphlet, "We Know Who We Are," which Seidman refers to, assumed that AIDS was the product of "immune overload," a thesis which has long since been discredited (although previous and simultaneous infections might, of course, affect the likelihood of someone who is HIV-positive becoming ill).

"The existence of a virus" is not "the currently more accepted theory": it is the explanation for AIDS held by almost every reputable scientist in the world, Unfortunately, the peculiar paranoia of a once great paper, the *New York Native*, means that every crackpot theory which contests this view gets aired, and is seized upon by those people who desperately want an explanation—any explanation—for AIDS which denies the consensus of the great part of the scientific community. I do not deny that it is *possible* that the world scientific community will be proved wrong. But it is dishonest—or ignorant—of Seidman to write as if the "overload" theory and the existence of HIV (the internationally recognized term) were somehow equally reputable theories.

It is equally puzzling to me how someone can comment on the social construction of AIDS in 1987 and totally ignore the widespread existence of the disease in Africa and the very strong evidence that it originated there.[3] It is, of course, true that early perceptions of AIDS lead to it being conceptualized as a homosexual disease—this is one of the main themes of my own book. But, at least outside New York, that perception has been considerably modified over the past few years as reports of its extent in Africa have become common. Other forms of stigma are brought into play—as is also the case for the existence of AIDS among drug-users—but at least we need acknowledge how these complicate the metaphorical uses to which the disease can be put.

The stress on discourse that runs through this article is somewhat apolitical—one would not know from Seidman's article that the "gay community" has created considerable structures to respond to the epidemic, and that in many parts of the United States, including cities the size of Dallas and Miami, these provide virtually the only arenas for AIDS education and information. If there is a new discourse on gay sexuality being created it is often through the educational work of groups like the San Francisco AIDS Foundation and Gay Men's Health Crisis, who have deliberately set out to find ways of eroticizing "safe sex" (and whose programs are deemed unsuitable in many areas of the country where governments give greater priority to respectable language than to saving lives; Seidman's article reads as if written before the appearance of the Report of the Surgeon General).

I strongly agree with Seidman (that if AIDS is not to unleash greater homophobia, it requires a gay political mobilization) but this point needs much greater elaboration. Here, again, the peculiarity of New York comes into play; the gay movement in New York has long been noticeable as having far less impact on city politics than that of cities such as San Francisco, Washington, Boston, etc. An examination of how San Francisco responded to the epidemic will immediately make clear that "making homosexuality a public issue" is hardly the crucial point—rather it is recognizing homosexuals as a legitimate community, with access to governmental decision-making. Without this, the fact that "AIDS has forced public officials to gather and publicize knowledge about homosexuality" is just as likely to lead to a new anti-homosexual vigilantism.

Even more striking is the difference on a national level between the United States on the one hand, and, say, Australia or the Netherlands on the other. In both of these latter countries, the gay movement has had a major input into government decision-making on AIDS which could well serve as a model for the United States. If Seidman had spent a little time reading about the response to

AIDS outside the United States—not one of his references comes from elsewhere—he might have recognized the sad irony that the western country with the highest caseload is also one of the least responsible in developing a national program of public education on the transmission of AIDS.

This comment probably sounds harsher than I would want to be about this particular article. Maybe the harshness is born out of a sense of frustration at both the academicism and the New York centrism of Seidman's approach. By concentrating so heavily on the media—indeed on the New York media—he seems to me to miss the political significance of the role of gay/AIDS community organizations in responding to the challenge of the epidemic, and their impact on both the lived experience and the discourse of sexuality.

NOTES

1. For a discussion of the issues raised, see Steven Epstein, "The Limits of Social Constructionism," *Socialist Review* 93, no. 4 (1987).

2. "The Impact of AIDS in the Developed World," *British Medical Bulletin* **44**, no. 1 (1988), and "Legitimation Through Disaster," in *AIDS: The Burdens of History*, ed. E. Fee and D. Fox (Princeton: Princeton University Press, 1988).

3. See R. Shilts, *And the Band Played On* (New York: St. Martin's Press, 1987), for a popular account of this theory.

The Motives of Gay Men for Taking or Not Taking the HIV Antibody Test*

KAROLYNN SIEGEL, *Memorial Sloan-Kettering Cancer Center*

MARTIN P. LEVINE, *Bloomfield College*

CHARLES BROOKS, *New York University*

ROCHELLE KERN, *Columbia University*

This paper analyzes the motives for taking or not taking the HIV antibody test among a sample of 120 gay men. The motives were forged from prevailing cultural constructions of the HIV test. The most commonly cited motives for taking the test were: to take medical treatments for HIV infection, to become motivated to make needed health and lifestyle changes, to clarify an ambiguous medical condition, to inform sexual decision making, and to relieve psychological distress associated with not knowing HIV status. The most frequently reported motives for not taking the test were: to avoid the adverse psychological impact of a positive test result, to avoid social discrimination and repressive governmental actions, to avoid an ambiguous or unreliable test result, and to avoid having to make undesired lifestyle changes.

The present paper explores the motives given by gay men for taking or not taking the HIV (Human Immunodeficiency Virus) antibody test. Following Mills (1940), we conceptualize these motives as reasons, explanations, or justifications for taking or not taking the test. Moreover, we also conceptualize HIV antibody testing as problematic behavior, mainly because of the momentous psychological and social risks and benefits associated with testing. As one noted chronicler of the AIDS (Acquired Immune Deficiency Syndrome) epidemic put it,

> To test or not to test clearly would become the most important personal decision most gay men would make in their adult lives. To be tested meant learning that you might at any time fall victim to a deadly disease; it was a psychological burden few . . . could imagine. However, not to be tested meant you might be carrying a lethal virus, which you could give to others (Shilts 1987:540).

Other risks include stigmatization, discrimination, and disrupted social relationships (Miller 1987). Among the benefits connected with testing are the opportunity to learn of one's seropositive status and obtain available treatments, a reduction in the anxiety of individuals who test seronegative, the opportunity to plan more effectively for the future, and support for a differential diagnosis when HIV infection is suspected (Goldblum and Seymour 1987).

To date, not much is known about gay men's motives for taking or not taking the test (Coates et al. 1988). What little data that are available indicate that gay men's motives frequently refer to perceived consequences of learning test results or taking the test. For example, Lyter et al. (1987) used fixed choice mail questionnaires to investigate the reasons why participants in the Pitt Men's Study (the Pittsburgh component of the Multicenter AIDS Cohort Study) did or did not ask to be informed about their antibody test results. These men had their blood tested as part of the research protocol. Out of a total of 2,047 gay and bisexual men, 61 percent chose to learn their results. The chief reasons offered for learning test results

* This research was supported in part by a grant from the National Institute of Mental Health (MH42275). The authors acknowledge the assistance of Shona Brogden, Douglas Oliver, and Lisa Rosen. Correspondence to: Siegel, Department of Social Work, Memorial Sloan-Kettering Cancer Center, 1275 York Avenue, New York, NY 10021.

were curiosity about possible infection with HIV and the belief that knowledge about antibody status would help them cope with fears of AIDS and reduce high-risk sexual practices. Conversely, the primary reasons for not learning test results were concerns that positive results would be psychologically harmful (in the sense that it would increase anxiety, depression, and worry), and the belief that the test does not predict the development of AIDS.

Another study directly tapped motives for not being tested among a community sample (N = 213) of gay and bisexual men living in the San Francisco area (Research and Decisions Corporation 1986). About three-quarters (73%) of the respondents were untested. The major reasons reported for not taking the test included concerns about emotional reactions to the test, uncertainties regarding the utility and meaning of the test, and fears about the confidentiality of the test.

This paper expands our understanding of the motives of gay men for taking or not taking the antibody test. In what follows, we discuss the research methods used to collect our data on gay men's motives, report the motives cited by our respondents, and close with a discussion of how the major cultural definitions of the HIV test are reflected in the respondents' reports.

Method

The data presented below come from an ongoing qualitative study of sexual decision-making among gay men in the context of the AIDS epidemic. The study was undertaken in response to a recognition that, although self-identified gay men have participated in a number of survey studies concerning the extent to which the AIDS epidemic caused changes in their sexual lives and emotional well-being, there was a notable lack of research on the meaning of AIDS as it is phenomenologically and pragmatically experienced by the men themselves. The research was designed to address this gap in understanding by using a primarily qualitative methodology that includes participant observation, the use of a brief self-administered questionnaire, and relatively unstructured but focused group and in-depth individual interviews.

Respondents for the study were recruited through fliers distributed and posted at a variety of gay service, political, and social organizations (including the large Gay and Lesbian Community Center which serves the organized gay community in New York). In addition, recruiting announcements were run as advertisements in gay newspapers, as public service announcements on gay cable television, announced at various gay organizational meetings, published in a range of gay newsletters, and distributed through a constantly growing recruitment network.

To participate, respondents had to be between 18-65 years of age, live in the greater New York metropolitan area, have not used intravenous drugs in the past six months, and not have been diagnosed with AIDS. Seventeen men participated in initial group interviews. A total of 150 gay men eventually will participate in two, two-hour individual interviews. All interviews were conducted as relatively unstructured open-ended discussions led by the project's interviewer. Interview sessions began with a nine-minute videotape produced by the study team as a projective stimulus for discussion. The video contained five vignettes in which actors portray gay men articulating their diverse views about safer sex and AIDS. The vignettes included men who have adopted safer sex practices and express differing feelings about their choice as well as men who justify continuing to engage in risky sex. By presenting varying views about safer sex, the video was designed to give respondents permission to express themselves candidly (e.g., to acknowledge disagreement with safer sex recommendations or involvement in unsafe sexual practices). Interviews were audiotaped and transcribed verbatim.

The material presented here was derived from individual unstructured focused interviews (Merton et al. 1956) with a total of 120 men. Of these, 41 percent were untested, 22 percent were seropositive, and 37 percent were seronegative. One hundred and eleven of the respondents were white, four were Hispanic, three were black, and one was Asian. The mean age of the sample was 34.6 years and the median age was 33 years (range = 18 to 63 years of age). Eighty percent of the sample was between ages of 18 and 40 years. Respondents were well educated: 69 percent had at least a college education; about 26 percent had completed some college; and the remaining 5 percent were high school graduates. Approximately 22 percent of the respondents earned less than $20,000; 29 percent earned between $20,000 and $29,000; 19 percent earned between $30,000 and $39,999; and 30 percent earned more than $40,000. All interviews were conducted between May 1988 and May 1989.

The data reported below were either spontaneously volunteered by respondents or offered in reply to a general query by the interviewer asking them to discuss what led to their decision to or not to be tested. Because the interviews were unstructured there were no standardized probes as a follow-up to their responses. That is, the interviewer did not systematically probe about the possible importance of factors other than those reported by the respondent. In this way, we believe that we captured the respondent's subjective perceptions and definition of the situation and insight into what factors were personally most salient to him in arriving at his decision. For the purposes of exposition the reasons offered by men for their decisions are segregated. In reality, however, men frequently expressed more than one reason for their decision, and one reason would seem to potentiate another. All of the motives reported below for undergoing testing were cited by men who were actually tested. Similarly, all of the motives presented for not being tested were offered by untested respondents.

In presenting the findings we have pooled tested men regardless of their test results. Because the decision to be tested obviously temporally precedes knowledge of one's antibody status, the latter should not be causally implicated in explaining decisions about whether or not to be tested. Still, it must be recognized that, as reports regarding why one was tested are in fact retrospective accounts, it is possible that a respondent's test result influenced his reconstruction of his earlier decision to take the test. In describing the experiences of respondents who have been tested, their antibody status will be noted.

Motives for Taking the Test

The men who said they had taken the test told us they did so primarily because of the medical and health consequences they believed might follow from knowing their serostatus (whether positive, meaning that the HIV is present, or negative). In addition, they sought to know their test status in order to make more informed decisions about their sexual and social lifestyles. We have grouped their comments into five categories of motives: (1) to enable medical treatments for HIV infection, (2) to become motivated to make needed health and lifestyle changes, (3) to clarify an ambiguous medical condition, (4) to inform sexual decision making, and (5) to relieve the psychological distress associated with not knowing HIV status.

To Enable Medical Treatments for HIV Infection

Most men who underwent testing reported being previously opposed to taking the test. At first, they believed that nothing could be done to help HIV infected individuals or prevent the disease from running its inexorable course. In addition, they believed that learning that one was seropositive carried grave psychological dangers. In this sense, "ignorance was bliss" under conditions of helplessness. Some further rationalized not being tested on the grounds that they practiced only safer sex, and therefore did not place any partners at risk. They viewed their decision not to be tested as socially acceptable rather than as selfish, self-protective, or irresponsible because they did not engage in practices that could potentially infect partners.

However, the perceptions of these men changed over time. Many came to believe that there were effective medical therapies for HIV diseases. These included prophylactic treatments (e.g., aerosol pentamidine) for some of the more common opportunistic infections and antiviral drugs (e.g., Azidothymidineor AZT) that slow the replication of HIV. Accordingly, they recognized that these treatments provided a means of exerting some control or influence over their future health and said or implied that this recognition motivated them to take the test. One 32-year-old seropositive man said,

> Up until a few weeks before I took the test, which is in December, I had a couple of the opinions that I heard on your videotape. And that was, "No one really knows what they're talking about", and "There's nothing that can be done anyway" And I didn't hear this on the tape, but you know it's in line with that—ah, my feeling that the HIV test is just a blood marker and not an indication of whether or not one will get AIDS. I was thoroughly ignorant until December. And then I came upon information that was not consistent with what I had thought up until then. Someone told me that the HIV test is not just a marker any more. That is old information. Now there are prophylaxis measures that one can take if one tests positive, and you can keep, you can possibly keep your T-4 cells from dropping. So I . . . got as much information as I can. And I found out that untreated HIV, the current wisdom is that untreated HIV will progress to AIDS in like 76 percent of the cases over six and a half to seven years time. And there's no other information . . . right now. That is the current wisdom, and things can be done. Things can be done to possibly halt the degeneration of one's immune system.

Another, 26-year-old, who was tested but had not yet received the results, said,

> Until recently, for myself, I thought that . . . testing positive would just scare me. And that I was behaving, or trying to behave, you know, in my sex life, just as if I was positive and not putting other people at risk. And that I didn't see, I didn't see what I would gain from learning I was positive. Just seemed like there wasn't much I could do. You know unless I wanted to, you know, like go on a macrobiotic diet; or, you know, start swimming every day; or, you know, just do general things which make me healthier—which, you know, if I had the will to do, I would do anyway. Ah, but just recently, it just seems like there's a lot more people can do. I mean whether it's, you know, taking low dose AZT when it's in a symptomatic stage, or whether it's getting your T-cells monitored and doing aerosol pentamidine. Ah, you know, as well as nutritional and general health maintenance things. It just seems like there's enough, enough that people can do that it seemed like a rational decision.

A seropositive man, 41 years old, told us that:

> Up until recently, I didn't feel that there was any prophylactic treatment. And now I'm encouraging people to go get their diagnosis because I think now with aerosol pentamidine, and we're doing experiments with AZT being given to people with ARC. And there are a couple of new drugs on the market that are AZT analogues with less side effects that I think more and more is gonna become, it's becoming advantageous to be diagnosed earlier. But until recently, I don't think this was true.

Some men also recognized that early implementation of these treatments could prolong health and life. They felt that those who did not take prophylactic actions were likely to be diagnosed when it was "too late," at an advanced stage of the disease, with a poorer treatment outlook and consequently shorter survival time. One man, 40 and seropositive, said,

> I feel that I'm better taken care of by my doctor. And the old saw, the old line used to be, "What difference does it matter if the doctor knows because there's nothing they can do." Well, now there are things they can do. Granted, not in terms of giving you ten years, but there are things they can do in giving you one and half years versus two years and a certain amount of quality time. Ah, someone who doesn't know whether he's HIV positive or not might very well go right up to getting a

> full-blown case of AIDS, without any prophylactic medication whatsoever. And I think that's regrettable because then it is indeed much harder to treat the person.

And a 34-year-old seropositive respondent said,

> I think gay men need to hear in a clear, concise, and convincing way that if their HIV status is known it could benefit them. It could in fact make the difference in years, added to or taken off of their life. 'Cause I believe that's the case. Ah, not knowing your HIV status, I think is very dangerous—psychologically as well as physically. I think it's a bad medical decision to have, if you're a homosexual and you've been sexually active over the past ten years, or maybe fifteen, you should have your status determined. . . . It's gonna, there are gonna be two situations. There will be those who, like myself, have sought help before they needed it. 'Cause I think in this it, when it's too late, it's too late. You wait too long and that's it. Ah, whereas those like myself who seek out the help, have their bloodwork done, and work with their health care professionals, and also work with their, work on their head too, you know, psychologically keep themselves healthy in every way, that they can influence—I think we can do quite well. Maybe I'll live to be 60 years old. You never can tell. But I think those on the other scenario, the other extreme, they're gonna die very quickly.

The diagnosis and subsequent rapid death of friends and acquaintances reinforced some men's perceptions of the medical benefits of early intervention. A few men previously felt they could adopt a "wait and see" stance, delaying the decision to take the test and/or the decision to take recommended medical treatments until the appearance of HIV-related symptoms. The experience of seeing untested and seemingly healthy gay men suddenly become very sick and diagnosed with AIDS altered this stance and motivated them to be tested. Knowledge of their serostatus would allow them to take appropriate medical treatments. For example, a 51-year-old seropositive man told us:

> I feel it's better to take it. If you know the results you can explore ways you can deal and cope with it. And there are support groups and so there someone can go for help. And then rather than not know about it, because there have been cases of friends of mine who did not take the test and suddenly were diagnosed and died instantly in about a few months. Whereas those who have taken the test a long time ago and have been practicing safe sex and using preventive measures, as well as vitamins, and a non—, ah, antitoxic drugs have been able to survive and are doing very well.

A man, 26, recently tested but who had not gotten the results, said,

> So I've been thinking for the past few months that I wanted to do it [get tested] and I was just a little nervous about actually doing it. Ah, but then, someone who I knew a little bit, a friend of a friend, just about three or four weeks ago, after I mean having no indication that he was HIV positive or had any health problem, you know. He had a cold which became a cough and it persisted. And it turned out he had pneumocystis pneumonia. And so, you know, he was diagnosed as having AIDS, just like that. And he is certainly someone with, you know, access to medical information and medical care. And, you know, like he could have been doing pentamidine, you know, if there was any reason for him to. Ah, and that sort of like jolted me into realizing that, you know, I really ought to do it.

Nearly all the men citing the possibility of medical treatments as the motive for undergoing testing, described their decision as one they made for themselves. Nevertheless, several reported that their personal physicians played an important role in influencing them. These men were obviously impressed that their doctors, who had previously shared their opposition to testing, had altered their stance in light of recent scientific data and clinical experience indicating the potential efficacy of available treatment options. One 29-year-old seronegative man commented:

> When I saw him [my doctor] a year and a half ago he did not recommend taking the test. He recommended *not* taking the test. And then, then six months ago, it's really more like more like eight months ago, . . . I knew my former lover had ARC, so was positive—HIV positive. And I went to the doctor just for a general check up and told him this. He said at this point he was very insistent

that his patients, people who think that there might be the possibility or just for—you know, he recommends the test because he now feels with AZT if you're symptomatic, but not diagnosed, there may be time to start treatment if necessary. . . . And he explained, he took out charts and he took, you know, he had articles about it and we talked about it. He was just, you know, he was very level-headed about what he was saying to me.

Another seronegative man, 34, said,

> Yeah, it was actually a hard decision. And I, I thought about it for probably two or three years before I did it. Ah, I have a doctor who is gay, who treats a lot of people with AIDS. And he, a lot of my decision was based on his recommendations. Ah, there was obviously a natural curiosity all through the years. Ah, I think that only after I was convinced primarily through his telling me so, that there would be good, there could be good to come from having taken the test and finding out that you were positive, in terms of there being certain medical things that could be done. . . . Previous to that he was a strong proponent of *not* taking the test because medically there was nothing that could be done.

To Become Motivated to Make Needed Health and Lifestyle Changes

Some men said they took the test to become motivated to make desired health and lifestyle changes. Although aware of the desirability of safer sex, sound nutrition, reduced alcohol and drug consumption, they said they were insufficiently motivated to initiate and maintain these behaviors in the absence of knowing they were positive. They felt that a positive result would represent a concrete and certain threat to their health and to their partners, which would motivate them to make appropriate behavioral changes. For example, a 31-year-old seropositive man said, "I also knew that I was really not taking proper care of myself—physically, safe sex speaking, and just everything [like] nutrition . . . and somehow I thought that it might give me just the jolt I needed." And a 28-year-old seronegative respondent said,

> I defended my own reluctance to take the test by saying, much like one of the guys in here [on the videotape], "If I have it, I don't want to know. And if I don't have it it's not gonna change anything about me anyway because I can't, ah, there's no cure. There's nothing to do." You know, I'm a sitting duck. And then some friends of mine . . . had taken the test and their doctors began to—they tested positive—and then the next step was to be, to have the T-4 cells counted and all this other stuff. And it became clear to me that, if in fact I was positive, there were things I could do to protect myself. I could give up the alcohol I was drinking. I could give up the marijuana I was smoking. I could worry more about my diet. I could, ah, be more honest with myself and my future. Ah, whatever future I would have. Ah, it became . . . really a question of honesty and courage. And, and protecting myself to the extent that I could."

Another man, 51 and seropositive, believed a positive result would stimulate him to adopt holistic health practices:

> I'd given it thought and I wanted to know whether I had the virus and that if I did, what I was going to do to help myself. And what preventative measures that it's gonna take to protect my life. And this is exactly what I did. I'm exercising. I wake up at five to do some meditation for half an hour. I do the Hatha Yoga exercises. I eat macrobiotic food cause I feel that's helped people in the past. [I take] minerals that inhibit the virus from manifesting itself, and I do megadoses of vitamin C like 10,000 grams per day.

To Clarify an Ambiguous Medical Condition

In some cases, the appearance of possible HIV-related symptoms motivated respondents to be tested. Where the prevalence of HIV infection is assumed to be high, as in New York City, physicians caring for gay men often consider this as a possible cause of an ambiguous medical condition, since the symptoms of HIV infection are often similar to those of other illnesses. Therefore, to arrive at a definitive diagnosis of a patient's condition, physicians treating gay men may recommend antibody testing. This was commonly reported by our respondents. Nevertheless, in a few instances respondents took the initiative and proposed to their physicians that they be tested. A 26-year-old seropositive respondent said he took the test "because I got really sick with a kidney infection. And it did not clear up with the antibiotics right way. And I knew I was gay. I knew that my sexual activity would definitely put me in that risk group." Another man, 27, and also seropositive, said,

> I had been seeing a physician for an unrelated problem [anal warts] that he was treating. And as he treated it, the recurrence he said was possibly indicative that I was HIV positive. . . . He said the recurrence of the warts were possibly had to do with HIV positive. I didn't believe him. I wanted to [take the test]. I wanted to find out and prove to him and myself that I was negative.

A man, seronegative and 44, said, in response to the question of why he decided to take the test,

> Oh 'cause I think when I had I had this little basal cell carcinoma . . . I got very paranoid about it 'cause when it first showed up, it's this little red rash. Right on my clavicle. I was in St. Thomas when it happened. And I thought, "Oh well" and I ah—"Who knows what it is?" And then two weeks later it opened, you know, it bled, it ulcerated, it didn't close. And I thought, "Well, cancer." I knew enough about KS [Kaposi's sarcoma] to know that these lesions don't ulcerate that way. But it still, you know, the unconscious grip is much stronger than the rational one.

And a 36-year-old man who said he was seropositive commented:

> I found out I had a form of muscular dystrophy, so I went to the doctor; went to the hospital for ten days to find out exactly what it was, 'cause I, at the same time, I had bruises and everything. I thought it might have been AIDS. Ah, I found out I was just anemic. I had low platelets, and muscular dystrophy and everything. About six months later he [my doctor] decided to, "Let's try it [the HIV antibody test], if you want. Let's try to take the test 'cause I want to know if this is gonna, if this is related or not."

To Inform Sexual Decision Making

Some men explained that they had taken the test so that they could make more informed and responsible decisions about their sexual behavior. There were two subgroups among these respondents. The first consisted of those who felt a negative result would allow them to expand their sexual activities, such as one 27-year-old seronegative man:

> Well I did it [took the test] because I was in a relationship. The one that I'm in now. It's been going on for eleven months. And I just, I tested negative twice. And he tested negative twice. But he had just recently been tested negative. And I just, we were having, we were pretty much having safe sex. I mean we blew it a couple of times. And so we were trying to decide if we wanted to have unsafe sex. And we knew we wanted to be mutually exclusive. And so I just wanted to do it one more time to make sure.

Another 34-year-old seropositive man, citing similar motives, commented:

> I was sure I was negative. . . . In [the] autumn of 1986, I had a boyfriend and this guy was very hypochondriac. He had the test at least twice and he was negative. But he set very strict sex rules for us. And I thought that one of the reasons of our problems was that he couldn't have a relaxed sexual life because of that. Turned out that I was wrong. But, I couldn't know that. I thought, well, if I take the test, too, and I, of course, I'll be negative, then we'll be both negative. We'll make a pact of mutual total fidelity, sexual fidelity. And so we will be able not to have, not to follow safer sex guidelines anymore."

And a seronegative man, 26, said, "I think it [a negative test result] allowed me to perceive myself as being at less a risk, and to have fewer qualms about having unprotected oral sex."

The second subgroup was motivated to be tested because they wanted to know if their sexual activities presented any risk of infecting their partners. They believed that if they tested negative, they posed no risk to others, regardless of their behavior. One 27-year-old seronegative man said he took the test "for a variety of reasons. First off, I really thought I was going to be negative. But I also didn't want to pass it on to anybody else. I mean I was having—I, I didn't want to pass it on to anyone else." Another man, 25 and who had tested negative, told us:

> Well, what basically led up to it [getting tested] was in September I met my lover. And I felt something I had never really felt for anybody else before. And he told me I guess about a month into our relationship that he has been tested negative three times, because there was someone he had been with that told him afterwards that he had it. So he was quite upset from that. So he went and told me, you know, he took it three times. And he was negative all three times. And I just felt that this was something that was very important to me. And this was something that I really cared a great deal about. And I didn't want to be in the dark about it and risk something happening at some point. Ah, so I decided, you know for myself, but also for him that I wanted to try it out [be tested].

Another respondent, also negative and 24, spoke of the "responsibility" he felt to others:

> But anyway, the reason I got tested was mainly because I wanted to know. It's a big responsibility. Ah, this is my counter to the argument of "I don't want to get tested." Because you have a responsibility to the person you are going to sleep with. You have a responsibility to make sure they are healthy when they leave you. And that's something that I take very seriously. I mean in terms of whether or not you want to know for yourself, doesn't hold up if you are going to endanger the life of somebody else. And that's basically my argument. So I really wanted to know for that.

To Relieve Psychological Distress Associated With Not Knowing HIV Status

Virtually all respondents recognized that they may have been infected through past sexual behaviors. Even those who had consistently practiced safer sex during the last several years and expected they were negative realized that they could have acquired the virus through their earlier behavior. Furthermore, even those who had remained asymptomatic for several years after stopping unsafe behavior worried about infection because they knew that the disease had a long incubation.

The ambiguity of their status left them psychologically vulnerable to persistent fears and suspicions that any symptom might be HIV related. To relieve this psychological distress, some respondents were motivated to take the antibody test. A 30-year-old man who had taken the test, with negative results, about a year earlier said,

> I knew about the test I guess since it's been out. What was happening up until that point, you know, every time I'd be sick, I would think "Is this AIDS?"... [And] for a long time I was able to live with that fear. What I realized was that, you know,the stress of every disease that was coming up, every common cold—anything—the stress that I would put myself through by not knowing if I was exposed to the virus was just outweighing me getting a positive result back. You know it came to that point where I finally realized that if I got a positive result back it'd probably be less stressful than not knowing. So I went and took the test at that point."

For many men, learning that past partners or close friends tested positive or were diagnosed with AIDS heightened their own sense of vulnerability and finally raised their anxiety to an intolerable level. These men experienced a kind of "closing circle" effect as the illnesses of past partners and friends personalized the threat of the disease, making it harder to deny the immediacy of the peril to own health. A 63-year-old man who said he was seronegative described these feelings:

> I was worried, I was very worried. . . . Ah, several partners, previous partners, got AIDS and died with AIDS which scared the hell out of me. . . . And each time I heard that someone got AIDS and subsequently died of AIDS, I used to say, "There but for the grace of God go I." Ah, then ah, anytime I'd see something on my skin or something unusual in my physical make-up, I'd get frightened. Uh oh, here's a symptom coming up. Ah, it was two years ago, I was on the beach in the, down in Florida in the wintertime. And I saw three spots on my calf I had never seen before. Holy shit! KS [Kaposi's sarcoma]. Ah, and I was living with those fears, and I just didn't like it. I felt if I was positive, I could cope with it, but I just wanted to know. Ah, I wanted to push paranoia aside or whatever.

A 28-year-old man with a seronegative test result said,

> I had three good friends who died of AIDS. And it was all over the papers and all over everything. And I, in my mind I kept saying to myself, "Well, gee that it could be that chance that I have it." And it was just getting to me. And it was getting the best of me. And I don't usually let anything get the best of me, but it, it kind of was. And I said, "Well, fuck it. Let me go for my [test], just to see. And I did.

One 31-year-old respondent initially had chosen not to be tested, justifying his decision by saying that he felt that knowing he was positive would be like walking around with a "time bomb" inside of him. However, eventually he decided to be tested (obtaining a positive result) because he felt not knowing his status was equally psychologically distressing:

> Then what happened was I, I think I started walking around with that anxiety and that time bomb feeling even without taking it [the test]. . . . AIDS was something I was always able to keep at a comfortable distance. You know even though I volunteered at GMHC [Gay Men's Health Crisis, a community-based AIDS service organization], I could still go home and forget about it. Ah, most of the people that I—all of the people that I knew that had become sick were acquaintances, not close friends. And over the past year and a half, it started to hit closer to home. Closer friends, just people in my social circle. And, ah, so I suppose I started feeling the time bomb syndrome anyway, and then really wanted, you know, the anxiety level was high and I wanted some affirmation either way.

Motives for Not Taking the Test

Respondents who had not taken the test spoke of the anticipated negative psychosocial consequences that a seropositive result might have. We organized these responses into four categories: (1) the desire to avoid the adverse psychological impact of a positive test result, (2) the desire to avoid social discrimination and repressive governmental actions, (3) the desire to avoid an ambiguous or unreliable test result, and, (4) the wish to avoid having to make undesired lifestyle changes.

To Avoid the Adverse Psychological Impact of a Positive Test Result

Respondents most frequently cited the wish to avoid negative psychological consequences as their reason for not taking the test. The men feared a devastating emotional impact if they learned that they were infected and expected they would become severely depressed and even potentially suicidal if confronted with that knowledge. Some said they would feel that their lives would "be over," "destroyed" by such an awareness. These fears were usually based on the belief that most, if not all, infected individuals would eventually develop AIDS and die and that available medical treatments could not prevent that eventuality. A 39-year-old said,

> As far as the test is concerned, I just feel for myself, I am not, I haven't taken it and I don't intend to.

I sort of agree too, very much, that if you test positive, it seems now that just about everybody who tests positive is gonna get it, you know. And that if you know that, first of all your life, your life is destroyed; even if not physically, just as much destroyed."

And a man, 26, spoke of how knowing that he was positive would "destroy" him:

> I would never get tested. I mean it. It would take a lot for someone to convince me to be tested. Ah, if I found out that I was positive, it would destroy me. Whether you could tell me I was gonna live for seventy or five hundred years. I think I would start, I would really feel, start to think really negatively. As it is, I think I probably have the HIV virus. But I don't know. So it's almost like it's better for me living for me that way. I mean I go back and forth. It would be great to find out it was negative. But if I found out it was positive, it would be devastating. And that's too great a risk for me to take. Basically, it's—I feel that if I found out I was positive on a piece of paper, my life would be over. I would, I would think every day, "Well, I just wonder when it's gonna happen." Not *if* it's gonna happen. When. I'd wonder if it will happen, you know, like a year from now, or two years. I mean it would totally wreak havoc.

Another, about the same age, said,

> Ah, I know myself well enough to know that I'm not the sort of person who would respond well to that kind of information. So, ah I would rather not know. I don't take it because I conjecture that I would be really debilitated by it. I wouldn't be able to function well, knowing that I would worry. I would live a life of default. Ah, but at the same time, it's hard not to know. I mean if I were in the circumstance and at that point were faced with no option, but to cope with it or kill myself, I don't know. I don't know which I would do.

Other men saw the immediate psychological impact as less acute and devastating, but felt knowing they were positive would become a chronic stressor which would significantly compromise the quality of their lives. They felt they would become morbidly preoccupied with their health and possible death if they knew they were infected. They expected they would be continually anxious about the specter of the appearance of the first HIV-related symptoms and be alarmed by even innocuous symptoms and ailments. Most described themselves as already riddled with anxiety about their antibody status and future health. They believed that the certain knowledge that they were infected would only serve to heighten their worries and fears.

One 38-year-old respondent, who described himself as already in a panic because a former live-in lover had died of AIDS, said if he found out he was positive he would "be even more frightened. I'd think of when would it come. . . . What I would do. . . . It's a death sentence." Another man of the same age said he thought about being tested "every single day. . . . Will finding out I'm positive or not change what I do? No. Will it make me worry more? Yes. . . . And I don't need to worry more." And a 19-year-old respondent also said he preferred not to know:

> But I wouldn't take the test because if, God forbid, the results were positive, I, I couldn't take that. I'd feel like I'm a time bomb and I'm going to explode soon. I just wouldn't want to know. If I have it, I have it. Ah, and I don't—now I haven't been doing any sexual practices that would, you know, harm anyone that I'm in sexual contact with.

Several men recognized that their past sexual behavior placed them at high risk for exposure to the virus, and even presumed themselves to be seropositive. Still, they felt that not having definitive knowledge that they were positive permitted them to maintain a modicum of hope that they were uninfected and that was psychologically protective. One 33-year-old man described the importance of this hope as something that could "sustain" him:

> [If positive] I would worry, you know. I'm more, kind of a hypochondriac in a lot of ways. And I think that ah, I worry enough as it is. And that thing, that little point zero one percent hope that I might be negative, you know, may sustain you sometimes. . . . I don't want to deal with the fact that I'm probably positive.

When we asked him about the difference between assuming he is positive and knowing it, he responded, "Just that difference. That little bit of, you know, there's a little bit of hope there." Similarly, a 36-year-old man who said he assumed he was positive, spoke about how not knowing for sure gave him "that little five percent that says maybe I'm not. And so, ah, rather than be told, "Yes, you are", and having to deal with that." He preferred not to be tested.

A number of men felt that learning they were positive could have adverse physical consequences. These men believed that psychological stress damaged the immune system's functioning. A 39-year-old said, "I feel good. If it's gonna happen, it's gonna happen. Ah, if I got the test and it was positive, I would probably worry about it and make matters worse. So if I don't know, then I'm gonna proceed on a healthy way of life." A man, 36, said knowing he was positive could result in "damaging stress" to his immune system, and he thus avoided the test. One 27-year-old, who had gone to be tested in the midst of what he described an "incredible anxiety attack" but decided not to return to learn the results, explained his decision this way:

> At that time it seemed so certain that you were going to die very soon if you had it, that I just didn't want to face that information. And I guess I believe in the holistic idea that a healthy mind can help a healthy body. I do believe that ah, if you are infected, if you worry about it constantly, it's much more likely to sort of undermine your immune system than if you don't have worry about that very real solid fact.

To Avoid Social Discrimination and Repressive Governmental Actions

Another motive mentioned for not being tested was to avoid social discrimination and repressive governmental actions. Many men doubted that their test results would remain confidential or be truly anonymous and thus feared that testing positive, or even just taking the test, could result in loss of jobs, insurance coverage, and civil liberties. While the dangers of repressive government actions against infected individuals were typically discussed as something that could happen in the future, fears about loss of insurance or employment were usually based on stories they had heard of the past experiences of others and were perceived as an immediate threat. These men seemed to put little credence in assertions by various institutions or officials that results would be kept confidential or that testing was anonymous. Our respondents expressed distrust of public officials, employers, insurers, and even the general public. One 46-year-old man spoke of his fear of "getting on somebody's list":

> You know, I think politically, I mean in pure politics, that we see our country frequently shifting into a real conservative bent. And when they are in power, there is nothing to stop them. And once you've been tested, I really think you're probably on somebody's list, whether it's the doctor's list or public health's list or something like that. . . . I'm also concerned about the insurance question, medical insurance. People being refused it or dropped. Ah, I don't trust the American public. Especially when something selfish comes, I don't trust any public . . . I just, I feel that panic that we've seen at times. And it will probably get worse because there are all indications that it's going to go into—it's broadening its spectrum in terms of the number of people and kinds of people that it's hitting. But I would be fearful of getting on some list.

Another man, 35, also doubted the anonymity of the test results:

> I think of a few of the horror stories about test results, about test results being released to insurance companies, to employment agencies, to these kinds of things. Unfortunately I don't believe we are at a point where these things are totally anonymous. I don't feel I'm being overly cautious. If I felt it was something, that being tested was going to save my life, I wouldn't care. But the idea that somehow my insurance would be dropped or something based on the fact that some worker in a health department somewhere was convinced by an insurance company employee that for X amount of money that certain records could be left open or copies could be made. I've heard many horror

stories of men with AIDS who have been dropped from insurance programs, and it's pretty horrible. I don't think knowing whether I have the HIV virus or not is worth right now taking that risk.

A 26-year-old man who said he "worked in government relations" commented that he didn't

trust public authorities with any kind of information regardless of what they say about confidentiality, including this. Public policy advocates will use information in any way that they can to advance their cause. And those advocates are not always going to be people who are sympathetic to those people who have taken the test. And even though right now the balance of power may be such that you have nothing to worry about now, that doesn't mean it will be so in the future.

To Avoid an Ambiguous and Unreliable Test Result

The perceived ambiguity of and/or unreliability of the antibody test results, the significance of HIV as a "cause" of AIDS, and the meaningfulness of a positive or negative test for anticipating future health were also offered as reasons not be tested. These respondents seemed to feel that tolerating the uncertainty of not knowing their status was possibly no worse than submitting to the ambiguity of a potentially unreliable or inaccurate test result. A few men remained unconvinced that HIV was the etiologic agent in AIDS or that seropositivity was a useful predictor of future health. One man, 37, said he thought taking the test was "like flipping a coin":

I have friends who tested negative up until the day they died. . . . I have heard it's as high as 40 percent false positive, false negative, for example. 40 percent on the ELISA [an initial test to screen blood for HIV antibodies]. The Western Bloc [a more precise confirmatory text for the antibodies] is 70 percent, fairly accurate. . . . [My roommate's second lover] hung himself in his hospital room. . . . One day his test was positive and the next day negative, right up until the end. And it was like, "Oh no, it's just lymphatic cancer you lucky dog," you know. Really, every couple of days it was "you've got it, you don't have it, you've got it, you don't have it," you know.

Another man, 24, spoke of his understanding that the test was not "100 percent accurate":

It doesn't mean that you don't have it [HIV infection] if it comes out negative. So I guess that would be the main thing. So what would be the sense of you taking it and then it coming out negative, and then having sex and end up catch, you know, contracting AIDS anyway.

The men recognized both the dangers inherent in a false sense of security that a "false negative" can provide and the psychological devastation that a "false positive" can bring. A respondent, 26, said,

So I get a negative? Great. Well, maybe it's a false negative. You know, who knows? Or then I have to go get tested again. If they come up with a sure-fire test that says, "you are definitely, 100 percent." Until then I don't really think it would do that much for me. And I think getting a positive, which again could be false, is actually worse than not being sure and sort of assuming you have it. I think that would be, that would be worse.

To Avoid Having to Make Undesired Lifestyle Changes

Other men had decided not to undergo testing because they felt a positive result would require changes in their lifestyle that they did not want to make. Ignorance of their status seemed to make it at least personally acceptable to maintain current practices. A man, 29, said,

I kind of like, well I do like the way I live now. And I know my personality. And if someone were to tell me that I tested positive for this, I wouldn't live my—I know I'm pretty sure I wouldn't live

> my life the same way. I would worry. I'd be in fear. At the same time, if I tested positive it would probably be the end of my sexual activities.

Like this man, others said that learning they were positive would obligate them to modify their sexual behavior or lifestyle, something they did not feel compelled to do in the absence of certain knowledge they were positive. A man, 27, spoke of the "moral issue" involved:

> if I found out I tested positive, it's not real for me to say that I would stop having sex. It's not real for me to say I would find a lover who has AIDS and only have sex with him. Ah, so I would continue to not practice safe sex, but I would continue to have sex—a great deal of anonymous sex. And that's wrong.

We asked him why he thought that was "wrong":

> Because you know that you are in effect poisoning people. . . . I agree with the first person [on the videotape] who said every person that has sex with you without asking you first [if you're infected] is taking a risk, and that's his responsibility, not yours. And it's an implied risk and so you're off the hook. Well yes, if you don't *know* you're going to contaminate this person. If you know you're infected, you know that you will contaminate him if what you do is unsafe. And that's, morally that's wrong. Worse [to me] than actually having the disease and dying would be to live the rest of my life and not be able to have sex with anyone or knowing I was killing whoever I was having sex with.

And finally, a 38-year-old man speculated about how knowing he was positive might affect his relationships:

> I don't think that would necessarily stop me from having a relationship with another person. But I know that it would really curtail the sexual activity because of what I may contribute to the person's development. Who knows, it may be multiple infections or whatever, so it would probably be better not to have any, you know, contact with his semen. You know it would probably be bad for both of us.

Discussion

The motives our respondents offered for taking or not taking the HIV antibody test both reflect and constitute prevailing social constructions of the test. In this final section of the paper, we characterize these cultural constructions more broadly and comment on changes in the motives offered over time.

Within the broader culture there are three competing definitions of the HIV test, which can be labeled the public health, psychosocial, and medical constructions. The men we interviewed discussed their motives for taking or not taking the test by drawing on these definitions, applying them to their own circumstances, and thus revitalizing them as cultural constructions. An analysis of public health and gay literature shows that the first two, what we call the psychosocial and the public health definitions, emerged shortly after the development in 1984 and subsequent licensing in 1985 of a test for serum antibodies to HIV. The third, the medical definition, appeared following the growing recognition in 1987 and 1988 that HIV causes a spectrum of diseases that culminate in AIDS. All three constructions differ in regard to the meaning and anticipated consequences of the test.

The psychosocial construction of the test depicts it as a grave threat to individuals' basic human rights and psychological well-being. A perception of pervasive homophobia in the United States prompted gay community leaders and civil libertarians to become the main proponents of this perspective (Shilts 1987, Bayer 1988). According to this construction, all but anonymous testing procedures presumably are associated with the creation of registries of infected people or provide the potential for such registries to be established. Although assurances of confidentiality may currently exist, it is recognized that future laws or court orders could overturn these protections. Subsequent breaches of confidentiality could be exploited by anti-gay interest groups, possibly leading to employment and housing discrimination against registered individuals as well as loss of their health and life insurance protection.

This construction also holds that test results may be emotionally and socially disruptive to individuals in a number of ways. First, positive results can have profound adverse psychological consequences, including depression, anxiety, suicide, and the disruption of social relationships. Second, the technical limitations of the test, including the existence of a period after infection during which antibodies cannot yet be detected, can lead to inaccurate or inconclusive results. False positive results can engender the same adverse emotional consequences as accurate findings, and, of course, false negatives can allow those infected to unknowingly transmit the virus.

The campaign against testing within the gay community in New York City conveyed the psychosocial construction. The leading gay newspaper and AIDS organizations published editorials, advertisements, and informational brochures discouraging gay men from being tested for technical, social, and psychological reasons (Shilts 1987, Bayer 1988). A widely distributed GMHC pamphlet was typical of these campaign materials. Written in alarmist tones, this brochure warned gay men that test results were unreliable and ambiguous and could cause them to "lose their jobs or health insurance."

The motives cited in the interviews for not taking the test drew heavily upon the psychosocial definition. Most of the men reported avoiding being tested because they feared social discrimination, repressive governmental actions, and the adverse psychological impact of positive results. Many men feared that hostile groups would gain access to test results and use them for discriminatory purposes. In addition, they believed that a positive result, even if it was inaccurate, would leave them emotionally traumatized and devastated.

The medical construction views the test as a valuable tool for planning the most efficacious and appropriate clinical management of at risk individuals. AIDS clinicians, researchers, and treatment activists have been the major supporters of this perspective (Redfield and Burke 1988, Institute of Medicine 1988, Helquist 1989, Delaney 1989). In this definition, HIV is presumed to cause a sequence of disease conditions, ranging from acute infection to seropositivity to chronic HIV infection and, finally, to AIDS. Furthermore, the antibody test is regarded as an acceptably reliable indicator of HIV status, with a positive result indicating the presence of the virus and infectivity. Therefore, a positive test result is considered to be grounds for initiating medical treatments. Moreover, it is presumed that if left untreated seropositivity will inexorably progress to AIDS, and hence early intervention is considered central to prolonging health and survival.

Prominent gay clinicians and treatment activists began to articulate this definition in New York City in early 1988. At public forums and in articles in the gay press and the newsletters of AIDS organizations, they encouraged gay men to get tested in order to take advantage of emerging medical treatments for HIV infection. They recommended that seropositive men practice sound health maintenance, participate in holistic therapies, and take either antiviral drugs or medicines that can either boost the immune system or prevent opportunistic infections.

The men's motives for undergoing testing largely embodied the medical definition. Many of the men stated that they took the test in order to more effectively monitor their health status and plan medical interventions. Knowledge of their test results would allow them to determined whether or not they should take drugs that could either slow the replication of HIV or forestall opportunistic infections. Others stated that they needed this knowledge in order either to become motivated to lead a healthier lifestyle or to arrive at a definitive diagnosis of a problematic medical condition.

The public health definition views the test as an effective mechanism for controlling the spread of the HIV epidemic. Public health officials and policy makers were the principal advocates of this construction, with most favoring widespread, voluntary, and confidential testing (Bayer 1988, Brandt 1987, Koop 1986, Centers for Disease Control 1986). According to this interpretation, the antibody test is an acceptably accurate and reliable indicator of HIV infection. Hence, individuals who test positive are regarded as being infected and presumably infectious.

Furthermore, testing, especially among high risk populations, is regarded as an effective strategy for reducing HIV transmission. First, testing is believed to locate infected individuals who are unaware of their status; these people can then be counseled to cease behaviors associated with the transmission of the virus and to adopt health maintenance practices. Second, some proportion of the asymptomatic infected population who are currently unaware of their status and unknowingly infecting others will learn of their seropositivity and be motivated to cease practices that spread the virus. Finally, widespread testing presumably provides more accurate surveillance data concerning the geographic and demographic spread of the virus, enabling more intensive educational efforts to be targeted to those regions and groups with high rates of infection.

The motives offered in the interviews for taking or not taking the test drew slightly from the public health construction. For the most part, the men saw little personal benefits in the public health rationale for testing. Some commented that the civil liberties and psychological risks associated with testing far outweighed the public health need for more accurate surveillance data. Others felt that education, not testing, was what was needed to motivate gay men to practice safer sex.

Only one of the motives cited for being tested reflected the public health construction. A few men reported that they took the test in order to alter current sexual practices. They felt that knowledge of their test results would allow them to either expand their range of sexual practices to include risky behavior or restrict their conduct to practices that posed no risk of infecting others.

The interviews indicate that over time there was a shift in men's definitions of the consequences of the test. When testing initially became available, most respondents subscribed to the psychosocial construction of the test. Accordingly, they perceived it as having potentially far-reaching adverse social and psychological consequences while offering no meaningful benefits. With the emergence of the medical construction in 1987 and 1988 some men redefined their perception of the anticipated consequences of being tested. Testing came to be viewed as providing a means of learning one's HIV status, and if infected, initiating medical treatments that could prolong health and life. Conversely, most of the respondents who have remained untested continue to adhere to the psychosocial construction of the test.

The respondents' accounts suggest that the medical construction is likely to take on increasing importance in gay men's motives for testing. For example, if evidence continues to accrue demonstrating the efficacy of treatments for HIV infection and the benefits of beginning treatments early, more men will be strongly motivated to be tested. Furthermore, as the data indicating that HIV infection is the first stage of a progressive disease that will culminate in AIDS proliferates, the value of learning early that one is seropositive is likely to be viewed as greatly increased. Nevertheless, the psychosocial construction continues to present formidable barriers to testing. As our study and others cited above indicate, anticipated psychological distress and discrimination are among the most frequently reported motives for not taking the test. To overcome these barriers, gay organizations, public health agencies, and AIDS commissions and community-based organizations have repeatedly called for the availability of anonymous testing procedures and laws safeguarding the confidentiality of and prohibiting discrimination against tested individuals (Bayer 1988, Institute of Medicine 1988). Without these protections, it seems likely that many gay men will continue to regard the risks of testing as unacceptable.

References

Bayer, Ronald
1988 Private Acts, Social Consequences: AIDS and the Politics of Public Health. New York: The Free Press.

Brandt, Allan
1987 No Magic Bullet: A Social History of Venereal Diseases in the United States from 1880. New York: Oxford University Press.

Centers for Disease Control
1986 Additional Recommendations to Reduce Sexual and Drug-Abuse Related Transmissions of Human T-Lymphotorophic Virus Type III Lymphadenopathy-Associated Virus. Morbidity and Mortality Weekly 35:152-55.

Coates, Thomas, Ron D. Stall, Susan M. Kegeles, Bernard Lo, Stephen F. Morin, and Leon McKusick
1988 "AIDS antibody testing: will it stop the AIDS epidemic? will it help people infected with HIV?" American Psychologist 43:859-64.

Delaney, Martin
1989 "Staying alive. making the ultimate political statement: new reasons to consider taking the antibody test." The Advocate February 28:33-37

Goldblum, Peter and Neil Seymour
1987 "Whether to take the test: counseling guidelines." Focus: A Guide to AIDS Research 2:1-3.

Helquist, Michael
1989 "Update on getting tested" The Advocate June 6:36.

Institute of Medicine
1988 Confronting AIDS: Update 1988. Washington, DC: National Academy Press.

Koop, C. Everett
1986 Surgeon General's Report On Acquired Immune Deficiency Syndrome. Washington, DC: U.S. Department of Health.

Lyter, David, Ronald O. Valdeserri, Lawrence A. Kingsley, William P. Amodoso, and Charles R. Rinaldo Jr.
1987 "The HIV antibody test: why gay and bisexual men want to know their results." Public Health Reports 102:468-74.

Merton, Robert K., Marjorie Fiske, and Patricia L. Kendall
1956 The Focused Interview. Glencoe, IL: The Free Press.

Miller, David
1987 Living with AIDS and HIV. London: Macmillan.

Mills, C. Wright
1940 Situated actions and vocabularies of motive. American Sociological Review 5:904-13.

Redfield, Robert and Donald S. Burke
1988 "HIV infection: the clinical picture." Scientific American 259:90-99.

Research and Decisions Corporation
1986 Designing an Effective AIDS Prevention Campaign Startegy for San Francisco: Results from the Third Probability Sample of an Urban Gay Male Community. San Francisco, CA: The San Francisco AIDS Foundation.

Shilts, Randy
1987 And the Band Played On: Politics, People and the AIDS Epidemic. New York: St. Martin's Press.

Archives of Sexual Behavior, Vol. 20, No. 1, 1991

Plethysmography in the Assessment and Treatment of Sexual Deviance: An Overview

Walter T. Simon, Ph.D.[1] **and Peter G. W. Schouten, M.A.**[2]

Theoretical and practical implications of previous research on plethysmography in the assessment and modification of sexual preferences has been limited by insufficient attention to definitional and procedural issues and sample heterogeneity. This paper reviews current theory and research on the use of the penile plethysmograph to diagnose or predict sexual deviance and to monitor therapeutic change in the modification of sexual preferences. Phallometric tests are discussed in terms of the basic components of the measurement technique, evidence of technical adequacy, and general principles underlying their use. The review points to a need to guard against false expectations and erroneous conclusions about sexual deviance based on this measurement technique. A case is made for closer attention to previously untested working assumptions and issues of definition, etiology, and measurement. Directions for future research are proposed.

KEY WORDS: sexual deviance; assessment; penile plethysmograph.

INTRODUCTION

The physiological aspects of the human sexual response have been the focus of research on normal sexuality, sexual deviation, and sexual dysfunction. The physiological measurement of arousal was an important component in the pioneering work of Masters and Johnson (1966, 1970) and subsequent research on male sexuality (Quinsey and Marshall, 1983; Rosen and Keefe, 1978). The parameters of sexual arousal are of interest in the

[1]Darrow Clinic, 777 Grant Street, Suite 605, Denver, Colorado 80203.
[2]Focus Research, 3960 Vallejo Street, Denver, Colorado 80211.

0004-0002/91/0200-0075$06.50/0

scientific study of human sexuality, and also in clinical and legal responses to alleged or known sexual deviations.

The penile plethysmograph provides a measure of tumescence in response to fantasy or laboratory stimuli. Early research with this instrument focused on sexual preferences as to the age or sex of partner and specific sexual activities (Freund, 1963). Quinsey (1973) emphasized its potential in discharge decisions regarding institutionalized child molesters. Freund *et al.* (1979) later argued its value in the diagnosis of "non-admitters." Although routinely used for clinical purposes, particularly with forensic populations, basic theoretical premises underlying this measurement paradigm have not been clarified and its technical adequacy remains in question. Drawing upon recent research, this paper reviews major conceptual and methodological problems in plethysmography for the evaluation and treatment of sexual deviation.

THEORETICAL AND CONCEPTUAL BACKGROUND

Use of the plethysmograph in the diagnosis and treatment of sexual deviance reflects an implicit, but not necessarily accepted, theoretical explanation of sexual deviance. The individual is thought to act upon a sexual aim (a pattern of behavior) or chooses a sexual object which then becomes a target. Overt sexual acts presumably reflect sexual arousal that is elicited by the individual's fantasy of the act or object (Freund, *et al.*, 1979). Certain preferences are thought to have specific behavioral consequences. Further, distinct erotic interests can presumably be inferred from laboratory measures of penile responses to normal and deviant stimuli. These premises warrant closer examination.

Working Assumptions of Phallometric Testing

Plethysmography in the assessment of sexual deviance assumes a natural operational linkage between stimulus-specific penile arousal patterns and overt sexual acts. This view is the presupposition of the use of phallometric tests to diagnose sexual deviance and predict dangerousness. The assumption of arousal–behavior relationship is also central to a behavior modification doctrine which emphasizes direct attempts to modify the penile arousal patterns that are thought to lead to deviant behavior (Abel and Blanchard, 1976; Earls and Marshall, 1983; Laws and Osborn, 1983; Quinsey, 1973; Quinsey and Marshall, 1983; Rosen and Kopel, 1978). The goal of this treatment approach is reduced arousal to deviant sexual stimuli and increased arousal to appropriate stimuli (Bancroft, 1970, 1974). Given this therapeutic goal, the plethysmograph might appear to be a logical choice as a measure of treatment effectiveness.

Available evidence does not provide unequivocal support for the hypothesized relationship between sexual arousal in the laboratory and overt sexual acts. Furthermore, to explain sexual interests and acts strictly in terms of categories of stimulus specific arousal is to ignore the role of individual differences variables in mediating relationships between these distinct, though related, aspects of the human sexual response. Examples would include an impotent pedophile whose deviant acts involve fondling rather than actual or attempted intercourse or exhibitionists who expose themselves without accompanying erection. Rosen and Kopel (1978) pointed out that "In such cases it appears that the inappropriate behavior is functionally independent of genital response" (p. 1520). In these and other cases, phallometric measures would not be relevant to either assessment or treatment. Individual differences variables that may mediate the relationship between physiological measures to overt behavior must be considered in evaluating the validity of plethysmography in the assessment of sexual preferences.

TEST AND MEASUREMENT PARADIGM

Empirically derived assessments of deviance have a statistical basis for confidence in diagnosis and prediction (Gabor, 1986). In plethysmography, evidence of the validity of conclusions based on test results must be evaluated in light of measurement issues. In this paradigm, sexual deviance has been operationally defined as a penile response pattern elicited in the laboratory. Philosophical issues aside, a basic question remains: Does the plethysmograph accurately assess male erectile responses? (Farkas, 1978; Farkas *et al.*, 1979; Freund *et al.*, 1988). To answer this question, the basic components of the measurement technique and testing and scoring procedures must be evaluated.

TRANSDUCERS AND RECORDING EQUIPMENT

Phallometric measures are commonly obtained using a strain gauge (Barlow *et al.*, 1970) or mercury-in-rubber gauge (Bancroft *et al.*, 1966). Circumferential measures are contrasted with penile volume measures. The latter are designed to assess complete volume changes in terms of both penis length and diameter. Volumetric devices and strain gauges have been compared (Wheeler and Rubin, 1987) and have been found to provide conflicting results (McConaghy, 1974; Freund *et al.*, 1974). The relationship between volumetric and circumferential measures is unclear due to differences in metrics. However, different types of circumferential measures may also yield conflicting results (Laws, 1977).

Increased sensitivity and precision in measurement may be possible with a better understanding of the operating characteristics of the penis, particularly at low levels of responding. Earls and Marshall (1983) found that in the initial stages of penile responding, the magnitude of increases in length (28%) is substantially greater than that of diameter change (2.5%). They noted that "at 10% of diameter-assessed arousal, almost half of the total length change had occurred" (p. 349). Earls and Marshall (1983) concluded that circumferential measures are inadequate because they fail to assess the lengthening of the penis during erection. Current phallometric techniques may also fail to tap other potentially important, but as yet unidentified, physiological dimensions of the human sexual response.

Laboratory Stimulus Materials

Plethysmography utilizes various media to provide erotic cues to produce sexual arousal in the laboratory. These include pictures of nudes, movies, erotic stories, and audiotaped narratives. Certain test stimuli presumably constitute "relevant inappropriate material" (Laws and Osborn, 1983; Quinsey *et al.*, 1981) suitable for eliciting deviant arousal. The importance of stimulus materials in phallometric assessment is apparent from evidence showing that subjects' ability to bring arousal under voluntary control is influenced by stimulus content (Malcolm *et al.*, 1985). However, the critical role of these materials in the laboratory assessment of sexual deviance has been largely overlooked. Few studies have directly compared the effectiveness of modalities or the impact of erotic cues within a single class of stimuli (Abel *et al.*, 1975; Abel, Blanchard, and Barlow, 1981). In fact, studies in this area have typically provided little descriptive detail regarding the stimulus sets used.

Recent research has underscored a lack of precision in the use of laboratory assessment of pedophilia (Fuller *et al.*, 1988). To confirm a diagnosis of pedophilia, a subject may be exposed to pictures of nude prepuberal children since this diagnostic category is defined by an erotic preference for children at this stage of development (American Psychiatric Association, 1987). Pedophilic stimuli have traditionally been selected on the basis of age. However, age categories are imprecise because persons within a given age range are characterized by idiosyncratic patterns of pubertal change and varying degrees of physical development (Fuller *et al.*, 1988). The distinction between developmental and age-graded categories has major implications for the assessment of sexual deviance. The distinction means that some pedophiles may be aroused only by child sexual stimuli which are defined by highly specific developmental aspects; others may be aroused by materials within much broader classes of child stimuli. It is not always possible to determine what type of stimuli are most effective.

The impact of laboratory stimuli is dependent not only on aspects of physical development or sexual maturity. For example, in a study reported by Wormith (1986), a blonde model elicited significantly greater arousal than a redhead. Interactions between model attributes (bodily shapes, facial features, skin color, extent of undress, posture, etc.), setting, the exact nature of sexual activity, or the quality of pictures may also contribute to variations in sexual arousal.

Still other aspects of the stimulus materials must be considered, namely, elements of consent and violence. Quinsey *et al.* (1984) found no differences in the phallometric responses of rapists and non-sex-offenders to audiotaped sadomasochistic stories. The appropriateness of sadomasochistic themes in the assessment of rapists is unclear.

Among pedophiles elements of consent have been linked to greater arousal to child stimuli (Hall *et al.*, 1988). Clearly, violence and consent are critical dimensions of laboratory stimuli used in the assessment of alleged or known sexual offenders and their treatment. In this context, it should be noted that standardized laboratory stimuli may not be useful for treatment applications of the plethysmograph. As Rosen and Kopel (1978) suggested, stimulus materials used in the modification of arousal patterns should be specifically developed to approximate an individual's unique erotic interest. Such an approach reflects a realistic appraisal of the idiosyncratic nature of sexual preference.

Duration of Stimulus Presentation

Duration of stimulus presentation may be an important factor in the accurate assessment of sexual preferences. The strength of penile responses may be influenced by how long a subject is exposed to stimulus materials. Examination of recent research reveals that duration of presentation may vary widely with stimulus modality, ranging from relatively brief exposures for individual slides to extended videotape or audiotape sequences (Marshall and Barbaree, 1988; Wheeler and Rubin, 1987; Wormith, 1986).

Some subjects may not achieve levels of arousal indicative of their true interests if given insufficient exposure. Longer exposure times may facilitate stronger responses, but may also give subjects more time to modify their responses. These issues are complicated by individual differences in responsiveness, with some subjects achieving full erection much sooner, and some much later, than others in the presence of certain stimuli. Attempts to determine optimum duration of stimulus presentation must take into account differences between modalities, the impact of specific content within modalities, and their interaction with individual differences in responsiveness.

Scoring Procedures

The penile response can be measured in several ways (Abel, Blanchard, Murphy, *et al.*, 1981; Earls *et al.*, 1987). Penile circumference change is the most common, and is assessed as amount of change in millimeters. In view of individual differences in penis size, the raw data may be transformed to percentage of full erection. Alternatively, because many subjects do not achieve full erection in the laboratory, the raw data may be transformed to reflect magnitude of change from baseline using *z*-score transformations (e.g., Wormith, 1986). For a sample of paid volunteers, Earls *et al.* (1987) found that *z* scores were more sensitive to differences in stimulus categories than raw score and percentage change indices. In addition, these researchers pointed out that unlike the percentage change index, the *z* score method does not require an upper limit (i.e., full erection). Data reported by Earls *et al.* (1987) indicate that the amount of variance accounted for within a sample is influenced by scoring method. Thus the validity and generalizability of individual and group data are qualified by the type of scoring method used.

A commonly used ratio index of deviant arousal is calculated by dividing arousal to inappropriate material (e.g., depictions of rape) by arousal to appropriate material (e.g., depictions of consenting sex). Quinsey and Marshall (1983) summarized the rationale for this ratio index: "What differentiates child molesters and rapists from non-sex offenders are their penile responses to the relevant inappropriate material in relation to their responses to appropriate material" (p. 268). As noted in our foregoing discussion of test stimuli, issues of definition relating to the appropriateness of stimulus materials are difficult to resolve. In addition, it is not clear how the ratio index would function in the assessment of individuals with mixed, rather than pure, erotic interests. For example, a nonexclusive pedophile may be equally aroused to child and adult laboratory stimuli. The individual may be interested in both children and adults, but no less deviant than an exclusive pedophile.

Controlling for Faked Responses

Erectile responses can be faked or suppressed to simulate a normal sexual response profile (Freund, 1963; Hall *et al.*, 1988). Voluntary control of penile tumescence appears to be mediated by both cognitive and mechanical processes. Mechanical distortions may involve muscle contractions or "pumping" behaviors (Freund *et al.*, 1988). The cognitive aspects may include elaborations of laboratory stimuli or inattention to those stimuli (Abel and Blanchard, 1976; Laws and Rubin, 1969). These processes in turn may be regulated by factors such as vividness of imagery (Smith and Over, 1987) and other individual differences in proneness to fantasy or subjective appraisal of sexual stimuli which are currently not well understood.

Concerns about the effect of voluntary control on test results have led to systematic efforts to identify key signs of faking and to devise means of offsetting it (Freund *et al.*, 1988; Malcolm *et al.*, 1985; Quinsey and Bergersen, 1976; Wydra *et al.*, 1983). This work has yielded a number of potentially useful and theoretically interesting findings about the conditions under which faking is more likely to occur, and has provided direction for determining the parameters of voluntary control and the study of individual differences in faking (Freund *et al.*, 1988; Malcolm *et al.*, 1985). For example, Freund *et al.* (1988) found evidence that age preference is easier to feign than gender preference. Malcolm *et al.* (1985) found that a forensic sample consisting primarily of rapists exhibited greater control of penile responses in the presence of nonpreferred sexual stimuli and less control in response to preferred stimuli.

However, there are at present no generally accepted procedures for estimating the probability of faking, detecting it, or controlling for it (Malcolm *et al.*, 1985). Available methods of minimizing or compensating for it are inadequate (Earls and Marshall, 1983). Rather than directly improving the accuracy of measurement, these strategies may only provide a basis for concluding that test results do not reflect an individual's true sexual preferences. Even what is considered the most obvious clue to faking is an ambiguous indicator. That is, if a subject shows no tumescence, this could mean either suppression of arousal or lack of interest (Earls and Marshall, 1983).

TECHNICAL ADEQUACY

The concept of internal validity relates to methodological soundness and the extent to which findings are free from the confounding effects of extraneous factors (Campbell, 1957). Farkas (1978) noted two major threats to internal validity, namely, subjects' ability to exert voluntary control over their penile responses and the weak relationship between self-reports of arousal and phallometric indices. Additional challenges to the internal validity of these indices are apparent with respect to reliability, the discriminability of sexual preference, classificational accuracy, sample selection, and procedural and contextual confounds. Threats to external validity are also noted in this review of recent research findings.

Reliability

Campbell (1969) pointed out that "instability" is a threat to internal validity. This is an issue given the common practice of repeated phallometric assessment to monitor treatment efficacy. It is also an issue in view of the state–trait distinction (Zuckerman, 1971). Sexual arousal as measured by the plethysmograph may reflect a temporary state of sexual tension rather than a stable, trait-like tendency to become aroused to a special class of sexual stimuli. An individual's arousal pattern must be sufficiently stable across time to serve as a basis for determining sexual preferences or for predicting future activity.

As Eccles *et al.* (1988) have pointed out, although reliability is central to the notion of sexual preference, few studies have directly addressed this issue. Evidence of temporal stability for penile response patterns has been mixed and is qualified by the length of the test–retest interval (e.g., Freund *et al.*, 1979) and by selection bias (e.g., normal volunteers vs. offenders) or inadequately defined selection criteria. Further, reliability is influenced by stimulus content. For example, Wormith (1986) reported a wide range of reliability coefficients for a relatively large sample of sex offenders and non-sex-offenders presented with male and female adult and child stimuli.

In previously published research, reliability coefficients for phallometric scores have ranged between .38 and .94 (Earls and Marshall, 1983; Wormith, 1986). Uncontrolled-for differences in test procedures and environmental conditions (e.g., laboratory stimulus materials, instructional set, examiner characteristics and demand characteristics), may account for variations in reliability.

In addition, reliability coefficients may vary considerably with different scoring methods (e.g., Wormith, 1986). Test–retest reliabilities of penile responses calculated using standard scores have been found to be lower than those of self-reports of sexual interest (Wormith, 1986). This finding is interesting in view of the controversy regarding the relative merits of phallometric and self-report measures in the assessment of sexual preferences (Barbaree and Marshall, 1989; Quinsey, 1973; Zuckerman, 1971).

An issue of statistical conclusion validity (Cook and Campbell, 1979) should be noted here. Specifically, estimates of the temporal stability of an individual diagnosis should be expressed in terms of classificational accuracy rather than correlation coefficients. It is necessary to determine the proportion of subjects consistently classified at different times.

Classificational accuracy is also relevant in determining agreement consistency between independent judges in the assessment of sexual deviance. Interjudge agreement studies are needed to justify confidence in diagnostic classifications that are based on phallometric findings. But classification decisions must be both accurate and consistent. Meaningful use of an agreement index presupposes optimum cutting scores (Rorer *et al.*, 1966). However, there are presently no generally agreed-upon guidelines as to normal and deviant phallometric response ranges.

The clinical assessment of sexual arousal to monitor treatment progress in terms of deviant and nondeviant response levels may call for repeated measurement. Treatment effects may easily be confounded with habituation. Researchers and clinicians are therefore concerned about the impact of repeated measurement on reliability. In a sample of college students, Eccles *et al.* (1988) found no evidence of habituation for college subjects who were tested on the plethysmograph up to nine times in a 3-week period. Interestingly, in a previous study with college volunteers, O'-Donohue and Greer (1985) found evidence not only of habituation to both constant and variable stimuli but successfully unconfounded it from physiological fatigue.

Repeated testing has also been linked to increased potential for faking through familiarity with the procedures and stimuli (Quinsey *et al.*, 1983) and practice in controlling arousal (Earls and Marshall, 1983). Faking, rather than habituation, is particularly of concern in pretrial evaluations and the assessment of offenders involved in court-ordered treatment who are motivated to demonstrate progress.

The Discriminability of Sexual Preferences

Clear evidence of differences in the penile response patterns of normals and sexual deviates would support the utility of the plethysmograph in the assessment of deviance. Evidence along these lines has been mixed. Normal volunteers have been found to respond with arousal to slides of 8- to 11-year-old girls and to slides of the buttocks of prepubescent boys (Freund, 1972). Furthermore, non-sex-offenders also become aroused in response to slides of pubescent females (Barbaree and Marshall, 1989; Freund *et al.*, 1972; Quinsey *et al.*, 1975), and men in the general population may exhibit arousal patterns similar to those of rapists (Barbaree *et al.*, 1979; Malamuth *et al.*, 1986; Quinsey *et al.*, 1981). These findings do not show that most nondeviants are as attracted to deviant stimuli as are deviants. Rather, the findings indicate that arousal to deviant themes does not unequivocally confirm sexual deviance.

Plethysmography presupposes the ability to differentiate sexual deviates and normals as well as deviant subtypes on the basis of arousal. Evidence of discriminant validity has been ambiguous. In a study reported by Freund *et al.* (1986), rapists could not be distinguished from an entire family of deviant sexual preferences, including exhibitionism, frottage, and voyeurism. Hall *et al.* (1988) found no differences between rapists and molesters (victims to age 16) in terms of penile responses to four categories of stimuli (consensual sex with an adult, consensual sex with a child, sexual assault of a child, and nonsexual assault of a child).

Classificational Accuracy

Statistical conclusion validity, specifically concerning the use of appropriate statistical methodology, is a special case of internal validity (Cook and Campbell, 1979). In plethysmography, this issue has so far been largely overlooked with respect to the use of correlational techniques to relate phallometric indices to diagnostic group criteria. Correlational data are inadequate evidence of validity because such data do not indicate the probability that a test will accurately identify individuals in terms of the proportion of subjects accurately classified (Meehl and Rosen, 1955). Evidence of classificational accuracy must be evaluated independently because in some distributions high rates of misclassification may occur even when correlational data suggest substantial concurrence between predictor and criteria. The validity of phallometric findings with respect to group criteria cannot be evaluated without classificational statistics.

Wormith (1986) reported a discriminant analysis of the phallometric data of rapists, pedophiles, and convicts incarcerated for nonsexual offenses. The results indicated misclassifications of up to 36%. Inspection of the classificational results reveals that 42% of the pedophiles were classified as having normal sexual preferences and 33% of those with normal sexual preferences were erroneously assigned to the rapist group. Also of interest in this context are the Barbaree and Marshall (1989) findings. Specifically, 40% of incest offenders and 68% of matched nonoffenders exhibited a normal adult profile. Another 40% of incest offenders exhibited nondiscriminating patterns. A subset of incest offenders and nonfamilial child molesters responded with arousal to both child and adult stimuli. Only 35% of child molesters showed a pure "child" profile (Barbaree and Marshall, 1989).

Plethysmography has proceeded on the assumption that deviant sexual interest can be inferred from higher degrees of arousal to deviant stimuli relative to arousal to appropriate stimuli (Abel *et al.*, 1977). Hall *et al.* (1988) found that some between-stimulus category correlations either approached or exceeded the correlations within stimulus conditions for a large sample of sex offenders. They concluded that, contrary to the notion of stimulus-specific responding, arousal among sexual offenders occurs in a generalized manner.

External Validity

In plethysmography, evidence of external validity relates to the ability of laboratory findings to predict external criteria, such as history of deviance or recidivism (Earls and Marshall, 1983; Farkas, 1978). This type of validity overlaps with discriminant validity, which is the focus of studies that compare sexually deviant subtypes and normals. The external validity of phallometric data is also relevant in demonstrating change maintenance for interventions that are designed to modify penile response patterns. External validity is essential to justify clinical uses of the plethysmograph.

Studies have reported weak to moderate correlations between phallometric indices and actual sexual behavior. For example, in a study with 155 male volunteers, Malamuth (1986) found a correlation of .43 between physiological arousal to depictions of rape and self-reported history of sexual aggression. Thus the phallometric rape index accounted for about 19% of the variance in the criterion. In a study of long-term treatment effectiveness reported by Marshall and Barbaree (1988), unofficial records were better predictors of child molesters' recidivism than were phallometric data. Phallometric data permit stronger conclusions concerning sexual preferences when considered along with other predictor variables (Malamuth, 1986).

Sample Selection

Selection is a threat to internal validity and also places constraints on generalizability (Cook and Campbell, 1979). As in any research paradigm, a data set reflects a given sample. Evidence of the diagnostic and prognostic value of phallometric data has in large part been based on convicted offenders, homosexuals, and transvestites (Earls and Marshall, 1983). The use of such groups prevents generalization to college samples and also to other forensic samples (e.g., alleged or undetected offenders). For example, Saunders and Awad (1988) noted a dearth of phallometric research with adolescent sex offenders.

Selection bias may also be related to the use of groups of subjects who may be differentially influenced by demand characteristics. Offenders may be motivated to exhibit normal sexual interests. Such motivations may not be operative among college samples. Little is known about potentially important differences among diverse samples in this and other respects or about the impact of selection on clinical and research data. Indeed, studies in this area have often provided insufficient detail concerning sample selection and subject characteristics. For example, Malcolm *et al.* (1985) cited unpublished selection criteria for research with sexually deviant subtypes. Comparative statements about groups and individuals require meaningful criteria and precise definition.

A related problem stems from the practice of combining various subtypes of sexual deviates into a single group. For example, Barbaree and Marshall (1988) conducted a recidivism study with nonfamilial child molesters who had offended against male and female. This study did not control for possible differences between homo- and heterosexual groups (see Groth and Birnbaum, 1978). The practice of combining deviant subtypes in a sample threatens external validity because it obscures differential treatment responses and reoffense patterns. Follow-up research cannot accurately represent the prognostic value of deviant arousal with respect to future functioning without recognizing the heterogeneity of sexual deviates both within and between broad diagnostic categories (Marshall and Barbaree, 1988; Quinsey *et al.*, 1979).

One other selection-related issue deserves mention. Laboratory research subjects who exhibit no arousal are often dropped from the sample. For example, in an early study on faking, Laws and Rubin (1969) dropped three of seven subjects. More recently, Barbaree and Marshall (1989) excluded 11 extrafamilial child molesters and 11 incest offenders from their original sample because these subjects did not show at least 20% of full erection to age-graded stimuli. The practice of excluding nonresponders compounds the bias associated with the use of heterogeneous opportunity samples and compromises both internal and external validity.

Procedural and Contextual Confounds

Whether deviant response patterns are observed is determined not only by the complex stimulus materials used to elicit arousal, but by a variety of environmental contingencies. Test results may be influenced by the clinician conducting the evaluation, the setting, instructional set, and the circumstances leading to assessment or treatment. In addition, the impact of situational variables is likely to be potentiated by a variety of individual differences variables. For example, some subjects may respond with arousal to certain stimuli only under certain circumstances; others may be much less influenced by situational factors. Little is known about the nature of such confounds or their effect on phallometric findings.

CONCLUSIONS AND RECOMMENDATIONS FOR FUTURE RESEARCH

This review has focused on theoretical and methodological issues relevant to the validity of plethysmography in the assessment and treatment of sexual deviance. These issues are difficult to resolve, but can be discussed constructively in terms of the directions they offer for future research in this area.

True conclusions may be derived from false premises, but valid deductions require a valid basis. The use of phallometric findings for important clinical and legal decisions and scientific inquiry should reflect a full appreciation of the measurement technique and the assumptions underlying its use. This becomes possible given adequate empirical support and clear explication of general principles.

The validity and clinical utility of plethysmography in the assessment and treatment of sexual deviance remain to be established. At the same time, basic questions relating to the significance of physiological aspects of the human sexual response must be addressed. Future work in this area should focus not only on the appropriateness of plethysmography in typical clinical and research applications with forensic populations but also should respond to the need for empirical and theoretical knowledge about human sexuality in general.

The relationship of physiological arousal to other dimensions of sexuality must be further clarified. This calls for a better understanding of the variables that affect phallometric findings. Failures of replication and discrimination in this area may reflect important differences between studies in terms of the apparatus used (volume vs. circumference transducers), test stimuli, administration and scoring techniques, and sample selection bias. The effects of relevant and extraneous sources of variation must be determined to provide a basis for the development of practical guidelines and minimal standards of technical adequacy for phallometric testing. But attention to methodological considerations alone cannot ensure the integrity and usefulness of a scientific paradigm. Theory and research must be mutually complementary. Thus the theoretical ideas upon which a paradigm is based must also be evaluated.

Crawford (1979) observed, "Although it is too simple to view sexual deviance as consisting only of sexual arousal to deviant stimuli, it would be premature to suggest that deviant arousal is irrelevant or unrelated to the problem" (p. 155). Likewise, if sexual deviates do not uniformly become aroused in the presence of deviant stimuli, this does not mean that they are not motivated by deviant sexual interests. Thus more precise inferences about individual differences in sexual preference require other levels of analysis. An integrated approach to the assessment of sexual preferences will take into account aspects of an individual's functioning other than those of a purely sexual nature, as well as dimensions of an individual's sexuality other than genital arousal.

REFERENCES

Abel, G. G., and Blanchard, D. H. (1976). The measurement and generation of sexual arousal in male sexual deviates. In Hersen, M., and Miller, P. (eds.), *Progress in Behavior Modification*, Vol. 2, Academic Press, New York.

Abel, G. G., Barlow, D. H., Blanchand, E. B., and Guild, D. (1977). The components of rapists' and sexual arousal. *Arch. Gen. Psychia.* 34: 895-903.

Abel, G. G., Blanchard, E. B., and Barlow, D. H. (1981). Measurement of sexual arousal in several paraphilias: the effects of stimulus modality, instructional set and stimulus content on the objective. *Behav. Res. Ther.* 19: 25-33.

Abel, G. G., Blanchard, E. B., Barlow, D. H., and Mavissakalian, M. (1975). Identifying specific erotic cues in sexual deviations by audiotaped descriptions. *J. Appl. Behav. Anal.* 8: 247-260.

Abel, G. G. Blanchard, E. B., Murphy, W. D., Becker, J. V., Djenderedian, A. (1981). Two methods of measuring penile responses. *Behav. Ther.* 12: 320-328.

American Psychiatric Association (1987). *Diagnostic and Statistical Manual of the Mental Disorders*, 3rd ed., rev., APA, Washington, DC.

Bancroft, J. (1970). A comparative study of aversion and desensitization in the treatment of homosexuality. In Burns, I. E., and Worsley, J. I. (eds.), *Behavior Therapy in the 1970's*, Wright, Bristol.

Bancroft, J. H. (1974). *Deviant Sexual Behavior: Modification and Assessment*, Clarendon, Oxford.

Bancroft, J. H., Jones, H. G., and Pullan, B. P. (1966). A simple transducer for measuring penile erection with comments on its use in the treatment of sexual disorder. *Behav. Res. Ther.* 4: 239-241.

Barbaree, H. E., and Marshall, W. I. (1988). Deviant sexual arousal, offense history, and demographic variables as predictors of reoffense among child molesters. *Behav. Sci. Law* 6: 267-280.

Barbaree, H. E., and Marshall, W. I. (1989). Erectile responses amongst heterosexual child molesters, father-daughter incest offenders and matched nonoffenders: Five distinct age preference profiles. *Can. J. Behav. Sci.* 21: 70-82.

Barbaree, H. E., Marshall, W. I., and Lanthier, R. (1979). Deviant sexual arousal in rapists. *Behav. Res. Ther.* 17: 215-222

Barlow, D. H., Becker, R., Leitenberg, H., and Agras, W. S. (1970). A mechanical strain gauge for recording penile circumference change. *J. Appl. Behav. Anal.* 3: 73-76.

Campbell, D. T. (1957). Factors relevant to the validity of experiments in social settings. *Psychol. Bull.* 54: 297-312.

Campbell, D. T.. (1969). Reforms as experiments. *Am. Psychol.* 24: 409-429.

Cook, T. D., and Campbell, D. T. (1979). *Quasi-Experimentation*, Houghton Mifflin, Boston.

Crawford, D. A. (1979). Modification of deviant sexual behavior: The need for a comprehensive approach. *Br. J. Med. Psych.* 52: 151-156.

Earls, C. M., and Marshall, W. I. (1983). The current state of technology in the laboratory assessment of sexual arousal patterns. In Greer, J. G., and Stuart, I. R. (eds.), *The Sexual Aggressor*, Van Nostrand, New York, pp. 336-362.

Earls, C. M., Quinsey, V. I., and Castonguay, G. (1987). A comparison of three methods of scoring penile circumference changes. *Arch. Sex. Behav.* 16: 493-500.

Eccles, A., Marshall, W. L., and Barbaree, H. E. (1988). The vulnerability of erectile measures to repeated assessments. *Behav. Res. Ther.* 26: 179-183.

Farkas, G. M. (1978). Comments on Levin *et al.*, and Rosen and Kopel: Internal and external validity issues. *J. Consult. Clin. Psychol.* 46: 1515-1516.

Farkas, G. M., Evans, I. M., Sine, I. F., Eifert, G., Wittlieb, and Vogelmann-Sine, S. (1979). Reliability and validity of the mercury-in-rubber strain gauge measure of penile circumference. *Behav. Ther.* 10: 555-560.

Freund, K. (1963). A laboratory method for diagnosing predominance of homo- or hetero-erotic interest in the male. *Behav. Res. Ther.* 1: 85-93.

Freund, K. (1972). A note on the use of the phallometric method of measuring mild sexual arousal in the male. *Behav. Ther.* 2: 226-228.

Freund, K., Chan, S., and Coulthart, R. (1979). Phallometric diagnosis with "nonadmitters." *Behav. Res. Ther.* 17: 451-457.

Freund, K., Langevin, R., and Barlow, D. (1974). A comparison of two penile measures of erotic arousal. *Behav. Res. Ther.* 12: 355-359.

Freund, K., McNight, C. K., Langevin, R., and Cibiri, S. (1972). The female as a surrogate object. *Arch. Sex. Behav.* 1: 119-133.

Freund, K., Scher, H., Racansky, I. G., Campbell, K., and Heasman, G. (1986). Males disposed to commit rape. *Arch. Sex. Behav.* 15: 23-35.

Freund, K., Watson, R., and Rienzo, D. (1988). Signs of feigning in the phallometric test. *Behav. Res. Ther.* 26: 105-112.

Fuller, A. K., Barnard, G., Robbins, L., and Spears, H. (1988). Sexual maturity for classification of phallometric stimulus slides. *Arch. Sex. Behav.* 17: 271-286.

Gabor, A. N. (1986). *The Prediction of Criminal Behavior*, University of Toronto Press, Toronto.

Groth, N. A., and Birnbaum, H. J. (1978). Adult sexual orientation and attraction to underage persons. *Arch. Sex. Behav.* 7: 175-181.

Hall, G. C. N., Proctor, W. C., and Nelson, G. M. (1988). The validity of physiological measures of pedophilic sexual arousal in a sexual offender population. *J. Consult. Clin. Psychol.* 56: 118-122.

Laws, D. R. (1977). A comparison of the measurement characteristics of two circumferential penile transducers. *Arch. Sex. Behav.* 6: 45-51.

Laws, D. R., and Osborn, C. A. (1983). How to build and operate a behavioral laboratory to evaluate and treat sexual deviance. In Greer, J. G., and Stuart, I. R. (eds.), *The Sexual Aggressor*, Van Nostrand, New York, pp. 293-335.
Laws, D. R., and Rubin, H. B. (1969). Instructional control of an autonomic response. *J. Appl. Behav. Anal.*, 2: 93-99.
Malamuth, N. M. (1986). Predictors of naturalistic aggression. *J. Pers. Soc. Psychol.* 50: 953-962.
Malamuth, N. M., Check, J. V. P., and Briere, J. (1986). Sexual arousal in response to aggression: Ideological, aggressive and sexual correlates. *J. Pers. Soc. Psychol.* 50: 330-340.
Malcolm, P. B., Davidson, P. R., and Marshall, W. L. (1985). Control of penile tumescence: The effects of arousal level and stimulus content. *Behav. Res. Ther.* 23: 273-280.
Marshall, W. L., and Barbaree, H. E. (1988). Long-term evaluation of a behavioral treatment program for child molesters. *Behav. Res. Ther.* 26: 499-511.
Masters, W. H., and Johnson, V. E. (1966). *Human Sexual Response*, Little, Brown, Boston.
Masters, W. H., and Johnson, V. E. (1970). *Human Sexual Inadequacy*, Little, Brown, Boston.
McConaghy, N. (1974). Measurements of changes in penile dimensions. *Arch. Sex. Behav.* 3: 381-388.
Meehl, P. E., and Rosen, A. (1955). Antecedent probability and the efficiency of psychometric signs, patterns, or cutting scores. *Psychol. Bull.* 52: 194-216.
O'Donohue, W. T., and Greer, J. H. (1985). The habituation of sexual arousal. *Arch. Sex. Behav.* 14: 233-246.
Quinsey, V. L. (1973). Methodological issues in evaluating the effectiveness of aversive therapies for institutionalized child molesters. *Can. Psychol. Rev.* 14: 350-361.
Quinsey, V. L., and Bergersen, S. G. (1976). Instructional control of penile circumference in assessments of sexual preference. *Behav. Ther.* 7: 489-493.
Quinsey, V. L., Chaplin, T. C., and Carrigan, W. F. (1979). Sexual preferences among incestuous and nonincestuous child molesters. *Behav. Ther.* 10: 562-565.
Quinsey, V. L., Chaplin, T. C., and Upfold, D. (1984). Sexual arousal to nonsexual violence and sadomasochistic themes among rapists and non-sex-offenders. *J. Consult. Clin. Psychol.* 52: 651-657.
Quinsey, V. L., Chaplin, T. C., and Varney, G. (1981). A comparison of rapists' and non-sex offenders' sexual preferences for mutually consenting sex, rape, and physical abuse of women. *Behav. Assess.* 3: 127-135.
Quinsey, V. I., and Marshall, W. I. (1983). Procedures for reducing inappropriate sexual arousal: An evaluation review. In Greer, J. G., and Stuart, I. R. (eds.), *The Sexual Aggressor*, Van Nostrand, New York, pp. 267-289.
Quinsey, V. L. Steinman, C. M., Bergerson, S. G., and Holmes, T. F. (1975). Penile circumference, skin conductance, and ranking responses of child molesters and "normals" to sexual and nonsexual stimuli. *Behav. Ther.* 6: 213-219.
Rorer, L. G., Hoffman, P. J., and Hsieh, K. C. (1966). Utilities as base-rate multipliers in the determination of optimum cutting scores for the discrimination of groups of unequal size and variance. *J. Appl. Psychol.* 50: 364-368.
Rosen, R. C., and Keefe, F. J. (1978). The measurement of human penile tumescence. *Psychophysiology* 15: 366-376.
Rosen, R. C., and Kopel, S. A. (1978). Role of penile tumescence measurement in the behavioral treatment of sexual deviation: Issues of validity. *Journal Consult. Clin. Psychol.* 46: 1519-1521.
Saunders, E. B., and Awad, G. A. (1988). Assessment, management, and treatment planning for male adolescent sexual offenders. *Am. J. Orthopsychiat.* 58: 571-579.
Schwartz, M. F., and Masters, W. H. (1983). Conceptual factors in the treatment of paraphilias: A preliminary report. *J. Sex Marital Ther.* 9: 3-18.
Smith, D., and Over, R. (1987). Male sexual arousal as a function of content and vividness of erotic fantasy. *Psychophysiology* 24: 334-339.
Wheeler, D., and Rubin, H. B. (1987). A comparison of volumetric and circumferential measures of penile erection. *Arch. Sex. Behav.* 16: 289-299.
Wormith, J. S. (1986). Assessing deviant sexual arousal: Physiological and cognitive aspects. *Adv. Behav. Res. Ther.* 8: 101-137.

Wydra, A., Marshall, W. L., Earls, C. M., and Barbaree, H. E. (1983). Identification of cues and control of sexual arousal by rapists. *Behav. Res. Ther.* 23: 273-280.
Zuckerman, M. (1971). Physiological measures of sexual arousal in the human. *Psychol. Bull.* 75: 297-327.

THE POLLS—A REPORT
AIDS

ELEANOR SINGER
THERESA F. ROGERS AND
MARY CORCORAN

In 1981, a new, mysterious, and deadly disease known as AIDS was identified. At present there is no cure for it and no vaccine to prevent its transmission. Efforts to control the spread of AIDS are hampered by the long latency between infection and symptoms (an average of at least four years) and by the fact that once an individual is exposed to the virus presumed to cause AIDS, he or she can infect others without knowing it. The disease has been termed a pandemic; by 1986, 1.5 to 2 million people in the United States were believed to have been exposed to it.

To the best of our knowledge, the first survey of public opinion about AIDS was carried out in June 1983. Between then and November 1986, the cutoff date for this article, we identified 22 surveys on this topic. Four were carried out in 1983, nine in 1985, and another nine in 1986. Almost all have been nationwide, and they represent more than 200 questions that the public has answered about AIDS—what they know about the disease, how vulnerable they think they are, what they think the government should do, and what, if anything, they are doing to protect themselves. These data provide the best gauge we have of the public's knowledge about and reaction to AIDS and how their concerns and views may be changing.

In selecting questions for this article, our main criterion was the availability of trend data. In some cases, however, we have reported responses to items for which there are as yet no trends, because we believe they are likely to be asked again in the future.

We have organized this summary of the poll results in terms of six dimensions: awareness of the disease, concern about it both as a seri-

ELEANOR SINGER is a Senior Research Scholar at the Center for the Social Sciences. THERESA ROGERS is a Senior Research Scholar at the Graduate School of Business, and MARY CORCORAN is a graduate student in the Department of Sociology, Columbia University. The authors are grateful for the assistance of the Gannett Center for Media Studies at Columbia University, where the first author was a resident senior fellow during the preparation of this article.

Public Opinion Quarterly Volume 51:580–595 © 1987 by the American Association for Public Opinion Research
Published by The University of Chicago Press / 0033-362X/87/0051-04(1)/$2.50

ous medical problem in general and as a problem for one's own health, perceptions about the likelihood of its spread, beliefs about methods of transmission, attitudes toward measures for protecting the public, and reported changes in one's own behavior to avoid exposure.

Between June 1983 and August 1986, the percentage of the population who said that they had heard or read about AIDS increased from 77% to 99%. There are now virtually no differences among demographic categories in the percentage of those aware of AIDS. During the same period of time, the percentage who personally knew someone with AIDS increased only from 3% to 6%, though in cities with a high concentration of AIDS cases, the percentage was much higher. In New York City, for example, it was 16% in September 1985.

Media coverage appears to have obliterated the "awareness gap" between population subgroups, but other gaps in knowledge still exist. For example, those with the least amount of education are least likely to be well informed about methods of transmission. And those with less accurate knowledge about how AIDS can be transmitted are much more likely to express concern that they or someone they know will get AIDS, to say that they or someone they know avoids places frequented by homosexuals, and to favor government regulations, including quarantine for people with AIDS.

At the same time, those who are realistically at greater risk are also most likely to express concern about AIDS. Young people—those under thirty, single people, those living in urban areas in which a high number of cases has been identified, and blacks all express greater than average concern about contracting AIDS. They are also more likely to say they have changed their behavior, including sexual behavior, in order to avoid exposure to AIDS. Because of the lack of space, we have not shown these demographic breaks, but they are consistent across all surveys for which we have seen the data.

So far as the spread of AIDS is concerned, the data summarized below indicate no trend of increasing concern about AIDS as a problem for one's own health. But some (though not all) questions indicate increasing concern about the spread of AIDS beyond present at-risk groups to the general population.

The data on beliefs about transmission indicate widespread accuracy at the extremes, with some confusion about intermediate modes. For example, virtually everyone knows that AIDS can be transmitted by sexual contact, both homosexual and heterosexual, and by blood transfusions. At the other extreme, virtually no one believes that it can be contracted by being in the same room as someone who has AIDS. But with respect to kissing, sharing a drinking glass, and eating food prepared by someone who has AIDS, public opinion is divided. Substantial minorities express the belief that AIDS can be transmitted in these ways even though public health experts insist that it cannot. And as of late 1986 there did not appear to have been any increase in accuracy over time.

The evidence is mixed with regard to attitudes toward regulation. On some matters, such as fighting to have a child with AIDS removed from school, the percentage saying they would fight has decreased over time. On other matters, such as taking school employees with AIDS off the job, the percentage saying employees should be removed has increased. And on still other matters, such as favoring quarantine for those infected with AIDS, there appears to have been no change in aggregate opinion over time.

There is a slight increase in the number of those reporting that they are changing their behavior as a result of AIDS. Gallup, for example, finds a small but steady increase in the percentage saying that they or people they know avoid homosexuals, stay away from places where homosexuals may be present, and refuse elective surgery that would require blood transfusions. (Another behavioral indicator, not reflected in these opinion data, is the increasing recommendation of some doctors that patients donate their own blood prior to surgery.)

The data also provide evidence that the public credits the media as being an important source of information about AIDS. In response to questions by the *Los Angeles Times* (December 1985), 25% of the public said that they had been "paying most attention recently" to stories about AIDS in the media, and this figure was higher than that for any of the other seven topics they were asked about, including hijackings and the budget deficit. In fact, 72% reported hearing about or reading three or more stories about AIDS "in the last seven days." In the last half of 1985, a time when eight of the surveys whose findings are summarized here were conducted, the evening newscasts of the major networks were carrying an average of almost twenty stories per month on AIDS.[1]

One cannot, of course, say that the public's answers to poll questions mirror what the media have reported. The public remembers some things and not others, and they add to and subtract from what they have heard or read. At the same time, different media build up some stories and downplay or ignore others. Despite all of this selectivity and distortion, the poll data reveal that the general population is aware of AIDS and has some basic knowledge about how the disease spreads. In addition, those realistically at greater risk are the ones most likely to say that they are concerned about contracting the disease. There is variation from survey to survey in question wording and in the number and type of response categories, but, on balance, we see more

[1]As compiled from *Television and Abstracts: A Guide to the Videotape Collection of the Network Evening News Programs* in the Vanderbilt Television Archives. There was some variation among the three networks, but not a great deal.

agreement than disagreement across surveys in the public's answers.

Because information and education are the only means now available to control the spread of AIDS, the poll results are of interest to the public health community. From this standpoint, they provide good information about the public's awareness and level of knowledge. But the data are of limited utility in one important way: they are less informative than they might be about changes in behavior to avoid exposure to the AIDS virus. Only seven of the surveys asked specific questions about precautionary measures, if any, that the respondent was taking. The lack of such items and the paucity of trend data in this area are a weakness.

The poll results reported here were obtained from published and unpublished sources, the Roper Center, survey organizations, ABC, CBS, and NBC, *Newsweek*, and the *Los Angeles Times*. With the exception of two New York City surveys (ABC/DN 9/85 and Gallup 6/85), all surveys are based on nationwide samples. The sample sizes are at least 1,000 for all but the following six surveys:

Gallup	7/1983	$N = 767$
Gallup	8/1985	$N = 759$
Gallup	11/1986	$N = 756$
ABC/*New York Daily News*	9/1985	$N = 505$
CBS/*New York Times*	9/1985	$N = 762$
CBS	10/1986	$N = 823$

Responses totaling less than 0.5% have not been shown in the tabulations.

We wish to thank the organizations that shared unpublished data with us for this article. Further information about the surveys can be obtained from the appropriate organization.

ABC/DN—American Broadcasting Company/*New York Daily News*
ABC/WP—American Broadcasting Company/*Washington Post*
CBS—Columbia Broadcasting System
CBS/NYT—Columbia Broadcasting System/*New York Times*
Gallup—The Gallup Organization
Harris—Louis Harris and Associates
LAT—*Los Angeles Times*
NBC/WSJ—National Broadcasting Company/*Wall Street Journal*
Roper—The Roper Organization
YCS—Yankelovich, Clancy, and Shulman

Suggested References

Bayer, Ronald, Daniel M. Fox, and David P. Willis, guest eds. (1986)
The Public Context of an Epidemic. The Milbank Quarterly 64, supplement 1, pp. 1–182.

Bayer, Ronald, and Robert Hummel, eds. (1986)
AIDS and Public Policy Journal 1(1).

Feldman, Douglas A., and M. Johnson, eds. (1986)
The Social Dimensions of AIDS. New York: Praeger.
Institute of Medicine, National Academy of Sciences (1986)
Confronting AIDS: Directions for Public Health, Health Care, and Research. Washington: National Academy Press.
Siegel, Karolyn, guest ed. (1986)
"AIDS education: The public health challenge." Health Education Quarterly 13:285–427.

Contact: Direct and Indirect

Roper: Have you heard about the disease called AIDS that attacks a person's disease immunity system and is frequently fatal?

	8/83	*8/85*	*8/86*
Yes	91%	97%	99%
No	8	2	1
DK	1	1	1

Gallup: Have you heard or read about a disease called AIDS—acquired immune deficiency syndrome?

	6/83	*7/83*	*6/85*	*3/86*
Yes	77%	91%	95%	98%
No	23	9	5	2

ABC/WP, ABC/DN, CBS/NYT, LAT, CBS, Gallup: Do you personally know anyone who has AIDS?

	ABC/WP[a] *6/83*	Gallup[b] *8/85*	*ABC/WP*[c] *9/85*	*ABC/DN*[c] *9/85*	*CBS/NYT* *9/85*	*LAT*[d] *12/85*	*CBS* *10/86*	*Gallup* *11/86*
Yes	3%	4%	6%	16%	2%	5%	5%	6%
No	97	96	94	84	98	94	94	94
DK/No op.	—	—	—	1	—	1	1	—

[a] Do you know anyone who suffers from AIDS?
[b] Do you personally know anyone who has contracted the disease called AIDS?
[c] Do you personally know anyone, either living or dead, who contracted AIDS?
[d] Do you personally know anyone who has tested positive for AIDS, or has contracted AIDS? By "know," I mean someone who you would speak with at least once a month on the phone or in person.

Concern About AIDS as a Serious Medical Problem and Problem for Own Health

CBS/NYT, CBS: Think about some serious diseases or medical problems facing the country today. Which two or three do you think are the most serious?*

	CBS/NYT *9/85*	*CBS* *10/86*
Cancer	74%	75%
AIDS	51	55
Heart disease	41	38
Substance abuse	2	6
VD/Herpes	5	4
Diabetes	5	4

* Only the most frequently mentioned diseases are shown here. Multiple answers were allowed.

CBS/NYT, LAT, CBS: Now think about *your own* situation. Which two or three diseases or medical problems are *you* most concerned about getting?*

	*CBS/NYT***	*LAT****	*CBS***
	9/85	*12/85*	*10/86*
Cancer	59%	56%	64%
Heart disease	31	11	31
AIDS	13	12	12
VD/herpes	—	—	—
Diabetes	5	3	6

* Only the most frequently mentioned diseases are shown here.
** Multiple answers were allowed.
*** Alternatives were enumerated for respondents; only one response was allowed.

LAT: 12/85: What do you think is the most important problem facing this country today: crime, or AIDS, or government spending, or inflation, or the moral decline of society, or unemployment, or the possibility of war, or what?

	Knowledge of AIDS		*Fear of AIDS*		
	High	*Low*	*High*	*Low*	*All**
Crime	14%	18%	17%	15%	26%
Education	11	9	9	10	16
AIDS	5	5	9	4	8
Budget	19	18	15	20	30
Inflation	8	8	10	9	14
Morals	10	10	7	11	17
Unemployment	13	14	16	12	23
War	14	10	12	12	20
Others	5	5	3	6	8
Not sure	1	3	1	1	2
Refused	0	0	1	0	0

* Up to two responses were recorded for each respondent. Subgroup percentages are for most important problem only.

Gallup: Are there any new public health problems which especially concern you?

	7/83	*8/85*
Yes	41%	44%
No	58	55
DK	1	1
If yes, which ones?*		
AIDS	24	32
Herpes	14	4
Pollution/toxic waste	1	2
Other	13	12
DK	1	1

* Alternatives not enumerated for respondents; more than one response allowed.

NBC: How concerned are you about AIDS as a problem to your own health? Would you say you are very concerned, somewhat concerned, or not at all concerned?

	11/85	1/86*
Very concerned	27%	26%
Somewhat concerned	32	35
Not at all concerned	40	38
Not sure	1	1

* No difference by whether or not respondent has homosexual friends.

Concern About Spread

Gallup: Lately there has been some discussion in the news about the disease called AIDS. How worried are you that you or someone you know will get AIDS?

	8/85	*11/86*
Very	14%	19%
A little	27	25
Not very	27	25
Not at all	31	30
DK	1	1

ABC/WP, ABC/DN, CBS/NYT, Harris, CBS: Are you afraid that you might get AIDS?

	ABC/WP[a] *9/85*	*ABC/DN*[a] *9/85*	*CBS/NYT* *9/85*	*Harris*[b] *11/85*	*CBS* *10/86*
Yes	26%	42%	17%	10%	15%
No	73	57	79	87	83
DK/no opinion	1	1	4	3	2

[a] Are you afraid that you might pick up the AIDS virus yourself or aren't you afraid of that?

[b] Do you think that *you* run any risk of catching AIDS, or not?

CBS/NYT, NBC: So far, most of the people with AIDS have been homosexual men and intravenous drug users. Do you think AIDS will spread beyond those groups who already get it so that many people in the rest of the population will get AIDS, or don't you think so?

	CBS/NYT *9/85*	*NBC*[a] *1/86*
Yes, will spread	61%	76%
No	20	15
Depends (vol.)	7	—
DK	12	9

[a] As of now, most of the people with AIDS in the U.S. are homosexual men and intravenous drug users. Do you think AIDS will spread beyond these groups so that other people in the country will get AIDS, or don't you think so?

ABC/WP, ABC/DN: So far three-quarters of AIDS victims have been homosexual males. The rest of the victims have mainly been drug addicts or recipients of blood transfusions. Do you think that AIDS is spreading so that it is now a threat to the general public in the U.S. or not?

	ABC/WP	*ABC/DN*
	9/85	*9/85*
Yes	79%	79%
No	18	17
DK	4	4

Gallup: At the moment, cases of AIDS are largely confined to homosexuals, hemophiliacs, other people receiving blood transfusions, and intravenous drug takers. How likely do you think it is that AIDS will eventually become an epidemic for the public at large?

	8/85	*11/86*[a]
Very likely	27%	36%
Somewhat	35	37
Not too likely	26	18
Not at all	7	5
DK	5	4

[a] How likely do you think it is that AIDS will eventually become an epidemic for the public at large?

ABC/WP: To the best of your knowledge, is the number of diagnosed cases of AIDS in the U.S. closer to a million or closer to 10,000?

	9/85
Closer to a million	29%
Closer to 10,000	63
DK/no opinion	8

LAT: From what you have heard and read, how many people in the United States have been exposed to the AIDS virus and will therefore test positive for the presence of AIDS antibodies? Just your best guess.

	12/85
To 2m	49%
To 26m	12
To 50m	4
To 74m	2
To 98m	1
To 122m	2
To 146m	1
To 170m	0
To 194m	0
To 218m	0
To 240m	1
Refused	28

Methods of Transmission

I'm going to read you a list. For each item, please tell me if you think that it is or is not a way for someone to catch AIDS from someone who has it. Can you catch AIDS from:

(The introduction and precise wording of the mode of transmission varies slightly from survey to survey.)

	Gallup 7/83	*ABC/ WP 9/85*	*ABC/ DN 9/85*	*CBS/ NYT 9/85*	*NBC 11/85*	*LAT 12/85*	*NBC 1/86*	*Gallup 4/86*	*CBS 10/86*	*Gallup 11/86*	
Casual contact											
Yes	25%							6%[a]		17%[b]	
No	59							81		78	
DK	16							13		5	
Intimate sexual contact (having sex)											
Yes		95%	95%	91%			63%*		93%	79%[c]	91%[d]
No		2	3	2			25		1	10	3
DK		4	2	7			12		6	11	6
Blood transfusion											
Yes		95%	97%	95%			55%*				
No		2	2	1			33				
DK		2	2	4			12				
Sharing (using) intravenous (hypodermic) needles											
Yes		92%	95%	91%							
No		3	3	2							
DK		5	3	7							
Kissing											
Yes		50%	56%	32%					29%		
No		36	28	42					51		
DK		14	16	26					20		
Using same drinking glass											
Yes		28%	38%	47%	33%		38%		36%		
No		55	45	34	44		45		43		
DK		16	17	19	23		17		21		
Being sneezed on											
Yes		22%	33%				32%				
No		62	50				53				
DK		16	17				15				
Sitting on a toilet seat											
Yes		16%	26%	28%		24%			23%		
No		69	60	49		63			57		
DK		15	14	23		13			20		
Shaking hands (being touched)											
Yes		7%	7%	11%							
No		85	86	73							
DK		9	7	16							
Working (being) in the same office (room) with someone who has AIDS											
Yes				12%	5%				6%		
No				70	84				81		
DK				18	11				13		
Donating blood											
Yes							33%				
No							63				
DK							4				
Food handling or preparation											
Yes					29%	19%	31%*				
No					47	65	55				
DK					24	16	14				

* Asked only of those who think it will spread. Percentages have been converted to total sample.

[a] Do you believe a person can get AIDS by being in a crowded place with someone who has it?

[b] Casual contact, such as sharing a water glass, shaking hands, or riding in the same elevator with a person who has AIDS.

[c] Heterosexual contact with a person whose blood has tested positive for AIDS.

[d] Heterosexual contact with a person who has an active case of AIDS.

ABC/WP, ABC/DN: Assuming there is no intimate physical contact, do you think it is safe or unsafe to associate with someone who has AIDS?

	ABC/WP	*ABC/DN*
	9/85	*9/85*
Yes, safe	57%	46%
No, unsafe	36	44
DK	7	10

Gallup: I am going to read you some statements about AIDS. For each, please tell me if you think the statement is probably true or if you think it is probably false? Think it is probably true that:

		(NYC)
	6/85	*6/85*
Some people can get AIDS when they receive blood transfusions	92%	90%
Drug users who share needles have a high risk of getting AIDS	84	86
Most people who have AIDS are homosexual men	80	73
Some wives and girlfriends of drug users have gotten AIDS	68	71
There is a great danger that AIDS will soon spread to all kinds of people in our country	66	69
You can get AIDS by being in a crowded place with someone who has it	9	15

LAT, CBS: There is a test to determine whether or not a person has the AIDS virus. As far as you know, does everyone with a positive test for the AIDS virus get AIDS, or not?

	LAT[a]	*CBS*
	12/85	*10/86*
Yes	28%	10%
No	29	54
DK/no opinion	42	36
Refused	1	—

[a] Medical researchers have discovered a virus that is closely linked with AIDS, called HTLV Three. Like all viruses, this one causes the body's immune system to manufacture antibodies which fight the virus. From what you have heard or read, is it your impression that a person who tests positive to these antibodies will probably get AIDS?

Gallup: Next I have some questions about screening tests for AIDS. As far as you know, when someone without any AIDS symptoms tests positive for AIDS virus antibodies in the blood, does this mean the person . . .

	11/86
Has been exposed to the virus, but is not necessarily infectious to others or likely to develop the disease?	37%
Is infectious to others and may develop the disease?	29
Is infectious to others and is certain to develop the disease?	11
DK	23

Protective Measures: Regulation of Others

WORK

NBC: Do you think employers should be able to fire someone who has been diagnosed as having AIDS, or not?

	11/85
Yes	19%
No	64
DK/not sure/no opinion	17

NBC: Do you think people who have been diagnosed as having AIDS should be allowed to continue to work as long as they are able to, or don't you think so?

	11/85
Yes	67%
No	18
DK/not sure/no opinion	15

CBS: Should there be a law restricting where people with the AIDS virus can work, even though public health officials don't think that would control the spread of AIDS?

	10/86
Yes	28%
No	59
DK/not sure/no opinion	13

SCHOOL

ABC/WP, ABC/DN, CBS/NYT, CBS: Do you favor or oppose allowing students with AIDS to attend school if health officials say there is no danger?

	ABC/WP	*ABC/DN*[a]	*CBS/NYT*[b]	*CBS*[b]
	9/85	*9/85*	*9/85*	*10/86*
Favor	62%	39%	40%	56%
Oppose	31	55	27	17
DK/no opinion	7	6	17	15
Depends (volunteered)	—	—	16	12

[a] Recently, New York City public school officials allowed a 7-year-old child with AIDS to attend class in Queens. Do you favor or oppose . . . ?
[b] Should children who have AIDS be allowed to go to school, or not?

ABC/WP, ABC/DN, Gallup: If you thought a child with AIDS might be in your children's school, would you keep your children home or would you send them to school?

	ABC/WP	*ABC/DN*[a]	*Gallup*[b]
	9/85	*9/85*	*3/86*
Keep home	26%	48%	24%
Send to school	68	46	67
DK/no opinion	6	6	9

[a] Many parents in Queens protested allowing the child with AIDS to attend school by keeping their own children home. If you thought a child with AIDS might be in your children's school, would you keep your children home or would you send them to school?

[b] A 14-year-old Indiana boy who contracted AIDS through a contaminated blood transfusion was banned from attending school classes. After a county medical officer ruled that he posed no health threat to his classmates, he went back to school, but the parents of almost half the students at his school kept their children home. If you had children of this age, would you permit them to attend classes with a child who had AIDS, or not?

Gallup: If you learned that a child with AIDS was attending the same school as a child of yours, would you:

	8/85	*11/86*
Fight to have the AIDS child removed from school?	17%	10%
Keep your child at home?	8	7
Instruct your child not to have contact with the AIDS child?	25	27
Not worry about children passing AIDS to one another?	30	44
Don't know	20	12

ABC/WP, ABC/DN: School officials should tell parents if a child with AIDS is attending their child's school. Do you agree or disagree?

	ABC/WP	*ABC/DN*
	9/85	*9/85*
Agree	78%	79%
Disagree	19	18
DK/no opinion	3	3

Public school employees found to have AIDS should be taken off the job.

Agree	47%	66%
Disagree	45	26
DK/no opinion	8	9

HOUSING

ABC/WP, ABC/DN: If it was proposed that an AIDS patient treatment and housing center be located in your neighborhood, would that upset you a great deal, only somewhat, very little, or not at all?

	ABC/WP	*ABC/DN*
	9/85	*9/85*
A great deal	17%	19%
Only somewhat	27	28
Very little	23	20
Not at all	30	31
DK/no opinion	1	2

QUARANTINE

ABC/WP, ABC/DN, LAT, NBC: People with AIDS should be put into quarantine in special places to keep them away from the general public.

	ABC/WP	*ABC/DN*	*LAT*[a]	*NBC*[b]
	9/85	*9/85*	*12/85*	*1/86*
Agree	28%	42%	51%	31%
Disagree	65	48	40	57
DK/no opinion	7	10	9	12

[a] Would you favor or oppose adding "AIDS" to the list of diseases that must be quarantined?

[b] Do you think that people who are known carriers of AIDS should be separated from the rest of the population, or don't you think so?

REGULATION OF SEXUAL ACTIVITIES

NBC: Do you think governmental restrictions should be placed on the sexual activities of people who are known carriers of AIDS, or don't you think so?

	11/85	*1/86*
Yes	58%	51%
No	31	41
DK/no opinion	11	8

YCS: There should be no laws, either federal or state, regulating sexual practices—that's up to the individual to decide for himself or herself.

	1977	*7/86*
Agree strongly	45%	44%
Agree partially	25	25
Disagree	26	27
Not sure	4	4

TESTING

NBC, CBS: Do you think the U.S military should test its personnel to see if they have been exposed to AIDS, or not?

	NBC	*CBS*[a]
	11/85	*10/86*
Yes	78%	72%
No	16	21
DK/no opinion	6	7

[a] Do you think that testing for the AIDS virus should be required for people beginning military service, or don't you think so?

NBC: Do you think employers should test their employees to see if they have been exposed to the AIDS virus, or not?

	11/85
Yes	39%*
No	45
DK/no opinion	16

* Currently employed: 34%.

CBS: Would you favor a national policy that requires workers in general to be tested for the AIDS virus, or would that be an unfair invasion of privacy?

	10/86
Yes, favor	36%
No	53
Depends (vol.)	6
No opinion	5

CBS: Do you think insurance companies should be permitted to require people in groups with a high risk of getting AIDS to be tested for the AIDS virus before giving them insurance coverage, or is that unfair to people in these groups?

	10/86
Yes	40%
No	50
No opinion	10

EDUCATION

YCS: At what age do you think that children should *first* be taught about AIDS in school?*

	11/86
By the age of 8	23%
When 9 or 10	27
When 11 or 12	25
When 13 or 14	17
Or older than this	5
Not sure	3

Do you think that sex education courses for children who are eight should include information about:

	*Yes***	*No*	*Not Sure*
The dangers of AIDS	38%	56%	6%

Do you think that sex education courses for children who are twelve should include information about:

	*Yes***	*No*	*Not Sure*
The dangers of AIDS	93%	6%	1%

* Among those who agree that children should be taught about AIDS in school—83% of sample.

** Among those who think that sex education courses should be taught in school—86% of sample.

Gallup: Some people feel that an important way to combat AIDS is to provide more education in grade school about sex and sexually transmitted diseases, including the use of condoms, before students become sexually active. Others feel that this kind of education does more harm than good. Which comes closer to your view?

	11/86
More sex education	70%
Does more harm than good	25
DK	5

Protective Measures: Behavior Change

ABC/DN, ABC/WP, CBS/NYT, Harris, NBC, CBS: Is there anything in particular you have done to avoid getting AIDS?

	ABC/DN[a] 9/85	*ABC/WP*[a] 9/85	*CBS/NYT* 9/85	*Harris**[b] 11/85	*NBC**[c] 11/85	*NBC*[d] 1/86	*CBS* 10/86	*CBS*[e] 10/86
Yes	35%	22%	13%	41%	11%	7%	18%	11%
No	65	77	85	57	88	93	80	86
DK	—	1	2	2	1	—	2	3

* No follow-up questions asked

[a] Is there anything you yourself are doing to avoid exposing yourself to AIDS?

[b] Do you take any special steps or precautions to avoid catching AIDS, or not?

[c] Has public concern about AIDS caused you to change any part of your daily routine?

[d] Since you became aware of AIDS, have you changed your sexual behavior in any way?

[e] How about you personally? Have you changed your sexual habits because you are worried about getting AIDS?

If yes, what have you done?

	ABC/DN[a] 9/85	*ABC/WP*[a] 9/85	*CBS/NYT*[b] 9/85	*NBC*[c] 1/86	*CBS*[b] 10/86	*CBS*[b] 10/86
Limit number of partners	8%	6%	—	92%	—	—
Sex with one partner	8	10	—	—	3%	2%
Avoid homosexual acts/sex	—	—	1%	—	1	—
Cut down on sex	11	11	—	—	—	—
No sex	2	2	3	—	1	—
Use/partner use condom	2	2	—	49	—	—
Avoid homosexuals	13	17	1	—	—	—
Avoid people with AIDS	—	6	—	—	—	—
Avoid prostitutes	—	1	—	—	—	—
Socially careful	—	14	2	—	2	—
Careful who/what touch	—	—	1	—	3	—
Avoid needle drugs	—	6	—	—	—	—
Keep clean	—	5	1	—	3	—
Clean home/office more	—	1	—	—	—	—
Change public places I go	—	1	—	—	—	—
Avoid/more careful using public restrooms, etc.	—	25	1	—	—	—
Avoid/more careful using gyms, public pools, etc.	—	3	—	—	—	—
Use restrooms less	—	4	—	—	—	—
Avoid blood transfusions	—	11	1	—	1	—
Cut down/not giving blood	—	3	—	—	—	—
More careful/more careful selecting sexual partner	—	—	—	95	—	7
Other	77	12	—	—	4	1
No opinion	—	3	2	—	—	1

[a] More than one response allowed. Percentages are of those saying yes.

[b] Only one response coded. Percentages sum to those saying yes.

[c] Respondents were specifically asked if they had done these three behaviors. Percentages are of those saying yes, they had done.

Gallup: Have you personally or have people that you know taken any of the following precautions to try to reduce the chances of contracting AIDS?

		7/83[a]	*8/85*	*11/86*
Avoiding people you know or suspect to be homosexuals?	Yes		13%	18%
	No		77	72
	DK		10	10
Refusing elective surgery that would require blood transfusions?	Yes		21	27
	No		70	65
	DK		9	8
Taking any other precautions?	Yes		6	
	No		87	
	DK		7	
Using a condom?*	Yes			32
	No			55
	DK			13
Taking more care in choice of sex partners?*	Yes			58
	No			34
	DK			8
Avoiding certain places where homosexuals may be present?	Yes	21%	28	33
	No	67	65	55
	DK	12	7	8

* No trend information.

[a] Are you or other people in your community taking extra steps to avoid being in places where homosexuals are likely to be, or not?

Journal of Studies on Alcohol, Vol. 38, No. 11, 1977

Counseling Homosexual Alcoholics

Ten Case Histories

Edward J. Small, Jr.[1] and Barry Leach, Ph.D.[2]

SUMMARY. *The case histories of 10 male homosexual alcoholics are presented, and psychoanalytic theories about the link between homosexuality and alcoholism are reviewed.*

TWO MODERN STUDIES of homosexual men, discussed below, suggest a high incidence of alcoholism in that population. Our own clinical experience, moreover, is that almost one-third of the men seeking counseling or treatment for alcoholism are concerned about homosexuality.

For at least two reasons, it seems likely that an increasing number of problem drinkers seeking help in the future will identify themselves as homosexuals: growth of the "Gay Liberation" movement (1), and the American Psychiatric Association's removal of homosexuality from its official list of mental illnesses.

The case sketches that follow suggest that homosexuality and alcoholism in men are probably independent states, and that homosexuality need not be an obstacle to therapy or recovery from alcoholism under certain conditions.

Homosexuality has been linked to alcoholism or inebriety in theoretical formulations in the psychiatric and psychological literature for decades (2–6). Some of Freud's reinterpreters, linking oral tendencies to homosexuality, proposed that the etiology of alcoholism is homosexuality. Ferenczi (7, 8) and Knight (9) saw in compulsive drinking an attempt to allay anxiety over masculine inadequacy, resulting from an overindulgent mother, traumatic weaning, the father's emotional coldness, and envy of the father's penis. Bergler (10) offered a similar formulation, noting that an

[1] 99 East Fourth St., New York, NY 10003.
[2] 100 Bank St., New York, NY 10014.
Received for publication: 22 February 1974. Revision: 2 March 1977.

alcoholic's homosexuality is latent. Abraham[3] held that oral frustration resulted in overidentification with the father, amounting to latent homosexuality, and that alcoholics could express their "deviant" urges under the influence of alcohol within the "male" camaraderie of the saloon. Radó (12) declared homosexuality an irrational fear of being heterosexual, presumably dissolved by alcohol. In her extensive review of psychoanalytic views of alcoholism Blum (13) described love relationships established by an alcoholic as "supporting evidence for an oral fixation or regression," but also noted that fixation at the anal stage often results in "love for others, albeit of the same sex."

From many such formulations, it might be inferred that overt homosexuality averts alcoholism, or that no one can manifest both alcoholism and overt homosexuality. The emphasis on orality seems to define homosexuality almost exclusively as a drive to perform fellatio; none of the theories account for the frequency of manual masturbation, anal intercourse, flagellation or any other homosexual (and heterosexual) practices, not to mention observable enduring marriage-type or love relations between homosexuals. Psychoanalytic assertions do not constitute hard evidence, of course, nor do they account for all homosexuals, repressed or overt, who do not become alcoholics, for all women homosexuals, for all women alcoholics, for all heterosexual alcoholics, or for all "gay" male alcoholics who drink outside saloons.

As Saghir and Robbins (14), Madsen (15), and Weinberg and Williams (1) have noted, years of research have not led to agreement on either the definition or the etiology of homosexuality, or even whether there is indeed one such condition, personality type, or pattern of behavior which can be clearly delineated. Nevertheless, some investigators have tried to determine in small samples whether there is an association between alcoholism and what they consider homosexuality.

Landis (16) compared the personalities of 29 drinking and 25 remitted alcoholics and 21 nonalcoholic controls and found no relationships between homoeroticism and alcoholism; nor could Quaranta (17) find such a tie. Machover et al. (18) reported finding what they judged to be homosexual "trends" more in evidence among 29 drinking alcoholics, but did not find the tendencies more prevalent among men alcoholics than among nonalcoholic, pre-

[3] Cited in Fenichel (11).

sumed nonhomosexual, controls. McCord and McCord (19), in their longitudinal retrospective study of alcoholics, found that "overtly homosexual" pubescent boys ($N = 6$) were slightly more likely to become alcoholics than "feminine" boys (those who played with dolls, expressed the wish to be girls, or wore some feminine clothes), contradicting the pseudo-Freudian contention that latent homosexuals have greater vulnerability to alcoholism than overt ones. The McCords concluded that their research "does not support the belief that alcoholics have latently homosexual personalities" (19, *p. 32*). Prout et al. (20) found homosexuality in only 4 of 100 hospitalized men alcoholics. Botwinick and Machover (21), having searched for homosexuality, latent or patent, in alcoholics, concluded that "homosexuality cannot be an essential factor in alcoholism" (*p. 272*).

Gibbins and Walters (22) tested the psychoanalytic theory that alcoholism is linked to repressed or latent homosexuality, using three perceptual defense experiments on 179 men subjects, of whom 36 were manifest homosexuals ("arrested for homosexual offenses") and 43 were patients in an alcoholism clinic. The 100 controls, presumably neither alcoholic nor prealcoholic, neither overtly nor covertly homosexual, were men who regularly attended YMCA (Young Men's Christian Association) functions. Results of the first two experiments did not afford unequivocal support for the tested theory, the authors reported, and in the third, "responses of alcoholics were intermediate between those of homosexuals and normal subjects" (*p. 640*).

So, although sexual identity (not homosexuality *qua* homosexuality) can undoubtedly be a problem for some alcoholics as for some nonalcoholics, there is no clear evidence that alcoholism is caused by homosexuality. Factors which produce one may also sometimes produce the other, but evidence for this is also lacking. The only link or relationship between alcoholism and homosexuality may be their occasional occurrence within the same individual.

Nevertheless, two recent studies suggest there may be a relatively high incidence of drinking-related problems among men homosexuals. Although Barr et al. (23) concluded that recent evidence from studies of homosexuals who are not psychiatric patients suggests that homosexuals are not more neurotic than comparable heterosexuals they found problem drinking among 30% of their homosexual population and in only 20% of the heterosexual controls. Weinberg and Williams (1) studied 2497 male homosexuals (1117 in the United States, 1077 in the Netherlands, and 303 in Denmark) and found no differences in psychological problems between the homosexual and general population samples; they concluded that sexual orientation is not necessarily correlated with psychological problems. But they also noted that 29.4% of their homosexual sample reported "drinking more than they should," i.e., nearly "all the time"; another 31.3%, "pretty often"; and 30.4% reported frequenting a "gay" bar once or more a week. Other Weinberg and Williams findings could also correlate with drinking problems, although no direct relationship is shown. For example, subjects reporting seeing a psychiatrist, suffering from tremors, dizziness, nightmares, sweaty hands, guilt, depression, loneliness, job dissatisfaction and job changes could be revealing alcoholism.

The following case histories are believed to typify the coincidental occurrence of homosexuality in men in contemporary American culture. They appear to illustrate the hypothesis that the two conditions are most likely to coexist circumstantially rather than causatively, but as they do not constitute a representative sample of either condition their worth is only suggestive. The patients are all White men seen by us during a combined total of 15 years of working with alcoholics as an alcoholism counselor in an industrial setting and in a program for drinking drivers, and as a psychotherapist in private practice in association with a psychiatrist.

Cases

Case 1. J.B., an American-born man, presented for treatment at the age of 27. There was no family history of alcoholism.

He began experimental drinking and homosexual behavior in high school, where he was an athletic star, continuing through 4 years of college and 2 of voice study in Italy, with occasional periods of abstinence and continence. Alcoholism became severe during 3 years of professional singing in New York. He sought psychiatric treatment, convinced that a mental disorder caused the homosexual behavior and that this was at the root of his excessive drinking. During 3 years of group therapy he resisted suggestions to try Alcoholics Anonymous and found homosexuality in himself or others unacceptable. During times of abstinence he refrained from sexual activity, convinced he would "get over" being homosexual, marry and have children. Failure to fulfill a professional engagement because of drunkenness persuaded him to follow group advice and concentrate on abstinence by becoming an A.A. member. After a year of abstinence he began to feel comfortable with other "gay" A.A. members, entered into a homosexual marriage-type relationship with another A.A. member, and maintained continuous abstinence. The relationship has lasted 3½ years, and J.B. has terminated psychotherapy.

Case 2. J.M., an American-born Jewish advertising writer, at age 58 was referred by a county court to a rehabilitation program for "drinking drivers." He reported that both his parents were alcoholics.

After 4 weeks in the court program, J.M. announced that he was a homosexual, not an alcoholic. Sexual activity with both men and women had begun at age 14 and continued unabated after his marriage at age 21, which ended in divorce 10 years later. At that time he had never drunk except on ceremonial occasions, but after the divorce he became a heavy solitary drinker, isolating himself except during work hours and about once a month when he would get drunk and participate in homosexual orgies at a Turkish bathhouse. He called himself a "fag baiter and beater" and took elaborate pains to appear aggressively unattractive, masculine and hostile. He said he was stunned by a counselor's suggestion that he might be both homosexual and alcoholic, both happy and sober. "Being homosexual won't kill me, but drinking will," he finally announced. Highly intelligent and well motivated, he accepted referral to a psychotherapist in private practice, to A.A., and to a "gay" social club in which he never developed any interest. After 6 months in the driver program, he was discharged. Two and a half years later he is still abstinent, active in A.A. (in both homosexual and heterosexual groups), and says he leads a promiscuous "gay" sex life outside A.A. He has terminated psychotherapy. In the last year he has had dramatic professional success.

Case 3. R.C., an American-born Roman Catholic priest of Italian parents, was referred for counseling at age 42 by a priest friend after his third suicide attempt. His mother, a physician, became an alcoholic in middle age.

R.C. reported being a heavy user of alcohol and tranquilizers since seminary days. He speaks five languages, has two doctoral degrees and in his youth was considered a promising fiction writer. He was infuriated by the suggestion of alcoholism, saying he drank only because of fury at the superiors of his order who declined to let him practice an openly "gay" ministry. He had read widely about alcoholism, about A.A. and about homosexuality. He insisted he enjoyed being "gay," but admitted experiencing lengthy depressions. He saw each sexual contact as the start of a sort of "betrothal" which was sure to lead to "marriage," which would in turn make his homosexual behavior acceptable. He agreed reluctantly to attend "gay" A.A. meetings with another priest, also a homosexual alcoholic. Eight months later they formed a domestic partnership, and R.C. left the priesthood to enter business. He has now been abstinent 28 months, is successful in a highly structured commercial enterprise, is writing fiction again and is active in A.A. He believes his recovery began when he could accept identity first as an alcoholic, then as a homosexual. He believes he will eventually become a communicant in his faith again.

Case 4. G.M., a New York-born Puerto Rican, had begun recovery from alcoholism at age 36 with the aid of A.A. He said his father was a "reformed drunkard" who did not drink.

After 10 months of abstinence G.M. sought counseling through his employer's health program because he had fallen in love with a fellow laborer and was deeply depressed and fearful that he was a "queer." He had been a heavy user of wine and beer in high school, but alcoholism was not diagnosed until his foreman had urged him to go to A.A. He had had sexual experiences with many men and women, beginning in school days, but had been able to reach orgasm only with men. During the last 5 years of his alcoholism, however, he became impotent and said he had decided sex was highly overrated in America. Abstinence had restored his potency. He first described himself as "30% gay, 70% straight," but after 8 months of counseling he reversed the proportions. He is still abstinent, 5½ years after counseling terminated, and says he is content with a "gay" identity but still unhappy at what he feels is the necessity for hiding it. He says he used homosexuality as the excuse for heavy drinking.

Case 5. M.S., an American-born Irishman, at age 43 referred himself to his company's alcoholism program at the urging of A.A. friends.

Orphaned in infancy, M.S. was reared by foster parents who were prohibitionists. He was abstinent until age 29, when he got drunk after the break-up of his third engagement. His drinking has been periodic and pathological ever since. He reported being repeatedly raped by an older man in early childhood, and recalls no other sexual experience except solitary masturbation until after he began to drink, when he also began going to "gay" bars in a search for a homosexual lover, "in bitter resignation," he said. This was revenge for the broken engagements, he feels. At 35 he entered psychiatric treatment, and at 37 joined A.A. Until 8 months ago he had never remained abstinent longer than 2 months, always going on a binge at the break-up of a "love affair." Eight months ago, however, he began taking disulfiram daily, and he now seems delighted that he can have sexual experiences while sober and without emotional involvements. His attitude toward A.A. has become noticeably more positive.

Case 6. F.S., American-born of German parents, referred himself for group therapy at age 37 after a year of sobriety in A.A. There was no family history of alcoholism.

F.S. began intensive homosexual activity and heavy drinking in college, but neither prevented a rapid rise to financial success on Wall Street. At 35, depressed about failure to achieve any enduring homosexual love relationship, he entered a "gay" self-help group. The group persuaded him to go to A.A., but after a year's abstinence he was still unhappy, complaining of hypoglycemia, which no medical examination could confirm, and of migraine headaches. During 2½ years in group therapy he has remained abstinent and has begun to reassess his goals as a homosexual. He has become a leader in the "Gay Liberation" movement and is less concerned about so-called love affairs. He is active in A.A. and his somatic complaints have virtually disappeared.

Case 7. J.P. referred himself at age 45 for outpatient treatment for alcoholism. There was no family history of alcoholism.

Born in Kansas, the patient began drinking while working for his doctorate in economics, shortly before marrying a medical student. After 20 years of alcoholism he joined A.A., and after 2 years of abstinence sought psychotherapy. He described himself as asexual and said both he and his wife found sexual activity distasteful. However, after participating in some bisexual orgies, he began to wonder whether he could find a homosexual life satisfying as, he says, his wife now does. After 2½ years of group therapy he is still abstinent and says his life is 90% more productive than during drinking days. He has had four homosexual experiences in the past year and a half, but says that he finds A.A. Twelfth Step work and "gay" civil rights activities more important and satisfying than any sexual experiences.

Case 8. P.H., a third-generation Southerner, referred himself at age 34 for treatment for alcoholism. No known forebears were alcoholics.

Like his four heterosexual brothers, the patient began drinking in a Methodist college and, like them, was an alcoholic before graduation. All his sexual experiences in college were homosexual, but he married a classmate who was a Roman Catholic and was converted to Catholicism in the belief it would help him lead a heterosexual life. He became an airline pilot and lived a heterosexual life at home but away from home practiced homosexuality. He believes he drank to be able to perform homosexual acts, then used his "queerness" as justification for more drinking. Periodic binges finally led to affiliation with A.A. He became abstinent immediately, but 2 years later was divorced by his wife, who got custody of their daughter. The patient then sought psychotherapy. He has now been abstinent 40 months and is having a romance with a fellow pilot. He says sex still makes him feel sinful, but confession relieves him and he does not have to drink.

Case 9. H.H., a German-born graduate student, was referred at age 25 by a physician for counseling for alcoholism. His father was an alcoholic.

The patient had worked his way to this country at age 15. He says he had always been a heavy drinker and bisexual. In an East Coast university he had an affair with an older woman professor, but was a "gay" activist. He began to use distilled spirits and marihuana. A physician prescribed amphetamines, tranquilizers and barbiturates, and told H.H. that homosexuality was the root of his drinking problem. Upon graduation he became a chef to support further study. He was convinced that the use of drugs was an integral part of the "gay lifestyle," and frequently went to "gay" bars. After a nonproductive year of counseling he was persuaded to enter a hospital for detoxication, then to spend a month in a rehabilitation center for alcoholics. He has now been abstinent for 19 months, takes disulfiram and still uses marihuana but is discontented. He works as a chef while pursuing graduate studies, but has not achieved a satisfying social or sex life—that is, one which actualizes his fantasies. He has recently started group therapy.

Case 10. R.T., son of a Jewish father and an Italian mother, at age 55 was referred by his supervisor to his company's program for alcoholic employees. His mother had died of alcoholism.

This patient had begun both pathological drinking and homosexual experiences in high school. A technical writer, he lives with his father in the house where his father was born. Before alcoholism counseling began, his life had consisted only of work, barroom drinking, homosexual experiences in movie theaters, and watching television at home. He was hospitalized when he was 35, 40 and 45 for "nervous breakdowns," each following a painful encounter with his homosexuality. He was certain it caused his excessive drinking. Probably the last two hospitalizations were related in part to alcoholism, although it was not diagnosed. Referred to A.A., R.T. has now been abstinent for 29 months. All his friends and sexual liaisons are homosexual, but he insists he is not "one of those." He has lately begun to profess an interest in "gay" civil rights.

Discussion

None of the patients discussed above fits the stereotype of the male homosexual. None had any urges to transvestism or transsexualism, or appeared in any way feminine. Most are in occupations not commonly associated with homosexuality, and none displayed the mother fixation traditionally associated with male homosexuality. Half of them had no knowledge of parental alcoholism. Their personality types varied widely, as did both their homosexual activities and their drinking patterns.

Nevertheless, a dim pattern seems to emerge from the case histories. Those who were able to accept and live comfortably with the need for abstinence seemed also most likely to achieve relatively successful sexual function (Cases 1, 2, 3, 4, 7, 8, 10). Obversely, patients who had come to terms with their homosexuality seemed to find it easier to accept the diagnosis of alcoholism and the need for abstinence (Cases 5, 6, 9). So the traditional view that homosexuality causes alcoholism, as in Case 1, may well be erroneous, even antitherapeutic. Recovery from pathological drinking seemed to be within reach almost as soon as the patient could view alcoholism as a condition independent of homosexuality. At the least, these homosexual alcoholics responded to treatment for alcoholism when the therapy did not demand that they become heterosexual.

"Gay" alcoholics who insist that the "basic" problem is homosexuality, as in Case 2, may be trying to deflect attention from the drinking—a denial technique, noted by Fox (24), which can postpone the start of abstinence and recovery from alcoholism.

Socially conditioned feelings of discomfort about sexuality are often troublesome to these people, and reinforcement of such feelings by anyone who becomes an "enabler" (25) can exacerbate the unease and help the patient avoid recognition of alcoholism, since nearly all the alcoholics discussed here had used the fact of their homosexuality, or the "homosexual lifestyle," as a rationalization for drinking.

The 10 cases described here support Weinberg's (26) contention that many problems attributed to homosexuality are actually due to cultural traditions and society's reaction to perceived homosexuality. Such problems seem to lose much of their intensity when the homosexual's human environment is not, in Weinberg's (26) term, "homophobic."

Probably this was the case when many of these patients found themselves in the company of other "gay" alcoholics in A.A. The General Service Office of A.A. now lists meetings for such alcoholics in at least 15 cities in 3 countries[4] (although some homosexual alcoholics prefer to attend A.A. meetings not so segregated). In recent years *The A.A. Grapevine* has carried case histories of several recovered homosexual alcoholics, and A.A. World Services has just published a pamphlet (27) containing such an account.

REFERENCES

1. WEINBERG, M. S. and WILLIAMS, C. J. Male homosexuals; their problems and adaptations. New York; Oxford University Press; 1974.
2. WEYGANDT, W. Psychiatrische Begutachtung bei Vergehen und Verbrechen in Amt eines degenerativ-homosexuellen Alkoholisten. Arch. KrimAnthrop. **17**: 221–262, 1904.
3. NÄCKE, P. Alkohol und Homosexualität. Allg. Z. Psycht. **68**: 852–859, 1911.
4. DEUTSCH, H. Alkohol und Homosexualität. Wien. klin. Wschr. **26**: 102–103, 1913.
5. RIGGALL, R. Homosexuality and alcoholism. Psychoanal. Rev. **10**: 157–169, 1923.
6. NEVEU, P. Homosexualité apparue tardivement sous l'influence d'excés alcooliques. Ann. méd.-psychol. **107**^{2}: 36–37, 1949.
7. FERENCZI, S. Über die Rolle der Homosexualität in der Pathogenese der Paranoia. Jb. psychoanal. psychopath. Forsch. **3**: 101–119, 1912.
8. FERENCZI, S. Alkohol und Neurosen (Antwert auf die krilik Bleulers.) Jb. psychoanal. psychopath. Forsch. **3**: 853–857, 1912.

[4] Personal communication, 30 April 1976, from Box 459, New York, NY 10017.

9. Knight, R. P. The psychodynamics of chronic alcoholism. J. nerv. ment. Dis. **86:** 538–548, 1937.
10. Bergler, E. Contributions to the psychogenesis of alcohol addiction. Quart. J. Stud. Alc. **5:** 434–449, 1944.
11. Fenichel, O. The psychoanalytic theory of neurosis. New York; Norton; 1945.
12. Radó, S. An adaptational view of sexual behavior. Pp. 159–169. In: Hoch, P. and Zubin, J., eds. Psychosocial development in health and disease. New York; Grune & Stratton; 1949.
13. Blum, E. M. Psychoanalytic views of alcoholism; a review. Quart. J. Stud. Alc. **27:** 259–299, 1966.
14. Saghir, M. T. and Robbins, E. Male and female homosexuality; natural history. Compr. Psychiat. **12:** 503–510, 1971.
15. Madsen, W. The American alcoholic; the nature-nurture controversy in alcoholic research and therapy. Springfield, IL; Thomas; 1974.
16. Landis, C. Theories of the alcoholic personality. Pp. 129–142. In: Alcohol, science and society; 29 lectures with discussions as given at the Yale Summer School of Alcohol Studies. New Brunswick, NJ; Journal of Studies on Alcohol; 1945.
17. Quaranta, J. V. Alcoholism; a study of emotional maturity and homosexuality as related factors in compulsive drinking. Master's thesis, Fordham University; 1947.
18. Machover, S., Puzzo, F. S., Machover, K. and Plumeau, F. Clinical and objective studies of personality variables in alcoholism. *III.* An objective study of homosexuality in alcoholism. Quart. J. Stud. Alc. **20:** 528–542, 1959.
19. McCord, W. and McCord, J. Origins of alcoholism. Stanford, CA; Stanford University Press; 1960.
20. Prout, C. T., Strongin, E. I. and White, M. A. A study of results in hospital treatment of alcoholism in males. Amer. J. Psychiat. **107:** 14–19, 1950.
21. Botwinick, J. and Machover, S. A psychometric examination of latent homosexuality in alcoholism. Quart. J. Stud. Alc. **12:** 268–272, 1951.
22. Gibbins, R. J. and Walters, R. H. Three preliminary studies of a psychoanalytic theory of alcoholism. Quart. J. Stud. Alc. **21:** 618–641, 1960.
23. Barr, R. F., Greenberg, H. P. and Dalton, M. S. Homosexuality and psychological adjustment. Med. J. Aust. **1:** 187–189, 1974.
24. Fox, R. Treatment of the problem drinker by the private practitioner. Pp. 227–243. In: Bourne, P. G. and Fox, R., eds. Alcoholism; progress in research and treatment. New York; Academic; 1973.
25. Kellermann, J. L. Alcoholism; a merry-go-round named denial. New York; Al-Anon Family Group Headquarters; 1969.
26. Weinberg, W. Society and the healthy homosexual. New York; St. Martin's Press; 1972.
27. Do you think you're different? New York; A.A. World Services; 1976.

A New Sociobiological Theory of Homosexuality Applicable to Societies With Universal Marriage

James D. Weinrich
Department of Biobehavioral Sciences, Boston University Medical School

Several sociobiological theories have tried to explain human homosexuality. Adaptationally orthodox theories view it as a specific instance of reproductive altruism, in which the homosexual orientation in combination with a cross-gender identity is the emotional motivator of a nonreproductive role, leading to higher inclusive fitness for the individual displaying the trait in a particular environment. The nonreproduction is typically assumed to be complete—a large reproductive sacrifice. A new model is proposed in which human homosexuality remains a reproductively altruistic trait, but in which the magnitude of the altruism is much reduced, and so presumably is more likely to result in a net increase in inclusive fitness. The theory applies to societies in which social pressures require marriage of essentially all reproductively able individuals, and does not require gender nonconformity. Hence, the new theory fills some of the gaps left by the earlier orthodox theories, and in combination with them offers a consolidated set of hypotheses for testing.

KEY WORDS: Homosexuality; Bisexuality; Marriage; Sex roles; Altruism; Kin selection; Parent–offspring conflict.

INTRODUCTION

Readers of this journal will not need to be reminded that reproductive altruism and adaptation are central issues in sociobiology. Since the term "sociobiology" was popularized (Wilson 1975a), many sociobiologists have hypothesized that human homosexuality is of adaptive significance. The most common view (Wilson 1975a, p. 555, attributing the theory to R.L. Trivers and H.T. Spieth; 1975b, pp. 42–43; 1978, pp. 142–148) has been to see human homosexuality as a particular instance of reproductive altruism, in which homosexuals' sexual behavior

Received November 6, 1984; revised April 14, 1986.

Address reprint requests to: James D. Weinrich, Ph.D., Family Studies Laboratory, Department of Biobehavioral Sciences, Division of Psychiatry, Boston University Medical School, 85 East Newton Street, Boston MA 02118.

Ethology and Sociobiology 8: 37–47 (1987)

52 Vanderbilt Ave., New York, New York 10017 0162-3095/87/$03.50

with members of their own sex is the proximate cause of lower reproductive success (RS), which is hypothesized to redound to the reproductive benefit of relatives—thus possibly increasing the homosexuals' inclusive fitness (IF). In these theories, kin selection is the ultimate mechanism by which genes predisposing towards, or permitting the development of, a homosexual orientation spread under the action of natural selection.

This theory was investigated and elaborated upon by myself (Weinrich 1976, Part II; Weinrich 1978, 1980b) and others (Kirsch and Rodman 1977, 1982; Kirsch, manuscript in preparation), often in the context of a particular hypothesis: that there are many societies in which individuals acquire extra powers or knowledge by virtue of taking up a nonreproductive or less-than-fully-reproductive role that also necessitates or is customarily associated with homosexual behavior. Similarly, Trivers, in his parent–offspring conflict paper (Trivers 1974, p. 261), elaborated by suggesting that a general mechanism permitting the production of adaptively altruistic homosexuals would be subject to manipulation by parents who would be more likely than offspring themselves to increase their IF if the offspring increased kin-directed reproductive altruism. A homosexual erotic orientation, in the original theories and in these elaborations, is viewed as the emotional mechanism by which certain individuals are predisposed to choose (or allow to have chosen for them) such a nonreproductive role.

But this set of theories can be criticized on many grounds, and at least four others with a less orthodox sociobiological flavor have been proposed. G.E. Hutchinson (1959), writing in the presociobiological era, used what amounted to sociobiological logic in proposing that exclusive homosexuality may be the maladaptive but inevitable result of selection for a heterozygous bisexuality (see also Kirsch and Rodman 1977, 1982). Ruse (1981) described an unpublished theory due to R.D. Alexander in which homosexuality is viewed as a maladaptive result of strong selection for heterosexuality (a class of theories mentioned but not further investigated by myself: Weinrich 1976, Part II, p. 160). Gallup and Suarez (1983) proposed a theory not very different from this one in which homosexuality in both sexes was viewed as "a consequence of heterosexual frustration, dissatisfaction . . . , or both" (p. 315). And Symons (1979, chap. 9), later echoed by Gallup and Suarez, thought homosexuals' behavior to be what heterosexuals of corresponding sex would do if they were unconstrained by the reproductive strategies of the other sex. Symons refrained from speculating whether this behavior could be adaptive although his theory seems to suggest that it is not. I term these theories "nonorthodox" because they first attempt to explain homosexuality as a maladaptation.

A final characteristic of the orthodox theories is that they fail to show definitive parallels between human homosexuality and homosexual behavior in nonhuman animals, even though both kinds of behavior are widespread (Weinrich 1980a). This is not necessarily a weakness, if the particular hypothesis for the human case is compellingly tied to a unique human adaptation like language. But kin selection is not unique to humans—nor, for that matter, are the phenomena presumed by the other theories, including the nonorthodox ones (parent–offspring conflict, bisexual behavior, stringent selection for heterosexuality, juvenile males' inability to find willing female sexual partners, and sharply different sexual strategies selected in males and females). Indeed, it may simply be a mistake to search for an exact parallel in animals to human homosexuality (Weinrich 1980a, 1982). After all, we cannot find an animal species with a set of heterosexual behaviors precisely equivalent to human heterosexuality, and yet no one doubts that "animal heterosexuality" exists (imprecise as the term might be), and no sociobiologist doubts that animal and human heterosexuality are related (complicated though the relationship might be).

The orthodox kin-selection model (see, e.g., Weinrich, 1976) addresses this problem by tying homosexual orientation to desires for cross-gender status or sex-role inversion (a desire to take up the roles and/or occupations of the other sex). Animals are not known to transmit elaborate sex-role prescriptions to their offspring in socialization. This solution has been indirectly criticized with evidence that modern homosexuals are not markedly cross-gendered: most reputable sexologists, joined by Symons and by Gallup and Suarez, say quite rightly that the sexual behavior of homosexual women resembles the sexual behavior of heterosexual women far more than it does the behavior of men, with a similar statement holding for homosexual men.

But this is not to say that cross-gender behaviors can safely be ignored in modeling homosexual behavior, modern or primitive, psychologically or sociobiologically. In fact, an association between gender nonconformity *in childhood* and homosexuality *in adulthood* is by now so well supported it is undeniable (Bakwin 1968; Bell, Weinberg, and Hammersmith 1981; Green 1974, 1976, 1979, 1984, 1985, 1986; Lebovitz 1972; Money and Russo 1979, 1981; Whitam 1977a, 1980, 1983; Zuger 1966, 1978). In fact, childhood gender nonconformity is in some studies the strongest single predictor of adult sexual orientation not tautologically equivalent to it (Bell, Weinberg, and Hammersmith 1981; Pillard and Weinrich, unpublished data). For example, many adult gay men recall cross-gender-role wishes and acts in childhood, and a much larger proportion recall utter lack of interest in the rough-and-tumble, body-contact sports so prominent in American boyhood lore (although many prehomosexual boys are interested in other sports). Some workers have overlooked this evidence, pointing instead to the weak association between homosexual *behavior in childhood* and homosexual behavior in adulthood (e.g., Gallup and Suarez, 1983, p. 319). In fact, the orthodox kin-selection model is clearly justified in its attention to gender nonconformity.

On the other hand, there are children without particular gender nonconformity who grow up to identify themselves as homosexual (Zuger 1966), and many if not most of the childhood gender nonconformers drop much of their nonconformity in adulthood (Harry, 1983), at least in our society, and apparently in some others (Wikan, 1982, p. 180). Some social scientists (viz.,

Whitam 1977a, 1980), aiming at parsimony, have tried to include such children in the cross-gender-identified group by making *lack* of interest in stereotypically same-gender activities (such as sports for boys) part of the very definition of cross-gender identification. This short-circuits the question of whether such lack of interest is empirically associated with the active seeking of cross-gendered roles so typical of gender-nonconforming children (Green 1974). So although it is justified to attend to gender nonconformity in homosexuality, it is a mistake to become preoccupied with it.

Cross-gendering is related to another problem with the orthodox theory: it needs to explain why the reproductive altruism is implemented through the mechanism of homosexual attraction; wouldn't the perfect reproductive altruist be asexual rather than homosexual? I have addressed this criticism elsewhere (Weinrich 1976, Part II, p. 159), and so will only summarize my opinions here—and then propose a new theory that promises to relieve these difficulties.

From first principles, one should expect sexual attraction and/or bonding to serve more than reproductive purposes—an argument made by classical ethologists such as Wickler (1969/1973, Preface) and not a notion sociobiologists are likely to dispute (for example, Wilson 1978, chap. 6). Accordingly, homosexuality (sexual attraction to and/or bonding with a member of one's own genetic sex) can have, one presumes, some of the same not-directly-reproductive benefits that heterosexuality can (inheritance of property, for example, brideprice distribution, or the formation and maintenance of bonds between lineages). And perhaps it can have some benefits that seem unlikely for corresponding heterosexual acts (for example, applied sex education without the danger of pregnancy). Obviously, these benefits would vary as a function of social customs (see Conclusions), but they can exist; simple asexuality would forego these advantages. But just as obviously, same-sex sexual attraction and bonding need not *necessarily* be connected with cross-gender wishes. This is the pivot point of the new model, to be described forthwith.

THE MODEL

I have devised a simple theory that solves most of the difficulties with the classic kin-selection model of human homosexual behavior. It is not a replacement for the model but a supplement to it, and it begins with the observation that there are many societies in which the only people who fail to marry are the prematurely dead or the severely handicapped. In such a society, it might seem, sexual orientation would range not from heterosexual to homosexual, but rather from heterosexual to bisexual. Indeed, some of the most renowned "homosexuals" in history have married and had children (Oscar Wilde, Socrates, Margaret Mead); if they were reproductively altruistic, it was not to the extent of reducing their RS to zero.

Such societies have certainly existed in the past, and some exist today—even in regions where we might not expect them. Modern Saudi Arabia is an example of a deeply conservative culture in which little or no sex-role inversion homosexuality is said to exist [although it does exist in neighboring Oman (Wikan 1982)]. If modern Saudi men have homosexual desires, it is said, they satisfy them with boys or with Western gay tourists willing to play a receptive role. But an insightful modern account of gay life in Saudi Arabia (Traughber 1985, p. 36) makes it clear that this view is seriously incomplete:

> I was more curious than ever about this man who challenged all the myths about sex with an Arab. . . . Once, in response to one of my personal questions, he shook his head disgustedly, grabbing my mustache and then his own. "You are a man. See? I am a man. See? No problem. We like fucking. That's all. OK?" But as he dropped me off a few minutes later, he said with the moon in his eyes, "Oh, Habibi, I will dream of us making love all night." And then he kissed me.

Saudi Arabia is a society in which essentially everyone who is capable of marrying gets married. But as this account and others show, there are sex-role-typical men in that society who recognize a romantic and sexual attraction to other men. These two facts are all that are required for the theory to apply. Even people in societies that do not make strict linguistic distinctions between "homosexual" and "heterosexual" (such as the ancient Greece of Socrates) often recognize that people can have an *orientation* towards romantic attachments with one sex exclusively (Boswell 1982).

So my model begins by asking the following question: what does it mean to "be" homosexual in a society in which everyone marries? Evolutionarily, this question becomes: what is the effect on RS of homosexual as opposed to heterosexual romantic attachments in a society in which everyone marries?

Sociobiologically, one must first address a related issue: the evolutionary function of "limerence" (Tennov 1979): the ability to fall head-over-heels in love with another individual, an ability shared by heterosexuals, homosexuals, and bisexuals alike. To Desmond Morris (1967), this capacity for limerence seemed evolutionarily designed to motivate and strengthen the human pairbond—a theory that has not met with universal acceptance (e.g., Symons 1979, chap. 4). Others too numerous to cite have wondered whether the ability to become limerent might motivate and strengthen the desire to have affairs with people *other* than one's socially approved spouse. I suspect that human limerence might be complicated enough to serve both ends, but for the purposes of the present theory I only require that limerence *sometimes* function for the purpose of motivating extramarital, rather than marital, bliss.

If so, then one difference of reproductive significance between homosexuals and heterosexuals in a society in which everyone gets married would be that heterosexuals have extramarital affairs with members of the other sex, whereas homosexuals have them with members of their own sex. This possibility has an immediate consequence for RS: that heterosexuals in such a society are more likely to have children out of wedlock than homosexuals are. Hence, being homosexual in such circumstances can be, as in the orthodox theory, a reproductive altruistic act.

"Can be," rather than "is," because it is not clear on the face of things whether a particular instance of refraining from extramarital reproduction would be altruistic or not. All other things being equal, it would have to be; *some* extramarital reproduction results in higher RS than *no* extramarital reproduction. But all other things are never equal—perhaps especially so in this case, when a single extramarital affair in many societies could result in the participants being punished (perhaps with death). A careful reading of Trivers (1974), for example, shows that he withheld judgment as to whether extramarital affairs on average increased or decreased RS. A more detailed example is provided by Diamond (1985, p. 77), who also cited unpublished evidence that a substantial portion of RS is obtained extramaritally, at least in our society.

There is also the argument (posed by a reviewer of this paper) as to whether a homosexual orientation in a male would interfere with obtaining an investment-free copulation, were it to be offered to him by a passing female (ignoring for the moment the question of how often such fatherhood opportunities are expected to be offered according to evolutionary theory). What little evidence exists on this question suggests that modern homosexual men are willing to contribute to sperm banks and to father children by artificial insemination. Moreover, experiments show that many if not most homosexual men can be aroused by fantasies of physical sexual contact with females, though not by the preliminaries of meeting women and flirting with them (Freund 1974).

There is another sense in which being homosexual in universal-marriage societies can be considered reproductively altruistic. If one is homosexual, in most societies one cannot formally marry the object of one's love; if one is heterosexual, one sometimes can. If the society is one in which marriages are arranged by parents, or in which there is often conflict between parents and offspring concerning which member of the other sex one should marry, then many heterosexuals would face a conflict when the offspring wants to marry a beloved whom the parents regard with disfavor. Homosexuals in such societies, however, never expected to marry their beloveds, and so presumably would experience less conflict with their parents as to an appropriate marriage partner. (Societies which formally permitted homosexual marriage typically were those in which heterosexual marriages were simultaneously possible; homosexually-oriented members of such societies would not see the two as conflicting.) Trivers (1974, p. 261) has shown, entirely independently of this line of thought, that a tendency to agree to marry the person one's parents prefer—rather than the person the offspring itself would prefer—is a form of reproductive altruism; it is more likely to increase the parent's IF than the offspring's.

Accordingly, for a society in which nearly everyone gets married, there are two senses in which "becoming homosexual" could be (or is) an altruistic act—as it is in the orthodox theory. The magnitude of the altruism, however, is smaller, because RS is merely reduced somewhat, rather than being reduced to zero. It should accordingly be easier to fulfill the kin-selection inequality $B \times r > C$ (in which, as is customary, B denotes the RS benefit to relatives of the altruist, r is the degree of relatedness between the altruist and the recipient(s), and C is the RS cost to the altruist). Because C is smaller in the present theory, in practice it should be easier for $B \times r$ to be larger.

DISCUSSION

Good sociobiological theories of human behavior should not ignore social factors. This theory is specifically designed to take a particular set of social factors into account, and to do so in a nonsuperficial way. The theory cannot work in nonhuman species, the members of which do not arrange marriages (although many animal species have individuals who interfere with particular copulations), or exert social pressures to ensure that most individuals marry and reproduce. The kind of homosexuality proposed in this theory could begin to evolve only after the development of a society that had such social pressures. Of course, it does not address the preadaptation question of what caused the variability of sexual orientation in the first place, or the proximate questions of what mechanisms produce homosexuality in particular individuals and how deterministic these mechanisms are.

The theory remains adaptationist and kin-selectionist but does not tie homosexuality to sex-role inversion, although it partly shares the old theory's weakness in that it might better explain asexuality rather than homosexuality. I now regard this weakness as less important than I once did; homosexual and heterosexual couples alike report that the highly charged sexual excitement so prominent in early couplehood recedes to a more stable level of bondedness that is less "sexy" but retains an erotic tinge. It is a reasonable hypothesis that the highly charged component of sexual attraction could have functioned, as in preadaptation, as the initial emotional motivator of behaviors that lead to a same-sex bond; once the bond is formed, other bonding mechanisms (which need not include such genitally focused sexuality) can come into play. The situation may be analogous to the beginning of the evolution of a pairbond between adults using signals ethologically borrowed from parent–offspring relationships.

The new theory plugs gaps left by the first orthodox theories, but there remain many societies (Weinrich 1976, Part II, Tables 1-2) in which sex-role inversion's association with homosexual practices is clear. (To put this point provocatively, it seems that homosexuals act like members of their own sex rather than like members of the other sex, except when they do not.) The relative importance of the mechanisms proposed by the various theories would differ from society to society. If any of these mechanisms has a biological basis, then one would expect substantial heritability of homosexuality in more modern societies, in which the melting pot mixes the genes of the various ethnic strains more than they had been mixed in the past. That is, intersocietal genetic variation in sexual orientation mechanisms would be converted, over time, to interindividual genetic variation. The genotype-environment mapping (i.e., which environmental circumstances tend to promote which form of sexual orientation variability) could have a substantial genetic component, even while each individual's developmental history of sexual orientation was idiosyncratic.

This line of argument suggests some ways to test the theory—if not directly, at least as part of a set of theories that taken together might account for nearly all kinds of homosexuals and homosexuality. We ought to be able to develop a typology of sexual orientation—including heterosexuals in the typology as well—in which different sexual-orientation "types" were reliably passed on within families. To a first approximation, for example, the theory would be supported if cross-gendered and non-cross-gendered homosexuality seemed to be passed on independently of each other; it would be rendered less likely if these two types were expressed more as a function of cultural prescriptions than as a function of lineage.

Interestingly, the two twin studies of sexual orientation (Kallmann 1952a,b, which is methodologically poor—see the comments preceding Kallmann 1960—and Heston and Shields 1968, which is methodologically much better but based on a small sample) both found striking cases suggesting that "what is inherited" is much more specific than a direction to one's sexual orientation. It also appears that male homosexuality runs in families (Pillard, Poumadere, and Carretta 1981, 1982; Pillard and Weinrich 1986), and probably female homosexuality as well (Pillard and Weinrich, in preparation). There is little evidence that families with disproportionate numbers of male homosexuals have disproportionate numbers of female homosexuals as well (Pillard and Weinrich 1986).

The theory would also be challenged if it became impossible or embarrassingly difficult to construct a taxonomy of sexual orientation in the first place. After all, a trait cannot be considered "inherited" if taxonomists agree that the trait is not well-defined. In sexual orientation research, this question is called the "social constructionist/essentialist" debate (see Weinrich 1987, submitted for publication) or, as applied specifically to homosexuality, the "homosexual role" debate (Whitam 1977b, 1978; Omark 1978). However, a colleague and I (Pillard and Weinrich, 1987, in press) have such a taxonomy, and taxonomic questions have been prominently discussed by other sex researchers (see, for example, Freund 1967, 1974; Freund, Steiner, and Chan 1982; Langevin 1983; Langevin, Paitich, and Steiner 1977). Most sex researchers agree that such taxonomies are valid at least in their broad outlines.

And of course, the theory would be challenged if the patterns of homosexuality and bisexuality observed do not fit the details of the model. For example, if the empirical work supporting a taxonomy does not find that the less- or non-cross-gendered sort of homosexual exists in societies which insist upon universal marriage, or if parent–offspring conflict over the preferred marriage partner is just as (or more) intense among homosexually oriented offspring as it is among heterosexuals, then the theory fails in that case. Given enough such embarrassments, it will be rejected in general. Of course, if any of these traits were rare—on the order of a mutational equilibrium, say—doubt would also be cast on the adaptationist hypothesis.

CONCLUSIONS

I cannot pretend to have proven that this theory is true, or even to have made a direct empirical case for it. However, data-gathering must be motivated by good theory; it is hard to prove or disprove a theory using only data gathered before the theory was proposed.

Good theory, in turn, must be motivated by the proper fundamental principles. Adaptation is the central question in sociobiology, and some of sociobiology's greatest successes have been in demonstrating adaptation where others had found none. There is now a substantial body of experience backing up Trivers's early assertion that maladaptive explanations are explanations of last resort (Trivers 1972; 1985, chap. 2), so it is not by accident that the earliest sociobiological theories of homosexuality were adaptationist. It is unfortunate that some sociobiologists studying human reproductive strategy have overlooked adaptationist models as they approach the more taboo areas of human sexuality. In the absence of extrasensory perception, I cannot fairly attribute base motives or poor training to them, and even if I could their views may yet turn out to be the correct ones. But that cannot be agreed upon until more adaptationist theories have been proposed, criticized, and tested. Evolutionary biologists conclude that adaptation has been at work when there is a "good" fit between an adaptationist explanation and a set of well-documented traits. Unfortunately, in assessing whether "good" is good enough there are no absolute standards, and there is thus no substitute for logical argument by well-trained, intelligent experts considering the evidence of experiment. It is in that spirit that the present theory is put forth.

I thank John Kirsch for comments on an early version of the manuscript.

REFERENCES

Bakwin, H. Deviant gender-role behavior in children: Relation to homosexuality. *Pediatrics* 41: 620–629, 1968.

Bell, A.P., Weinberg, M.S., and Hammersmith, S.K. *Sexual Preference: Its Development in Men and Women*. Bloomington, IN: Indiana University Press, 1981.
Boswell, J. Revolutions, universals, and sexual categories. *Salmagundi* 58–59: 89–113, 1982.
Diamond, J. "Everything *else* you always wanted to know about sex* *but that we were afraid you'd never ask." *Discover* 6(4): 70–82, 1985.
Freund, K.W. Diagnosing homo- or heterosexuality and erotic age-preference by means of a psychophysiological test. *Behaviour Research and Therapy* 5: 209–228, 1967.
—— Male homosexuality: An analysis of the pattern. In *Understanding Homosexuality: Its Biological and Psychological Bases*, J.A. Loraine (Ed.). New York: Elsevier, 1974, pp. 25–81.
——, Steiner, B.W., and Chan, S. Two types of cross-gender identity *Archives of Sexual Behavior* 11: 49–63, 1982.
Gallup, G.G., and Suarez, S.D. Homosexuality as a by-product of selection for optimal heterosexual strategies. *Perspectives in Biology and Medicine* 26: 315–322, 1983.
Green, R. *Sexual Identity Conflict in Children and Adults*. New York: Basic, 1974.
—— One-hundred ten feminine and masculine boys: Behavioral contrasts and demographic similarities. *Archives of Sexual Behavior* 5: 425–446, 1976.
—— Childhood cross-gender behavior and subsequent sexual preference. *American Journal of Psychiatry* 136: 106–108, 1979.
—— Why the relationship between boyhood femininity and adult homosexuality? Paper presented at the joint annual meeting of the Society for the Scientific Study of Sex and the American Association of Sex Educators, Counselors, and Therapists, Boston, MA, June 7, 1984.
—— Gender identity in boyhood and later sexual orientation: Followup of 78 males. *American Journal of Psychiatry* 142: 339–341, 1985.
—— *"Sissy" Boys to "Gay" Men: A Fifteen Year Prospective Study*. New Haven: Yale University Press, 1986, in press.
Harry, J. Defeminization and adult psychological well-being among male homosexuals. *Archives of Sexual Behavior* 12: 1–19, 1983.
Heston, L.L., and Shields, J. Homosexuality in twins: A family study and a registry study. *Archives of General Psychiatry* 18: 149–160, 1968.
Hutchinson, G.E. A speculative consideration of certain possible forms of sexual selection in man. *American Naturalist* 93: 81–91, 1959.
Kallmann, F.J. Comparative twin study on the genetic aspects of male homosexuality. *Journal of Nervous and Mental Disease* 115: 283–298, 1952a.
—— Twin and sibship study of overt male homosexuality. *American Journal of Human Genetics* 4: 136–146, 1952b.
—— Discussion. *Psychosomatic Medicine* 22: 258–259, 1960.
Kirsch, J.A.W., and Rodman, J.E. The natural history of homosexuality. *Yale Scientific* 51(3): 7–13, Winter 1977.
——, —— Selection and sexuality: The Darwinian view of homosexuality. In *Homosexuality: Social, Psychological, and Biological Issues*, W. Paul, J.D. Weinrich, J.C. Gonsiorek, and M.E. Hotvedt (Eds.). Beverly Hills, CA: Sage, 1982, pp. 183–195.
Langevin, R. *Sexual Strands: Understanding and Treating Sexual Anomalies in Men*. Hillsdale, NJ: Lawrence Erlbaum, 1983.
Langevin, R., Paitich, D., and Steiner, B. The clinical profile of male transsexuals living as females vs. those living as males. *Archives of Sexual Behavior* 6: 143–154, 1977.
Lebovitz, P.S. Feminine behavior in boys: Aspects of its outcome. *American Journal of Psychiatry* 128: 1283–1289, 1972.
Money, J., and Russo, A.J. Homosexual outcome of discordant gender identity/role in childhood: Longitudinal follow-up. *Journal of Pediatric Psychology* 4: 29–41, 1979.
——, —— Homosexual vs. transvestite or transexual gender-identity/role: Outcome study in boys. *International Journal of Family Psychiatry* 2: 139–145, 1981.
Morris, D. *The Naked Ape*. New York: Dell, 1967.
Omark, R.C. A comment on the homosexual role. *Journal of Sex Research* 14: 273–274, 1978.
Pillard, R.C., Poumadere, J.I., and Carretta, R.A. Is homosexuality familial? A review, some data, and a suggestion. *Archives of Sexual Behavior* 10: 465–475, 1981.
——, ——, —— A family study of sexual orientation. *Archives of Sexual Behavior* 11: 511–520, 1982.

—— and Weinrich, J.D. Evidence of familial nature of male homosexuality. *Archives of General Psychiatry* 43: 808–812, 1986.

——, —— The periodic-table model of the gender transpositions: I. A model based on masculinization and defeminization of the brain. *Journal of Sex Research* 1987, in press.

Ruse, M. Are there gay genes? Sociobiology and homosexuality. *Journal of Homosexuality* 6(4): 5–34, 1981.

Symons, D. *The Evolution of Human Sexuality*. New York: Oxford University Press, 1979.

Tennov, D. *Love and Limerence: The Experience of Being in Love*. New York: Stein and Day. 1979.

Traughber, V. Arabian nights: Gay sex in the heart of Islam. *The Advocate* 416: 34–37, 1985.

Trivers, R.L. Parental investment and sexual selection. In *Sexual selection and the Descent of Man 1871–1971*, B. Campbell (Ed.). Chicago: Aldine, 1972, pp. 136–179.

—— Parent–offspring conflict. *American Zoologist* 14: 249–264, 1974.

—— *Social Evolution*. Menlo Park, CA: Benjamin/Cummings, 1985.

Weinrich, J. D. *Human reproductive strategy*. Doctoral dissertation, Harvard University, 1976. Dissertation Abstracts International, 1977, 37, 5339-B. (University Microfilms No. 77-8348.)

—— Nonreproduction, homosexuality, transsexualism, and intelligence: I. A systematic literature search. *Journal of Homosexuality* 3: 275–289, 1978.

—— Homosexual behavior in animals: A new review of observations from the wild, and their relationship to human homosexuality. In *Medical Sexology: The Third International Congress*. R. Forleo and W. Pasini (Eds.). Littleton, MA: PSG, 1980a, pp. 288–295.

—— On a relationship between homosexuality and I.Q. test scores: A review and some hypotheses. In *Medical Sexology: The Third International Congress*. R. Forleo and W. Pasini (Eds.). Littleton, MA: PSG, 1980b, pp. 312–317.

—— Is homosexuality biologically natural? In *Homosexuality: Social, Psychological, and Biological Issues*, W. Paul, J.D. Weinrich, J.C. Gonsiorek, and M.E. Hotvedt (Eds.). Beverly Hills, CA: Sage, 1982, pp. 197–208.

—— Is homosexuality a social construction or an essential reality? The answer is "yes." Submitted for publication, 1987.

Whitam, F.L. Childhood indicators of male homosexuality. *Archives of Sexual Behavior* 6: 89–96, 1977a.

—— The homosexual role: A reconsideration. *Journal of Sex Research* 13: 1–11, 1977b.

—— Rejoinder to Omark's comment on the homosexual role. *Journal of Sex Research* 14: 274–275, 1978.

—— The prehomosexual male child in three societies: The United States, Guatemala, Brazil. *Archives of Sexual Behavior* 9: 87–99, 1980.

—— Culturally invariable properties of male homosexuality: Tentative conclusions from cross-cultural research. *Archives of Sexual Behavior* 12: 207–226, 1983.

Wickler, W. *The Sexual Code: The Social Behavior of Animals and Men*. Garden City, NY: Anchor Press/Doubleday, 1973. (Originally published in German, 1969.)

Wikan, U. *Behind the Veil in Arabia: Women in Oman*. Baltimore, MD: Johns Hopkins University Press, 1982.

Wilson, E.O. *Sociobiology: The New Synthesis*. Cambridge, MA: Harvard University Press, 1975a.

—— Human decency is animal. *The New York Times Magazine* 125(42995): 38–50, October 12, 1975b.

—— *On Human Nature*. Cambridge, MA: Harvard University Press, 1978.

Zuger, B. Effeminate behavior present in boys from early childhood. I. The clinical syndrome and follow-up studies. *Journal of Pediatrics* 69: 1098–1107, 1966.

—— Effeminate behavior present in boys from childhood: Ten additional years of follow-up. *Comprehensive Psychiatry* 19: 363–369, 1978.

Acknowledgments

Chevalier-Skolnikoff, Suzanne. "Homosexual Behavior in a Laboratory Group of Stumptail Monkeys *(Macaca arctoides)*: Forms, Contexts, and Possible Social Functions." *Archives of Sexual Behavior* 5 (1976): 511–527. Reprinted with the permission of Plenum Publishing Corp. Courtesy of Yale University Medical Library.

Doyle, Dennis M. "The Meaning of AIDS." *Commonweal* 115 (1988): 343–346. Reprinted with the permission of the Commonweal Foundation. Courtesy of Yale University Sterling Memorial Library.

Eckert, Elke D., Thomas J. Bouchard, Joseph Bohlen, and Leonard L. Heston. "Homosexuality in Monozygotic Twins Reared Apart." *British Journal of Psychiatry* 148 (1986): 421–425. Reprinted with the permission of the *British Journal of Psychiatry*. Courtesy of Yale University Medical Library.

Fumento, Michael J. "The Political Uses of an Epidemic." *The New Republic* 199 (1988): 19–23. Reprinted by permission of *The New Republic*, copyright 1988 by The New Republic, Inc. Courtesy of *The New Republic.*

Grönfors, Martti and Olli Stålström. "Power, Prestige, Profit: AIDS and the Oppression of Homosexual People." *Acta Sociologica* 30 (1987): 53–66. Reprinted with the permission of the Scandinavian University Press. Courtesy of Yale University Seeley G. Mudd Library.

Herman, Ellen. "Getting to Serenity: Do Addiction Programs Sap our Political Vitality?" *Out/Look* (1988): 10–21. Reprinted with the permission of the *Out/Look*. Courtesy of Wayne R. Dynes.

Israelstam, S. and S. Lambert. "Homosexuality as a Cause of Alcoholism: A Historical Review." *International Journal of Addictions* 18 (1983): 1085–1107. Reprinted with the permission of Marcel Dekker, Inc. Courtesy of Yale University Medical Library.

Johnson, Susan R. and Jefri L. Palermo. "Gynecologic Care for the Lesbian." *Clinical Obstetrics and Gynecology* 27 (1984): 724–731. Reprinted with the permission of J. B. Lippincott Company. Courtesy of Yale University Medical Library.

Mohr, Richard D. "AIDS, Gays, and State Coercion." *Bioethics* 1 (1987): 35–50. Reprinted with the permission of Basil Blackwell Ltd. Courtesy of Basil Blackwell Ltd.

Money, John. "Gender-Tranposition Theory and Homosexual Genesis." *Journal of Sex and Marital Therapy* 10 (1984): 75–82. Reprinted with the permission of Brunner-Mazel, Inc. Copyright 1984. Courtesy of Wayne R. Dynes.

Murray, Stephen O., and Kenneth W. Payne. "Medical Policy Without Scientific Evidence: The Promiscuity Paradigm and AIDS." *California Sociologist* 11 (1988): 13–54. Reprinted with the permission of the California State University, Los Angeles. Courtesy of the Author.

Newmeyer, John A. "The Sensuous Hippie Part II: Gay/Straight Differences in Regard to Drugs and Sexuality." *Drug Forum* 6 (1977–78) 49–55. Reprinted with the permission of the author. Courtesy of Wayne R. Dynes.

Nye, Robert A. "Sex Difference and Male Homosexuality in French Medical Discourse, 1830–1930." *Bulletin of the History of Medicine* 63 (1989): 32–51. Reprinted with the permission of the Johns Hopkins University Press. Courtesy of Yale University Sterling Memorial Library.

Pargetter, Robert, and Elizabeth W. Prior. "Discrimination and AIDS." *Social Theory and Practice* 13 (1987): 129–153. Reprinted with the permission of the *Social Theory and Practice.* Copyright 1987. Courtesy of the *Social Theory and Practice.*

Ross, Michael W. "Understanding the Homosexual Patient." *Patient Management* (1985): 15–16, 19, 20, 22, 25. Reprinted with the permission of the Adis International Ltd. Courtesy of Adis International Ltd.

Seidman, Steven with Comment by Dennis Altman. "Transfiguring Sexual Identity: AIDS & the Contemporary Construction of Homosexuality." *Social Text* 19/20 (1988): 187–209. Reprinted with the permission of the *Social Text.* Courtesy of the *Social Text.*

Siegel, Karolynn, Martin P. Levine, Charles Brooks and Rochelle Kern. "The Motives of Gay Men for Taking or Not Taking the HIV Antibody Test." *Social Problems* 36 (1989): 368–383. Reprinted with the permission of the University of California Press. Copyright 1989 by the Society for the Study of Social Problems. Courtesy of Yale University Sterling Memorial Library.

Simon, Walter T. and Peter G. W. Schouten. "Plethysmography in the Assessment and Treatment of Sexual Deviance: An Overview." *Archives of Sexual Behavior* 20 (1991): 75–91. Reprinted with the permission of Plenum Publishing Corp. Courtesy of Yale University Medical Library.

Singer, Eleanor, Theresa F. Rogers and Mary Corcoran. "The Polls—A Report: AIDS." *Public Opinion Quarterly* 51 (1987): 580–595. Reprinted with permission of The University of Chicago Press, publisher. Courtesy of Yale University Sterling Memorial Library.

Small, Jr., Edward J., and Barry Leach. "Counseling Homosexual Alcoholics: Ten Case Histories." *Journal of Studies on Alcohol* 38 (1977): 2077–2086. Reprinted with permission from the *Journal of Studies on Alcohol*. Copyright by Journal of Studies on Alcohol, Inc., Rutgers Center of Alcohol Studies, New Brunswick, NJ 08903. Courtesy of the *Journal of Studies on Alcohol.*

Weinrich, James D. "A New Sociobiological Theory of Homosexuality Applicable to Societies with Universal Marriage." *Ethology and Sociobiology* 8 (1987): 37–47. Reprinted with the permission of Elsevier Science Publishing Co., Inc. Copyright 1987. Courtesy of Yale University Kline Science Library.

Index

For Product Safety Concerns and Information please contact our
EU representative GPSR@taylorandfrancis.com Taylor & Francis
Verlag GmbH, Kaufingerstraße 24, 80331 München, Germany